Lindsay R. Peat
DBMS Selection

Lindsay R. Peat

Practical Guide to DBMS Selection

Walter de Gruyter · Berlin · New York 1982

CIP-Kurztitelaufnahme der Deutschen Bibliothek

Peat, Lindsay, R.:
Practical guide to DBMS selection / Lindsay R. Peat. – Berlin, New York: de Gruyter, 1982.
ISBN 3-11-008167-9

Library of Congress Cataloging in Publication Data

Peat, Lindsay R., 1945–
Practical guide to DBMS selection.
Bibliography: p.
1. Data base management. I. Titel.
QA76.9.D3P4 1982 001.64 81-19533
ISBN 3-11-008167-9 AACR2

 Printing: Satzstudio Frohberg, Freigericht-Somborn. – Binding: Dieter Mikolai, Berlin. – Cover design: W.A. Taube, München. – Printed in Germany.

Preface

This book is aimed not only at EDP professionals, particularly those involved in selecting a DBMS, but also at informatics students who are interested in knowing how each DBMS implements its features and what this will imply.

Although the investigation has been concentrated on the IBM S/370 etc. versions of the DBMSs, these reports are applicable in general to the corresponding DBMSs available for UNIVAC and CDC hardware. Specific information is given in the introduction to each system report.

The original idea for this book resulted from an investigation to identify the most suitable DBMS for a large international organisation. Despite the fact that several such investigations have already been made into the characteristics and features of the available systems, they proved to be unsatisfactory, either because they are outdated, or because the individual reports on different systems are not comparable. The reports in this book are based on the versions of the systems which were available in the final quarter of 1980.

It should be recognised that no DBMS is 'better' than another, rather that each has its strengths and weaknesses; the object of the selection process is to find the system with the most advantages and fewest disadvantages for the envisaged EDP environment. Although each DBMS report concludes with a list of advantages and disadvantages as judged against the generalised requirements of an international company, these requirements may or may not apply to your specific environment.

During my work in this field, it has become apparent to me that there is a lack of centralised information in certain areas. I have attempted to fill the gaps by providing, in the appendices, the following: a dictionary of generalised DBMS terminology; a comprehensive list of DBMS publications ordered on specific areas; a list of contact addresses useful to those active in the DBMS field.

It should be noted that DBMS terms have throughout been printed in capitals, and clarification of these terms should be sought firstly in the relevant DBMS dictionary at the end of the chapter, and then in the appendix of general DBMS terminology. Diagrams have been numbered according to the number of the section in the text to which they relate.

Bad Soden, February, 1982 L.R. Peat

Acknowledgements

I would like to thank the following people in particular and their companies in general for the generous support and advice they have given me:

Herren Kepler & Jung of Software AG.,
Mr. L. Smith of Cullinane Corp.,
Hr. Schoon of ADV-Orga.,
Ms. Fox and Messrs. Armomi & Karbach of MRI Corp.,
Messrs. Cohen & Jacobs of ADR Inc.,
Ms. Tetzel of CINCOM Systems, Inc.

The following companies have given their kind permission for me to quote from their documentation and to use diagrams from their manuals:

Software AG,
Cullinane Corporation,
ADR,
CINCOM Systems,
MRI Corp.

The following companies have checked the veracity of the report on their products:

Software AG (ADABAS),
Cullinane Corporation (IDMS),
MRI Corp. (S2000),
ADR (DATACOM/DB).

Contents

List of Diagrams

SYSTEM 2000

ADABAS

IDMS

1. The Selection Procedure

There is no such thing as the 'best' database management system (DBMS) – only the best DBMS for a particular user. The object of this book is to help each user identify that DBMS which will most closely match his particular requirements.

The amount of money which will be invested in the DBMS and the associated application programs makes it imperative that a comprehensive selection process be followed. If the 'wrong' DBMS is selected, this will normally not be evident until too much time and money have been invested to make a change feasible. The cost, in both time and money, of the 'wrong' DBMS will be many times higher than the cost of the selection procedure.

The two initial problems connected with the selection of a DBMS are the vast number of systems available, and the fact that some Data Management Systems (DMSs) masquerade as DBMSs – although the distinction is rather blurred. In stage two, the DMSs will be disqualified because of their lack of facilities.
The first task is therefore to eliminate the majority of these systems, and this can most easily be done by considering just two essential features:

- the vendor must offer support in all the areas where the DBMS is to run
- the vendor must have at least 150 installed systems.

The number of 150 is only approximate, but it indicates that the vendor has reached a degree of financial maturity that will allow him to continue developing the product, and, in the unlikely event of a bankruptcy, the rental income would be sufficient to keep the development team together to provide support for the user base.

After applying these two criteria, it is unusual for more than six or seven DBMSs to be left in the race. This number can be further reduced by looking at the contenders in the light of your enterprise's detailed requirements. Although this step should ideally result in only one system being left, this is rarely, if ever, the case except when political aspects have a disproportionately large influence on the selection procedure. In fact, two or three systems will probably remain.

The first activity in this process is to prepare a preliminary document stating the enterprise's requirements of a DBMS. This should be done only in terms of the features required, the data volume to be handled, and the way in which data is to be handled. At this stage, database terminology should be kept to a minimum so as to avoid the possibility of misunderstanding between EDP personnel and management. Those DBMS terms used should always be accompanied by a detailed definition of their meaning. This statement of processing requirements is submitted to management for its approval.

Initially, identifying the DBMS requirements might appear to be a daunting task requiring detailed study of the standard works on DBMSs. To avoid this, the salient features of a DBMS are discussed in the following section. A number of points will be discussed which are not particularly relevant to the activity of identifying the processing requirements, but they do serve as a bridge to the next activity: gathering information on the remaining systems. However, for those readers who are totally unfamiliar with DBMSs and their terminology, it is recommended that they consult one of the standard introductory works listed in Appendix VI.

1.1 The Role of the Selection Team

The decision to install a DBMS must be supported by the board of directors because of the financial investment involved. It is equally important for the board to endorse the choice of DBMS. This means that the board should nominate the members of the selection team, and the team should report directly to that member of the board responsible for EDP. The board must also establish clerical and secretarial support for the selection team.

It should also be recognised by all involved that the recommendations of the selection team must be accepted. For the board to reject the team's recommendation and simply select some other DBMS is likely to lead to total demoralisation within the EDP department, since the board has, in effect, indicated its total distrust of the professional competence of the selection team in particular and the EDP department in general. It would be difficult to imagine a more inauspicious start for a DBMS.

1.1.1 The Composition of the Selection Team

The members of this team will form the nucleus of the DBA function after the installation of the DBMS. It is worth considering whether it might be necessary to recruit someone from outside the organisation who has DBMS experience, or to hire someone from a software house to help with the selection procedure, so as to avoid initial difficulties with an inexperienced team.

The majority of the team members must be employees of the enterprise. The longer they have been with the enterprise, the better, because the team should be acquainted with the processing requirements of the enterprise, and, because of their personal reputation they should be in a position to persuade the departments concerned to accept the selected DBMS.

The team should consist of about seven members and must be drawn from at least two separate sources within the enterprise: the EDP department and the user departments. The majority of the team members will be from the EDP department, and at least one systems programmer should be included. One of the members of the team should be versed in the procedure of cost/benefit analysis. Ultimately, the team members should be able to give competent judgement for each DBMS from the viewpoints of:

- computer operating
- the programmer
- the system programmer
- the end user
- management (at least as far as costs are concerned)

The team should be headed by the member of the board responsible for EDP, but since it is unlikely that he will be able to be involved in the daily deliberations of the team, the team must elect a manager who reports directly to the technical director. He will be responsible for coordinating the team meetings and the interviews with the vendors. Furthermore, the publication of the reports will be organised by the team manager.

Each team member cannot hope to be involved in the examination of each DBMS, nor can each system be examined by a single team member. The former would take too long and the latter be too prone to error. A healthy compromise is to have two members of the team examine each of the DBMSs. They should produce a common report, but if their opinions diverge markedly, the team manager should be called in to help resolve the conflict.

Every effort should be made to arrive at unanimous decisions: majority decisions lead to bad feelings and can endanger the whole selection process. Thus, the team manager should be chosen for his patience and objectivity, and should, if possible, be selected from outside the EDP department. This latter step should help avoid the accusation that the EDP department has forced its opinion onto the enterprise.

1.1.2 The Steps in the Selection Process

The first problem faced by the newly-chosen team is usually their lack of detailed knowledge of database technology. This problem is normally compounded by the unevenness of the knowledge of the different team members, and their possible commitment to different DBMS approaches.

The first problem can only be solved by attending relevant courses on basic database technology. The last problem can only be solved by intensive formal discussion sessions between the team members. These discussions must result in the team members agreeing on the important features of a DBMS as far as their enterprise is concerned.

The final preparatory activity before starting with the selection process is to produce a glossary of database terminology. This serves a double purpose:

- it is a final check that the team members have reached a large degree of agreement;
- it avoids misunderstanding within the enterprise when the selection team's reports are read.

If the team does not feel able to produce a glossary of DBMS terminology, the CODASYL glossary would make a very adequate substitute.

Armed with the common idea of what the important DBMS features are in terms of their own enterprise, the team members can take the first step in the selection procedure. The initial processing requirements present a formidable task, mainly because they require a formulation of the processing objectives for the next five to ten years. This is not necessarily limited to what the EDP department is planning, but must also include the wishes of the end-user departments.

Parallel to collecting the preliminary processing requirements, the team should be collecting information on the available DBMSs, so that as soon as the processing requirements are finalised, the elimination process can begin.

After having reduced the number of competing DBMSs to a short list of two or three, the team should update the preliminary processing requirements before going on to the final selection procedure. This is because new information will be available from the EDP and user departments, and the team will be in a better position to translate these requirements into database concepts because of the experience gained by this time.

The final step in the selection procedure will be very time-consuming, because each of the remaining DBMSs has to be analysed in great depth. The questionnaire in Appendix I is intended to support this step.

After each of the competing systems has been compared, and the team is agreed on the characteristics, advantages and disadvantages, the final report for the board of directors should be written. A short seminar of one to two days' duration should also be prepared, based on the final report. This seminar should be offered to all interested parties after the recommendations of the report have been accepted by the board of directors.

Benchmark tests should be avoided unless the board of directors insist. This is because such tests are far too time-consuming and the results seldom mean what the testers intend. (See also 1.4.8).

1.2 Factors Relevant to the Selection of a DBMS

The main factors which will influence the choice of a DBMS have been organised into four tables. The first table is concerned with the impact of the DBMS on the user, the other three examine the internals of the DBMS. This approach was taken because of the necessity of introducing the prospective user to the wide range of aspects which must be considered before the process of collecting the information on each DBMS begins.

1.2.1 User Related Aspects

These are the factors which will directly affect the whole of the EDP department. With all these features, contact with a current user can be both helpful and illuminating.

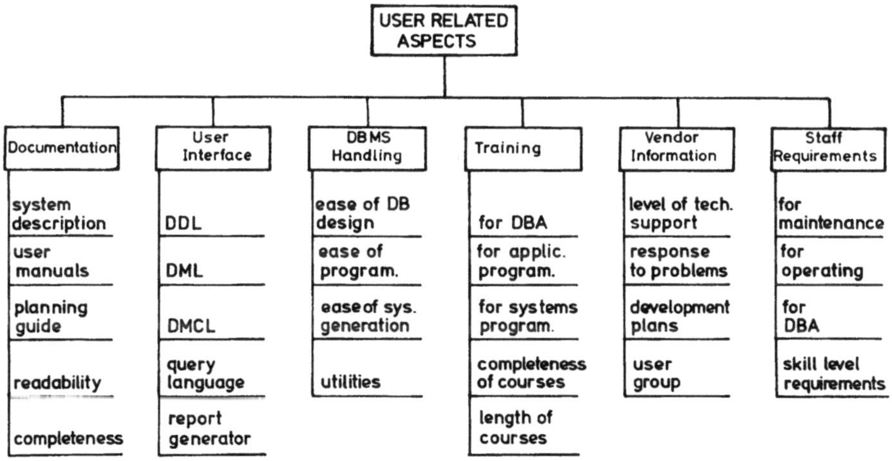

Fig. 1.2: User Related Aspects

1.2.1.1 Documentation

The documentation is the single most important aspect of the DBMS. A 'good' DBMS badly documented is next to useless. The system description and the planning guide are intended for a different group of people than the programmer's manual is intended for, and this should be borne in mind when examining the documentation.

Voluminous documentation does not necessarily mean good documentation; it may simply mean that the DBMS is very complex. The cross reference can often be a quick and telling guide to the quality of the documentation. Points to look for are: major topics that are dealt with piecemeal; major topics that are omitted.

Completeness of documentation can of course best be judged by reading it, but this is normally too time-consuming. The team should therefore make a list of about 10 topics, and judge the documentation of each DBMS on these.

1.2.1.2 The User Interfaces

The Data Definition Language (DDL) and the Device Media Control Language (DMCL) are for the exclusive use of the Data Base Administrator. The DDL will largely be dependent on the complexity of the structures which can be generated and the access methods available. The DMCL is often integrated within the DDL.

The Data Manipulation Language (DML) is the normal programmer interface to the DBMS and will be implemented either via subroutine 'CALL' statements, or via a preprocessor. The three aspects of interest are:

- the power of the DML commands
- the commands available
- the complexity of the formulation of a command

The commands needed to support the processing as outlined in the preliminary requirements must be available within the DBMS, and in addition, the following points should be considered:

- A LOCATE command should be available as well as a READ command. This avoids the unnecessary extra processing of transferring the record from the system to the program buffer. (For inverted files the saving is even greater since the record's presence can be identified in the index.)
- Commands should be available to process the database in both physical and logical sequence.
- When processing on non-unique keys, it is a great help if the answer to the query indicates the number of records fulfilling the criteria. This enables a decision to be made whether processing this number is feasible.

The power of the DML commands is in general directly proportional to their complexity. The experienced programmer tends to favour the DML which offers the greatest flexibility, while the beginner is inclined to favour simplicity. As most beginners turn into experienced programmers, it is sensible to choose that DML which offers the greatest flexibility. The beginner can then be limited to a subset of available DML command variations.

In many environments, end-user languages have relieved the pressure on the development personnel and made the users more sympathetic to the problems of the EDP department. Most EDP departments without experience of end-user accessing of the computer have a great, but unfounded, fear of it. DBMSs that have end-user facilities should be rated higher than those without, and those with true on-line capabilities higher than those limited to on-line input and batch processing of the request.

1.2.1.3 DBMS Handling

This is one of the most subjective parts of any DBMS investigation, particularly in terms of ease of programming and design. Ease of programming should not be confused with the DML commands available and their format – ie. ease of coding. Ease of programming is more concerned with the support the DBMS offers the programmer: whether or not the scope of the transaction is under programmer control; whether positioning (CURRENCY) is supported, which is particularly necessary when processing records without a unique key; whether the programmer can control when the positions are deleted, since otherwise extra coding may have to be included to re-establish a position.

It is essentially irrelevant whether the system chosen is based on network structures or on inverted file techniques. However, for rapid on-line processing, direct access methods should be available. In general, network-based systems are more complicated to design than those employing inverted file techniques and require far more preparatory work. With network (or hierarchical) based systems, the facility to order the record occurrences in a twin chain should not be underestimated.

If every small change to the DBMS requires a new system generation, then not only is this extremely inefficient in itself, but it also makes each slight modification the subject of a long discussion and decision process. This in turn hinders rapid response to changing requirements.

Another aspect of system generation is the number of functions of the system which can be influenced by the user. The more control the user can exercise on the configuration of the DBMS, the better, since the user can tailor the system more nearly to suit his requirements.

Utilities are a necessary adjunct to every system. Some DBMSs have the functions embedded in the system, others have 'stand-alone' utilities, which may be extra-cost items. The only sensible way to check on this is to list the subsidiary functions required and to check that they are available, however implemented. This list should contain most, if not all, of the following:

- DB Copy
- tuning, performance and design aids
- log file accumulation
- log file analysis
- reorganisation
- recovery: warm restart (often automatic)

- changes to the database: adding a new secondary index (if possible, without reloading the primary); adding/deleting a record type; adding/deleting a field to a record type; mass additions or deletions.

If a particular utility is not available, this need not automatically disqualify the system. The vendor should be approached with a view to his developing the required software at a moderate cost, and only if this fails should the DBMS be rejected.

1.2.1.4 Training

This is usually one of the least-investigated aspects of any DBMS. The training period is not just the time spent attending the formal courses offered by the vendor, but the time required before the DBMS is being competently used.

It should not be assumed that either the courses or the manuals contain all the relevant information. Remember that the initial contacts with the vendor are via his sales staff whose main aim is to persuade the prospective customer to buy the system, which may mean that disadvantages will be minimised, ignored, or even presented as advantages.

It is therefore necessary to assume – until the contrary is proved – that a course offered by a vendor is not complete, and that the complexity of the DBMS is directly proportional to the number of courses offered. To err on the side of caution, it should also be assumed that the number and length of courses is directly proportional to the time required afterwards to use the DBMS competently.

Contact with current users can give an indication of the time required to master the complexities of the system, and the general level of competence of the lecturers and the completeness of the courses. The complexity of the system can to some extent be judged by the number of manuals required to support the DBMS.

1.2.1.5 Vendor Information

Information regarding the vendor's attitude to the users cannot be reliably obtained from the vendor himself. The user group is probably the most reliable source of information, although it should not be forgotten that they themselves are interested in encouraging rather than discouraging new users. Nevertheless, they have a far more sober view of the DBMS than the vendor.

1.2.1.6 Staff Requirements

The points contained under this heading can be the source of the greatest cost within user related aspects.

Not only are there large differences in the personnel requirements between the different systems, but also the activities of the job functions vary greatly. This is particularly true of the DBA function. With some DBMSs, this function is strongly oriented to system maintenance, while with other systems, DB design and program support are the DBA's main task.

Particular attention should be paid to claims by the vendor, such as 'All complicated and complex tasks have been placed in the realm of the DBA, thus leaving the programmer free to program.' This may simply be a sales ploy meaning in reality that the DBMS is complicated to run.

The total number of staff required in maintaining and designing the database should be compared (programming should be excluded.) The skill levels required for the functions will be a deciding factor in the cost of the personnel. It should not be overlooked that difficulties could be encountered in recruiting personnel of the required qualitiy and quantity.

1.3 The External Technical Aspects

These are the aspects which describe the facilities offered by the DBMS. The internal technical aspects are concerned with how these facilities are implemented. Many of these aspects are not absolutely necessary, particularly for the new DBMS user. But remember that the DBMS will be used for a minimum of five years, and during this time the processing requirements will most probably grow to take advantage of any available facilities.

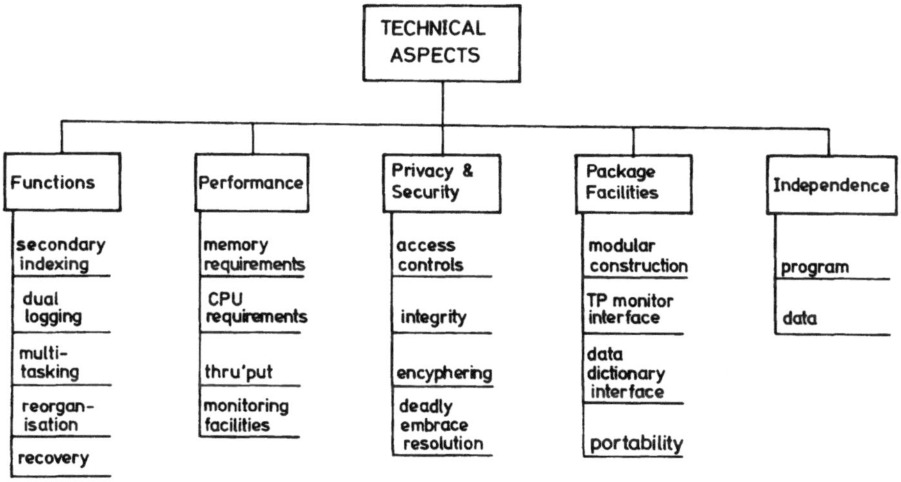

Fig. 1.3: External Technical Aspects

1.3.1 Functions

This section contains a number of unrelated facilities without which the product cannot claim to be a DBMS.

1.3.1.1 Secondary Indexing

Secondary Indexing should be implemented via inverted file techniques and should be capable of accommodating synonyms without having to chain them into overflow areas, or without making them unique by adding useless data to the key. It should moreover be possible to define a secondary index as being composed of a number of physically separate fields within a record. With two of the DBMSs examined, it was necessary to unload and reorganise the database in order to generate a new secondary index. This is an impossible situation, and can mean, for large databases, that it is simply too time-consuming a process to be used properly. The construction of a secondary index should simply require the primary database to be read.

1.3.1.2 Dual Logging

Logging is an absolute necessity for a DBMS. It must record all attempts to access the database – at least those attempts which are unsuccessful – and all changes to the database. Dual logging is simply a safety feature in that if one log unit breaks down, the other can continue until the operator shuts down the system. Similarly, if a log file is found to have a fault on it when the database is being reconstructed, the second one may be used. It is almost inconceivable that both have the same fault at the same place.

1.3.1.3 Multi-tasking

The DBMS should be programmed in such a way that the different DML commands can be serviced in parallel and that the same command type is serviced by a multi-threading module.

1.3.1.4 Reorganisation

The performance of every database begins to degrade as the contents are modified. The rate of degradation is dependent on many factors (see 1.4.2 Space Management). When the degradation becomes unacceptable, the DBMS must contain a function to reorganise the database so as to improve performance.

1.3.1.5 Recovery

Recovery is the process of returning the system to a physically intact state after a catastrophic failure. Failures fall broadly into one of two categories:

– program
– system (DBMS, OS, secondary storage, etc.)

Recovery procedures also fall into two categories, that is, Rollforward and Rollback.

Rollforward is almost always under the control of the operator as it entails taking a copy of the database and applying all changes made to the database from the time the database copy was taken to the chosen checkpoint. Rollback to the last checkpoint made (by each active program) is usually an automatic process. Rollback to an earlier checkpoint requires operator intervention.

1.3.2 Performance

Performance criteria can roughly be divided into two groups:

– DBMS design
– database design.

The first is something that the user can hardly influence and covers such points as the amount of memory required by the DBMS, the number of instructions that have to be executed by each DBMS request, and whether or not all the modules are reentrant.

Database design can be influenced by the DBA, but there are several areas in which the DBMS can be influenced only to a very limited degree, that is in reusing space released by deleted records; handling variable length records; handling synonyms; placing records in the data space, etc. The best the DBA can hope for is that a monitor is available which will deliver statistics indicating when a reorganisation is necessary.

1.3.3 Privacy and Security

Not only is it necessary to limit access to the database to authorised users, but also to limit their access in itself to those functions and record types that they require. Protecting the database from unauthorised access is implemented by one of two main methods:

– password
– encyphering (in some cases compression can also be considered to be encyphering).

Encyphering has the advantage that a dump of the database is also very difficult to read.

Most authorised users of the database are only interested in reading a few fields in the database. It is therefore sensible to limit each user's access to only that data which is necessary, and further, to allocate specific processing rights (read only, insert, delete, update).

The DBMS must also contain logic for resolving deadly embrace situations. This can be a simple timer mechanism or logic which identifies that deadlock will occur with a particular request.

Transaction-oriented processing should be available with every DBMS, with the unit of work that constitutes a transaction being under programmer control. This is necessary to guarantee the logical integrity of the database.

1.3.4 Package Facilities

Even those DBMSs which do not offer their own TP monitors and data dictionaries should offer an interface to such products, since it is almost certain that every user will require them to support the DBMS. The TP monitor must make synchronised checkpoints with the DBMS. Even better is a single log file complex.

An integrated data dictionary can be a powerful tool in supporting access control and data integrity.

Modular construction of the DBMS is a great help in tuning. It can also be economically advantageous if the modules are separately priced items. Portability is currently of interest to only a small minority of users, but the growing interest in distributed database technology means that the demand for portability is constantly growing.

1.3.5 Independence

It is of great advantage to be able to isolate all programs that are already in production from any changes made to the database structure. Changes to the database structure can be any of the following:

- a field can be added
- a field can be extended
- a field can have its characteristics changed
- a new record type can be introduced
- a record type can be removed
- a field can be deleted.

Removal of a field or record type from the database structure automatically requirès modification to each program that uses these items. However, any additions to the database structure (from the inclusion of a check digit to the introduction of a new record type) need not require any change to the currently running programs.

In addition to the absolutely necessary Record Level Sensitivity, Field Level Sensitivity should also be available. This feature should allow the user to receive and transmit fields in a different sequence and with different characteristics from those used to store the records. The security aspects of Field Level Sensitivity should not be ignored.

1.4 Internal Technical Aspects

This section is concerned with the ways that the DBMSs implement the functions and facilities. The points raised here are not a necessary part of the initial selection process, but will help to round off the essential background information before proceeding to stage three, the detailed evaluation.

It cannot be emphasised too strongly that the DBMS vendors may turn technical shortcomings into sales advantages and redefine standard terms to hide deficiencies in their products. This makes it imperative to confront the sales personnel with a questionnaire which specifies the subjects to be discussed and their order. Under no circumstances allow the salesman to give his prepared presentation; this will usually describe only the advantages of the DBMS. In some cases, claims are made for products which are demonstrably untrue.

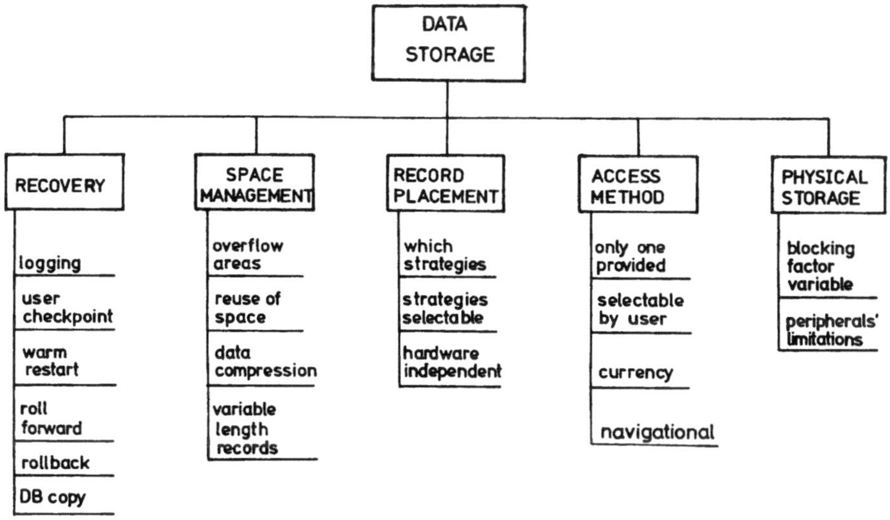

Fig. 1.4a: Internal Technical Aspects (I)

1.4.1 Recovery

Recovery facilities are offered by nearly all DBMSs, but the facilities differ dramatically in their nature and performance.

Logging is absolutely essential to a DBMS. The BEFORE and AFTER IMAGES of each modification are recorded for each database processed. Additonally, some systems log all DBMS access violations. DBMSs supporting transaction oriented processing must also log the start and end of each transaction.

For checkpointing, some systems allow the user to include his own information (needed for repositioning) on the log file with the checkpoint log record. Transaction-oriented processing requires a separate temporary log file to record all modifications to the database(s) until the checkpoint is reached, when the modifications are transferred to the permanent log file. All records modified by a program cannot be accessed by other programs until the modifying program issues a checkpoint. This can lead to a deadlock situation when more than one program is modifying the database. This possibility must be identified and resolved by the DBMS and not left to organisational measures of allowing only one program to modify the database at any one time.

The temporary log file is used in cases of system failure and if the program cannot, for any reason, complete a transaction, to return the database to the state applying at the beginning of the transaction. In the former case, the DBMS should automatically return the database to the last checkpoint, when a warm restart takes place after an uncontrolled shutdown of the DBMS. Returning the database to any earlier checkpoint usually requires DBA/Operator intervention and can use either ROLLFORWARD or ROLLBACK utilities. In the latter case the database should automatically return the database to the last checkpoint as soon as the program aborts.

The database must be periodically copied to backing storage. This should be done by copying the physical blocks in physical sequence – the fastest method. The log files contain modifications in a random order and may contain a series of modifications to a particular record. For speed of reconstruction (ROLLFORWARD) using the database copy and the log files, it would be advantageous to eliminate all 'duplicate' modifications and to sort the log records in ascending physical block sequence.

1.4.2 Space Management

Space management has a critical influence on performance. The type of space management required is dependent on the access method being supported. The direct access methods are far more sensitive to inefficient space management than those based on inverted file techniques, where a certain order is imperative.

The hashing routine indicates a physical block where a record should be stored, but if there is no space available in the indicated block, the record will be stored in a neighbouring block (or in the overflow area). It is largely irrelevant in which block a record is stored, if it is not the indicated one. Thus, if a record cannot be stored in its indicated block simply because of a record which has 'overflowed' from another block, the sensible approach is to remove the overflow record to make room for the 'home' record. This method is however adopted by no means all DBMSs.

Those DBMSs offering access methods based on inverted file techniques show large differences in their approaches, particularly in their handling of synonyms. The obvious approach – and the optimal – is to use variable length records, each holding the value, a series of pointers to those records holding the value, and a counter of these pointers. This common-sense approach is unfortunately not universal. Some DBMSs store all synonyms in the overflow area, or attach separate fields to the key values to make them unique, thereby wasting the space occupied by the extension of the key and also by having to repeat the key value. Both types of data organisation should release space resulting from record deletions and make it available for further insertions. Some DBMSs only set a flag in the record to show that the record may be removed at the next reorganisation.

There are two sorts of variable length record: firstly, a record type whose occurrences may have different lengths but any particular occurrence retains the initial length until it is deleted; secondly the true variable length record, where a record occurrence can change its length (increase or decrease) with each update. This second type requires a far more sophisticated handling because of fragmentation.

Data compression requires the DBMS to handle true variable length records efficiently. Those DBMSs which do not allow the record to move within the block are therefore incapable of handling true variable length records efficiently and of handling free space competently.

Data compression routines – and not simply a user exit – should be offered by the vendor. The compression routine should be capable of handling more than just repeated zeroes and blanks, and at least repeating double characters should be recognised.

1.4.3 Record Placement

Record placement is of secondary importance with storage methods based on inverted file techniques unless it is frequently necessary to process the database in a particular logical sequence. ADABAS offers a unique solution, which combines the advantages of direct access methods with a system based on inverted file techniques.

Hierarchical and network structuring DBMSs require sophisticated record placement strategies in order to reduce the I/O traffic on the most-used access paths. This is not particularly condusive to data independence. With hierarchical structures, the problem is limited because only the location of the root is normally considered important. Deep (ie. many levels of) hierarchical structures are normally avoided because this lack of placement strategy leads to poor performance. Networking systems should allow for different placement strategies for each record type. The problem which then results is that the design becomes too difficult and the resulting structure too rigid to easily accommodate processing pattern changes.

Twin chains produce an ordering problem. The DBMS should have the ability to order records on some key value (with synonyms being placed before the first or behind the last occurrence of that key value) in either ascending or descending order. When no key field is specified, the new insertion's placement should be under the programmer's control – at the front of, or at the end of the chain, or at some place in between, depending on the current position held by the programmer in the database.

The performance of databases using direct access methods is critically dependent on the randomizing routine. A selection of these routines should be offered, and the possibility available for the user to include his own routines.

If the database has to be redesigned and reorganised before it can be loaded onto a new secondary storage medium, then this might result in new cheaper storage types not easily being adopted because of the effort involved.

1.4.4 Access Methods

There is no necessity for the storage method to be the same as the access method. Randomly stored records can be processed directly, in a physical sequence and via a secondary index in a logical sequence. Data structures based on inverted file techniques can be processed in either logical or physical sequence. The physical sequence is used to process the whole database when the actual order of processing all records is irrelevant, because it is the most efficient way of accessing all records.

The concept of position is important in a database, particularly in hierarchical and network based systems, where the GET NEXT type instructions must be extended to include:

GET PARENT
GET PREVIOUS
GET CHILD
GET FIRST/LAST type instructions.

Without such instructions, traversing the data structure becomes difficult.

1.4.5 Physical Storage

Different parts of a database, ie. different record types, are processed differently, and it is useful to be able to vary the blocking factor to accommodate these differences.

For secondary index structures (and databases based on inverted file techniques) it is sensible to have different blocking factors for the primary and secondary files. It can be of great advantage to be able to place different parts of the database on different secondary storage devices in order to optimise cost/performance factors.

It is also very important to know whether there are any restrictions on the peripherals that are supported by the DBMS, particularly the more modern ones. Even if your installation has not been upgraded to the most modern peripherals, it is likely to be at some point in the future. Therefore, any contract should contain a guarantee that the vendor would provide the necessary support from some specified date.

1.4.6 Data Structures

In general, DBMSs are divided into two groups when discussing their structuring capabilities:

- hierarchical/network based systems
- systems based on inverted file techniques.

Hierarchies are only subsets of networks, therefore these two types are network based and should together be compared with the systems based on inverted file techniques.

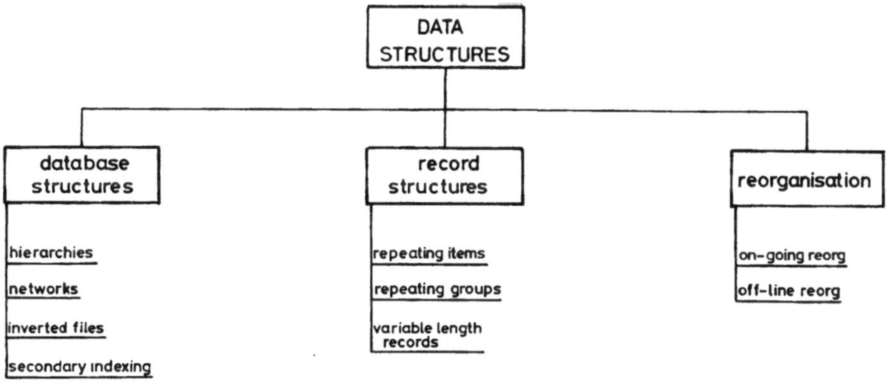

Fig. 1.4b: Internal Technical Aspects (II)

Networking based systems are characterised by the following properties:

- large initial design effort
- rigidity of structure (due to embedded pointers expressing the relationships)
- fast response along the designed paths.

Structures based on inverted file techniques, on the other hand, have these properties:

- low initial design effort before the first application is running
- great flexibility to changing processing requirements
- good response to processing on non-unique keys.

Had the distinction between the two groups remained so sharp, the choice would be simple. Unfortunately, processing is rarely on a single unique key, so that networking DBMSs have had to implement secondary indexing (usually using inverted file techniques) and those DBMSs based on inverted file techniques have implemented direct accessing techniques to speed up response which is especially necessary in an on-line query environment.

Thus, the essential difference remains between embedded physical pointers and symbolic keys: the former performs better in environments where little change in the structure and processing requirements is envisaged, and the latter in any other environment. The former requires more design and maintenance personnel; both types require the same level of programmer skills, although the areas requiring the skills are different.

1.4.7 Record Structuring

It is quite possible to have a hierarchical structure or a table contained within a record. In fact, such structures are far more common in traditional data processing environments than in a database environment. This is because the traditional record is 'broken down' into the constituent elements and each element is stored separately, and related via pointers to its associated elements.

Nevertheless, it can be advantageous to be able to express two or three levels of hierarchy, or a two/three dimensional table within a single record. This is particularly relevant to DBMSs based on inverted file techniques. This feature is implemented by allowing a field to repeat itself up to a specified number of times (REPEATING ITEM); the same construction can be applied to a group of items (REPEATING GROUP).

Care should be taken to ascertain if there are any restrictions on the number of times an item or group can be repeated. A DBMS which handles variable length records badly will not be able to use this sort of feature efficiently. If there are any restrictions on the number of fields that can be defined, or the definition of a large number of fields affects performance adversely, then the advantages of this feature will be largely negated.

In order to be able to handle variable length records, the location of a record must be moveable, at least within the block. This is irrespective of the storage organisation. If this is not possible, then fragmentation occurs – even when space is available within the block holding the record that has expanded.

The record's position can be variable because the pointer to it indicates only the block holding the required record. This has the advantage of using very little space for the relative address. The record's position within the block can be held in the block prefix, or can be found by scanning the block. In either case, the space available within the block can be used by any record, simply by shifting their positions.

If an expanded record cannot be accommodated within the block, then another block in the overflow area, or in the neighbourhood of the full one must be used to accommodate the expanded record, or the expanded part of the record. If a succession of expansions cause the expanded part to be stored in yet another block from the previous fragment, then performance will degrade, as record retrieval requires more I/O traffic.

If, however, the original part of the record, or at least a pointer, is held in the original location and the rest is held in one particular location, a maximum of two accesses is required to retrieve the record. This method is somewhat more expensive when updating a record, because when additional data causes a record to be moved to a new block, the pointer from the original block has to be modified.

This updating of the pointer in the original block can usually be accomplished at a minimum processing cost because the block is normally already in the I/O buffer. This is because it had to be retrieved to read the record that is being modified.

This problem can also be encountered in systems supporting hierarchical structures (even without variable length records!) It is a result of records being inserted into a hierarchy (after the initial load) and there being physically no space available within the block where the record logically belongs. Thus the record is accommodated in another block, which can result in excessive I/O traffic and require too frequent off-line reorganisation.

1.4.8 Reorganisation

Any database subject to modifications normally becomes progressively more disorganised. At some time, this disorganisation causes noticeable performance degradation and the database must be reorganised off-line to overcome this. During the off-line reorganising process, the database cannot be accessed by the users. Thus the time for the reorganisation should be held to a minimum, and the time between reorganisations should be as great as possible.

The first aim can be achieved by keeping the databases small, and the second aim is a parameter of the DBMS. Some DBMSs make little or no effort to stop the database from degrading, others make great efforts. (This is one reason why benchmark tests produce results of very questionable validity).

Since it is not always possible to keep the size of the databases to a minimum, it is important, in an environment which could cause disorganisation, to have a DBMS which makes a certain attempt at on-line reorganisation.

1.5 The Preliminary Elimination Process

The selection team should draw up a simple table listing those functions of a DBMS which they have identified as being important to the enterprise. Each of the DBMSs being examined will be evaluated on a scale 0–10, for each of the required functions. For particular key functions, a '0' will eliminate that DBMS automatically. Although this process would appear on first examination to be extremely long-winded and complicated, this is not usually the case since those DBMSs which do not support designated key functions are swiftly eliminated.

1.6 The Final Elimination Process

Appendix V contains a sample questionnaire for the final selection process. This final step should be sufficiently detailed to uncover the exact functioning of all the relevant features. This will require detailed interviews with the vendor's staff, as well as a careful scrutiny of the manuals. A second interview should be the last activity before the final report is written, and should be used principally to confirm the opinion formed by the team, and possibly to clear up any outstanding points.

The first interview with the vendor may have taken place during the earlier selection steps. Nevertheless, if the selection team feels it would benefit from a further interview, the vendor is normally only too happy to oblige. The main interview with the vendor will most probably take most of one day and will be used solely to elucidate the answers to the questions listed in the questionnaire.

The vendor should also be invited to give his opinion of the competing DBMSs. This serves a double purpose: it illustrates the kind of sales tactics adopted by that particular vendor; it allows the team to get a different – though not necessarily valid – view of the competing products. Each vendor tends to be scathing about their competitiors' products, and will obviously try to identify any weak points.

The features examined should, in this final stage, be weighted, whereas previously, the mere fact that a feature was available was sufficient to qualify the DBMS. Thus each feature should be weighted depending on its usefulness or necessity to the enterprise, and each feature should further be judged per DBMS as to how well it has been implemented, on a scale, say, of 1–5. For example, recovery is far more important than data compression – however desirable this latter feature may be – and there is a vast difference between the ways in which the individual DBMSs implement this feature.

The team should recognise that certain DBMSs possess a particular 'appeal'. The question is: should any effort be made to counteract this appeal? The answer is a simple 'no', since this appeal results from some aspect or from the logical construction of the DBMS, and as such, is an integral part of it. Thus in the allocation of points, this appeal should be rewarded. Each member of the team should be required to give an overall judgement of the DBMSs in the final stage, and list them in order of preference. This preference list should be included in the final decision matrix.

Reports on the six most popular DBMSs (on IBM and compatible hardware) have been included to ease the process of selection. For most users, the chosen DBMS will be one of these systems. The reports stem from the final quarter of 1980. Even if a particular vendor has made some significant extension to his DBMS (as can be expected from S2000), the validity of the reports still remains since the systems will not be radically changed, merely extended.

2. IMS (Information Management System)

IMS is IBM's principle database product for the S360/S370 and S30XX ranges of computer. It is composed of two separately priced products – the DC and the DB components. The DC product, IMS–DC is virtually never installed without the DB product, IMS–DB (or DL/1). The IMS–DB product has, however, been interfaced with a large number of TP monitors: IMS–DC, CICS, INTERCOMM, TASKMASTER, SHADOW II, ENVIRON/I.

IMS can trace its origins back to the early 1960s, when the Space Division of North American Rockwell was awarded the Apollo contract. IMS was developed jointly by IBM and North American Rockwell, and the first application was implemented using IMS on System/360 hardware during 1968. Later the same year, IBM released IMS–1 as a Program Product.

The initial requirements which led to the development of IMS were for an on-line generalised access method which could handle very large quantities of data. Data was considered to be hierarchical in nature. This hierarchical structure was supported by two storage organisations

– Hierarchical Sequential Access Method (HSAM)
– Hierarchical Indexed Sequential Access Method (HISAM).

In March 1971, IMS–2 was made available. This new version had a number of important improvements. Two new storage organisations were introduced:

– Hierarchical Direct Access Method (HDAM)
– Hierarchical Indexed Direct Access Method (HIDAM).

A further improvement was to separate the DB and DC components into two individually priced products. The third major enhancement was the most radical divergence from the original hierarchical storage concept: the facility to define and manipulate limited networks via LOGICAL pointers was introduced. (The user still saw his data structure in terms of hierarchies).

The next series of enhancements was introduced in February 1974 (IMS/VS) so as to coincide with the introduction of a virtual storage concept for the operating system (OS/VS). These included secondary indexing, variable length SEGMENTS, checkpoint/restart facilities and concurrent updating.

With IMS/VS 1.1.5 came the final improvement of importance: field level sensitivity was introduced, which considerably promoted data independence.

2.1 Classification

IMS is by far the most difficult DBMS, of those examined, to classify. This is partly due to the complexity, and partly due to the apparent lack of an all-embracing concept in the original design, which then dictated the evolution of the system. IMS was a system based purely on hierarchical structures, certainly until IMS–2 was introduced in 1971. Thereafter, a limited networking capability was available to the DBA, but the programmer was (and is) still limited to hierarchical structures in his LOCAL VIEW.

In order to process a network, the programmer has to use a series of LOCAL VIEWS, each representing a different hierarchical subset of the network. A further complication is that it is possible to generate a partially inverted file structure (similar to VSAM) using IMS. Nevertheless, IMS can best be described as a DBMS based on a hierarchical storage organisation with networking overtones.

Although this report is primarily concerned with DL/1 – the database component of IMS – it is in practice impossible to ignore the DC component because a number of functions necessary to the efficient execution of the system are contained within it.

Without the DC component, the DL/1 nucleus has to be loaded into each partition/region with the application program, so there is no protection against concurrent updating. The minimum CPU that will support DL/1 is a system 370/138 requiring ca. 125 Kb with typically 30–60 Kb for the I/0 buffers. Together with the DC component, a minimum of ca. 750 Kb would be necessary.

One further complication with IMS is that this system requires either ISAM/OSAM or VSAM as its basic access method. However, any new user would be well advised to choose VSAM, as its use offers many advantages, for example secondary indexing and variable length SEGMENTS. This report will only concern itself with VSAM, both for the sake of brevity and modernity.

Because of its complexity, IMS requires a larger team of DBAs than the other DBMSs examined, and the successful implementation of this system is more dependent on their skills than is the case with the competing DBMSs.

2.2 Data Item Definition

An IMS database consists of database records, each of which in turn is composed of a ROOT SEGMENT occurrence together with all its dependent SEGMENT occurrences. This concept of a database record is seldom used in IMS literature.

The SEGMENT (which can be thought of as one occurrence) of a repeating group, is of central importance to IMS. A maximum of 255 different SEGMENT types can be defined for any one database. Each SEGMENT is composed of one or more fields. There are two types of field. (A third type, the SYSTEM RELATED field, is relevant only when secondary indexing is used.)

All fields are characterised by three parameters:

- a start byte position within the SEGMENT
- a length (in bytes)
- the type of data to be held in the field, either hexadecimal, packed decimal or alphanumeric.

In addition to these parameters, it is possible to define one field per SEGMENT type as a SEQUENCE field, which is used to determine the order in which occurrences of the particular SEGMENT type are accessed. HISAM, HDAM and HIDAM databases must have a unique SEQUENCE field in the ROOT SEGMENT. With all other SEGMENT types the SEQUENCE field may or may not be unique. Whenever a SEQUENCE field is not specified, INSERT RULES must be specified. They cause the insertion of a TWIN SEGMENT occurrence at the beginning (FIRST), at the end (LAST), of the TWIN chain, or after the current position (HERE) within the TWIN chain. With non-unique SEQUENCE fields it is necessary to specifiy whether a duplicate key should be inserted before or after the SEGMENT(s) with the same value SEQUENCE field.

A database cannot contain more than 1000 field types, nor can a SEGMENT type contain more than 255 field types.

2.3 Data Storage Structures

IMS terminology has always been somewhat confusing, particularly because the terms PHYSICAL and LOGICAL when applied to databases had different meanings to those current in database literature generally. This was compounded by allowing the term LOGICAL DATABASE also to mean 'user view' – in keeping with normal database usage. IBM appears to have recognised this confusion and has now redefined the terms. 'PHYSICAL DATABASE' now includes those databases containing LOGICAL relationships as well as the mandatory PHYSICAL relationships. LOGICAL DATABASE is now reserved exclusively for the user view.

This change, while being a step in the right direction, is doubly unfortunate not only because the IMS manuals have not been updated, but also because there is no new term to indicate that a PHYSICAL DATABASE has been extended to include LOGICAL relationships.

Prior to explaining the various storage organisations and how they can be linked logically, it is necessary to explain the basic IMS terminology.

2.3.1 Basic Concepts and Terminology in IMS

The basic component of an IMS database is a SEGMENT, which consists of a series of fields. An IMS database consists of SEGMENTS structured hierarchically with up to 15 levels. It is possible to link one or more of these databases to create a new database containing structures more complex than hierarchies.

An IMS database must be based on one of the four basic storage organisations. The present discussion will limit itself therefore to the hierarchical structures in order to define the basic concepts of IMS, (see section 2.3.3.3 Logical Relationships, for the method of linking one or more databases to form complex structures.)

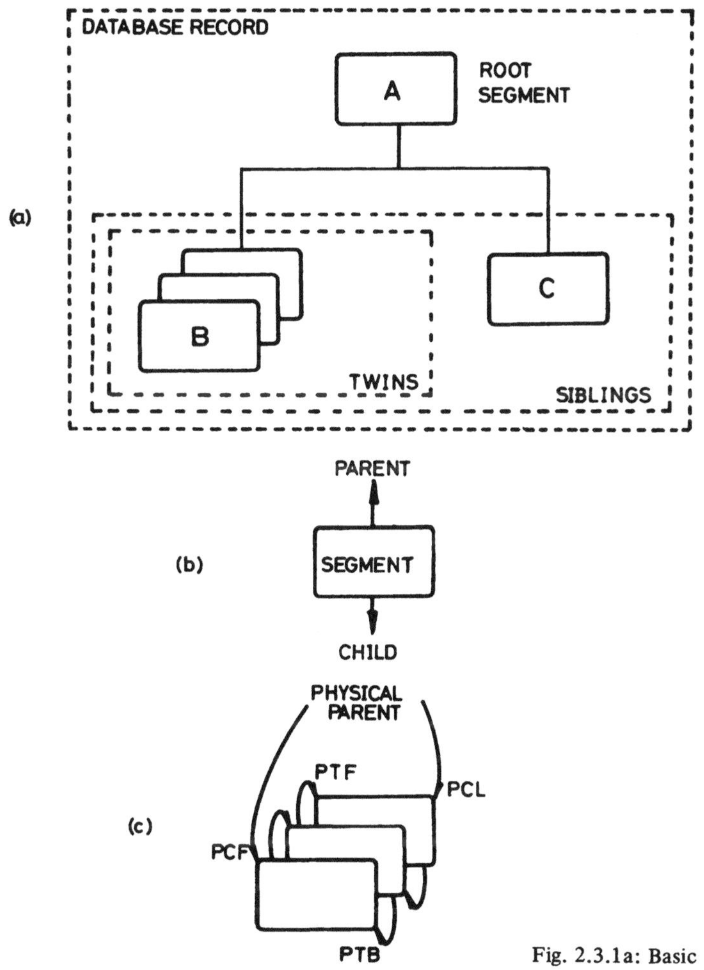

Fig. 2.3.1a: Basic IMS Terminology

A database record consists of a ROOT SEGMENT and a number of DEPENDENT SEGMENTS. The ROOT SEGMENT type is the highest level type in the hierarchy, all the other SEGMENT types, in the lower levels, being termed DEPENDENT SEGMENT types. Each DEPENDENT SEGMENT has a PARENT SEGMENT and is one element in a parent-child relationship. Multiple occurrences of the same SEGMENT dependent on one PARENT SEGMENT occurrence are termed TWINS. Multiple occurrences of different SEGMENT types all dependent on one PARENT SEGMENT occurrence are known collectively as SIBLINGS.

The Sequential Access Methods do not use pointers to link SEGMENT occurrences, but use physical adjacency to define the SEGMENTs' relationship to each other. The Direct Access Methods use PHYSICAL CHILD pointers to relate a PHYSICAL PARENT SEGMENT to its CHILD SEGMENTS and the TWIN SEGMENTS are also linked by PHYSICAL TWIN pointers or alternatively by HIERARCHICAL pointers, which will be discussed later in this section.

The PHYSICAL PARENT SEGMENT occurrence is linked to the first occurrence of a CHILD SEGMENT type with a PHYSICAL CHILD FIRST (PCF) pointer. Optionally, the last occurrence of the CHILD SEGMENT type can be linked using a PHYSICAL CHILD LAST pointer. The occurrences of a particular CHILD SEGMENT type are linked by PHYSICAL TWIN FORWARD (PTF) pointers. Optionally, the same SEGMENTS can be linked in the opposite direction using PHYSICAL TWIN BACKWARD pointers. All these points are illustrated in Fig. 2.3.1a and 2.3.1b.

The hierarchical structure of an IMS database is viewed as being from top to bottom, from front to back and from left to right. This is shown in Fig. 2.3.1b (ii), where the hierarchical sequence is shown by the numbers in each SEGMENT. SEGMENT No. 2 ie. the first occurrence of the type B has no C or D type occurrences dependent on it.

HIERARCHICAL pointers follow this same sequence. The disadvantage of these pointers is the long path to be followed to access some of the SEGMENTS eg. the single occurrence of the D type SEGMENT. This problem can be overcome by using a combination of PHYSICAL CHILD and PHYSICAL TWIN pointers in place of HIERARCHICAL pointers. This is demonstrated in Fig. 2.3.1c (ii). The D type SEGMENT can now be reached much more easily. The names of the pointers can be taken from Fig. 2.3.1a (c). In fact, HIERARCHICAL pointers are seldom, if ever, used.

With all pointer types, there is always a parallel pointer in the opposite sense which is optional, eg. TWIN FORWARD and TWIN BACKWARD, PARENT FIRST and PARENT LAST etc. These pointers improve IMS's delete performance. They do not provide the means to process a TWIN chain backwards for

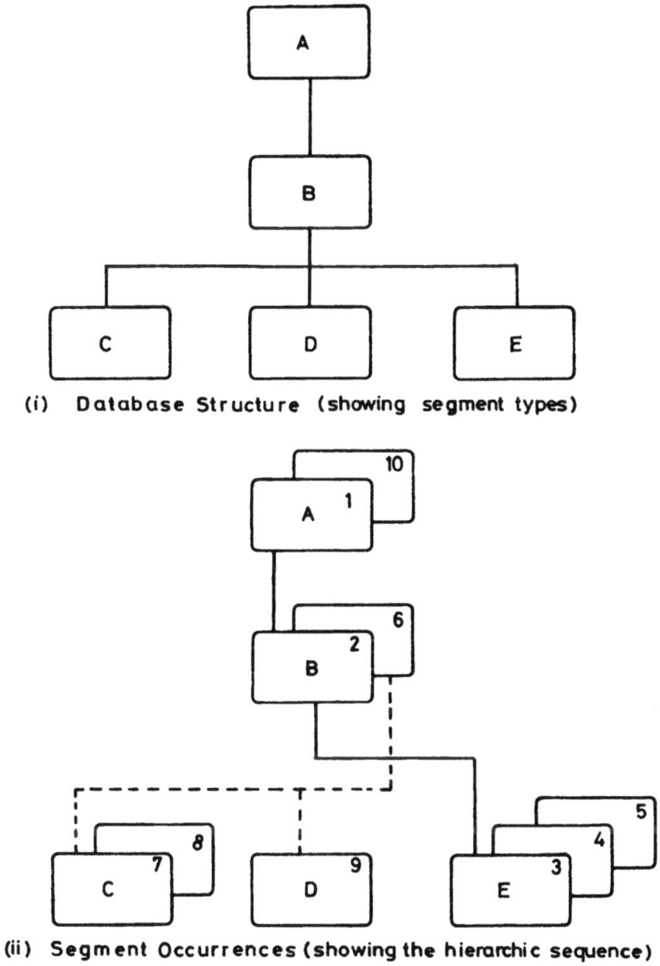

Fig. 2.3.1b: Basic IMS Concepts 1

example. This is generally not possible in DL/1, although there are a few partial exceptions – see section 2.4.

All these pointers, together with SEGMENT type and status information are held in a SEGMENT Prefix, (see Fig. 2.3.3d). Although this Prefix is totally under the control of IMS and totally transparent to the user view, the DBA needs to know the length of this area when calculating CI sizes etc.

Generally, IMS SEGMENTS consist of a Prefix and user data. The Prefix must contain at least a SEGMENT Code and a Delete Byte, see Fig. 2.3.3d. The

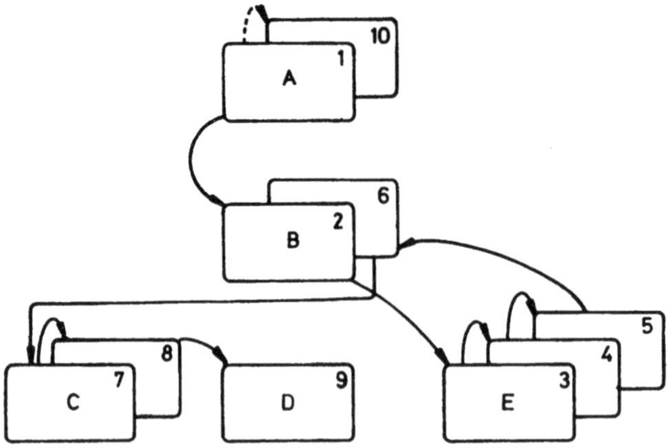

(i) Hierarchical Pointers

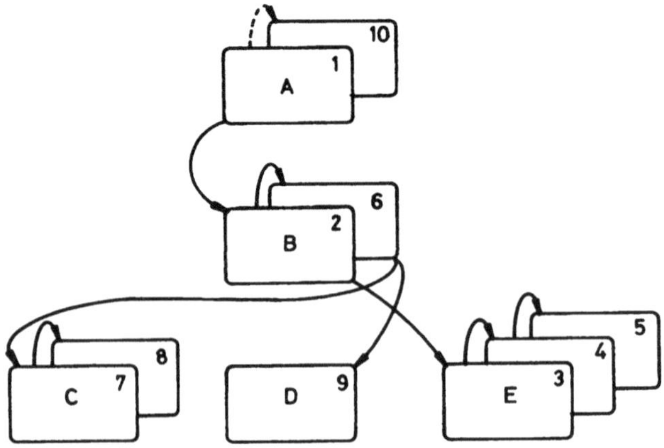

(ii) Parent / Child Pointers and Twin Pointers

Fig. 2.3.1c: Basic IMS Concepts 2

pointer and counter area will not be present in HISAM or HSAM databases for obvious reasons. Both HIDAM and HDAM databases relate SEGMENTS with direct points, so these SEGMENTS will contain one or more pointers in the Prefix. If a HISAM database is involved in logical relationships with a HDAM/ HIDAM database and the SEGMENTS in the HISAM database use direct pointers (instead of Symbolic pointers), then even a HISAM SEGMENT Prefix can contain pointers. Counters are only necessary in LOGICAL PARENT SEGMENTS under special conditions (see Section 2.3.3).

Each SEGMENT type is allocated a number between 1 and 255. This is called the SEGMENT Code, and uniquely identifies occurrences of this SEGMENT type. The number is allocated in ascending sequence starting with the ROOT SEGMENT type and continuing for all dependent SEGMENT types in their hierarchical sequence.

The Delete Byte is necessary because in most cases, a deleted SEGMENT occurrence cannot be removed immediately (and the space released) since it is either involved in other relationships, or with HISAM it is too complicated for on-line work. The meaning of each of the bits in the Delete Byte is shown in Fig. 2.3.3d.

2.3.2 Physical Databases

This section will describe the basic storage organisations available to the IMS database designer. The way in which the hierarchical data structures can be linked so as to avoid the problem of data redundancy will also be examined.

IMS databases can be constructed from one of four basic types of physical organisation. These are divided into two basic types of access method, namely DIRECT and SEQUENTIAL. Each access method offers two variants: indexed and non-indexed. The main difference between the two access methods is that with the SEQUENTIAL type, the hierarchical relationship between SEGMENT occurrences is defined by their physical adjacency in storage, whereas the DIRECT type uses pointers to define the hierarchical relationship.

1. HSAM (Hierarchical Sequential Access Method). A HSAM database may only be processed sequentially, no inserts or deletes being permissible unless the whole file is copied. For this reason, it is possible to hold a HSAM database on magnetic tape, as well as on direct access storage devices. A HSAM database consists of a number of fixed length blocks which are stored using BSAM or QSAM OS access methods. The hierarchical structure of the database is defined by the physical adjacency of the SEGMENTS (see Fig. 2.3.2a). Neither inserting nor deleting of records is possible. SHSAM, (SIMPLE HSAM) databases can be created with VSAM. These contain only ROOT SEGMENT types, hence the Prefix is not required, and they may be processed by the standard file management software. There would seem to be almost no place for HSAM in a database environment.

2. HISAM (Hierarchical Indexed Sequential Access Method). HISAM offers indexed sequential entry point access to ROOT SEGMENT occurrences. The method used is similar to VSAM itself, but does not have VSAM's exemplary key compression. Each ROOT SEGMENT occurrence must have a unique key (SEQUENCE field).

A HISAM database consists of two data sets. The first, the KSDS, is used for primary storage of SEGMENTS and for the index hierarchy. The second, the

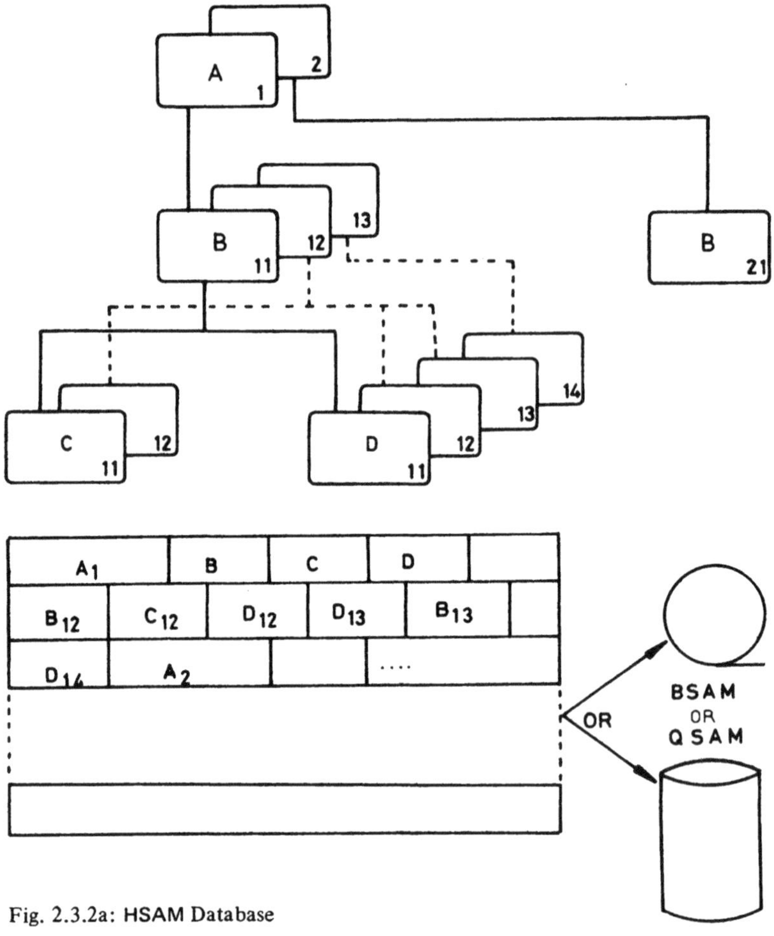

Fig. 2.3.2a: HSAM Database

ESDS, is to accommodate those dependent SEGMENTS which do not fit into the primary logical record. The terms used to describe the two data sets are 'primary' for the KSDS and 'secondary' for the ESDS.

Each KSDS logical record contains, in hierarchical sequence, one ROOT SEGMENT occurrence and as many dependent SEGMENTS as will fit. The remaining dependent SEGMENTS are stored, in hierarchical sequence in one or more logical records in the ESDS. All logical records containing SEGMENTS of the same database record are linked by direct address pointers, in hierarchical sequence. Each logical record is associated with only one database record and SEGMENTS are not split between two logical records. This is shown schematically in Fig. 2.3.2b.

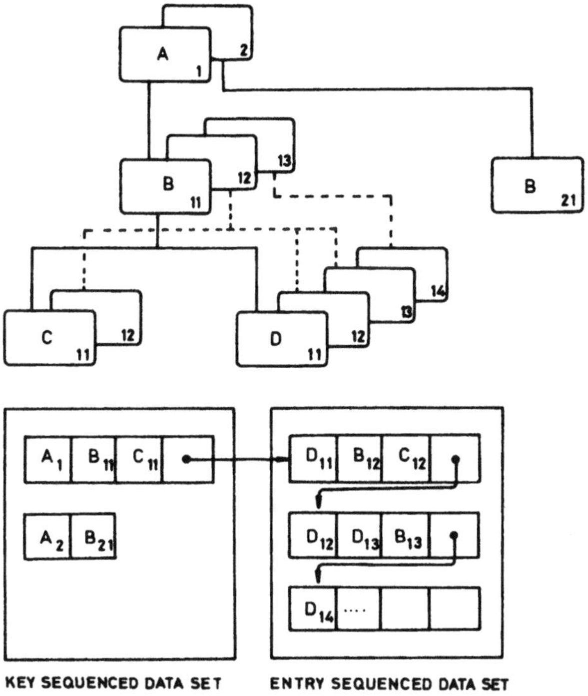

Fig. 2.3.2b: HISAM Database

The logical record structure is shown in Fig. 2.3.3d. The first four bytes are reserved for the direct address pointer. This pointer links all logical records of a database record in hierarchical sequence. Following the pointer are one or more SEGMENT occurrences of a database record in hierarchical sequence. A byte filled with zeros follows immediately after the last SEGMENT occurrence. One or more logical records are contained within a control interval, which is the unit of data transferred between an I/O device and main storage.

As all SEGMENTS belonging to a database record are related by their physical adjacency, any dependent SEGMENT added after the initial load must be accommodated by shifting all hierarchically lower SEGMENTS of the database record to make room for it. After the position for the new dependent SEGMENT has been identified, all SEGMENTS to the right of this position in the logical record are shifted to make room for the new SEGMENT. If, however, insufficient space is available, the contents of the logical record will be split and half moved into an empty control interval. The new SEGMENT will then be added to the C.I. (block) as described above. The same procedure is used to maintain the logical records containing the ROOT SEGMENTS in key sequence. The logical sequence of the database records is assured by the index in the KSDS.

The deletion of SEGMENTS is accomplished by setting the delete byte in the Prefix. The space is normally not available for reuse, except KSDS space when a ROOT SEGMENT is deleted during batch or 'exclusive' on-line processing. The associated ESDS space is not freed. Both ESDS and KSDS space is released during a reorganisation of the database.

Logical record size is a critical consideration for HISAM databases. Extremely long or short logical records tend to waste space, as do extremely large SEGMENT type length variations. Another source of performance degradation is high insert activity of dependent SEGMENTS. This can lead to the logical records associated with one database record being distributed over many control intervals.

3. HDAM (Hierarchical Direct Access Method). A HDAM database consists of an ESDS and either a user-written or IBM-supplied randomizing routine. The

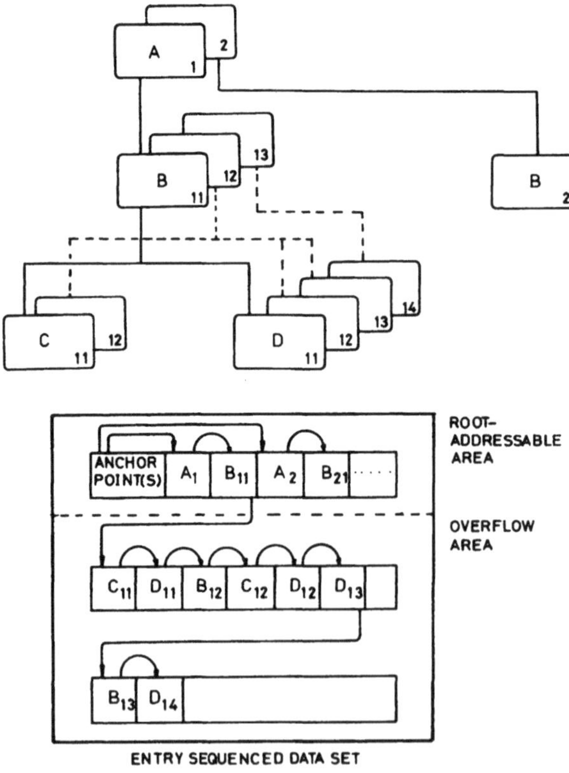

Fig. 2.3.2d: HDAM Database

new IBM-supplied randomizing routine will give good results in most cases. Should the user wish to write his own special randomizing routine, it should be remembered that the blocks used by the Bit Map have to be compensated for. It is possible to have a different randomizing routine for each HDAM database.

The randomizing routine operates on the key value (SEQUENCE field) in the ROOT SEGMENT to produce a RELATIVE BLOCK NUMBER and an ANCHOR POINT NUMBER. The RELATIVE BLOCK NUMBER indicates which control interval should be used to store the ROOT SEGMENT. The relative byte address of the SEGMENT will be stored in the ANCHOR POINTER AREA in a position determined by the ANCHOR POINT NUMBER. All SYNONYMS will be linked together irrespective of the CI they are stored in.

The ESDS is divided into two areas: the ROOT ADDRESSABLE AREA and the OVERFLOW AREA. The former holds the ROOT SEGMENTS. A number of dependent SEGMENTS can also be stored with the ROOT SEGMENT in the ROOT ADDRESSABLE AREA. The rest will be stored in the OVERFLOW AREA (see Fig. 2.3.2d). ROOT SEGMENTS can also be stored in the OVERFLOW AREA if no space is available in the RAA.

The randomizing routine used, as well as the sizes of the ROOT ADDRESSABLE and the OVERFLOW AREAS, and the number of ROOT ANCHOR POINTS per Control Interval are all dependent upon user-supplied parameters. The number of dependent SEGMENTS stored in the ROOT ADDRESSABLE AREA is also (to a limited extent) under user control. The user must specify the number of bytes of the database record to be stored consecutively in the ROOT ADDRESSABLE AREA by a series of INSERT commands (at load time or while processing the database). This can lead to fragmentation in the database, but this problem will be discussed more fully later.

The problem with any direct access method is the handling of synonyms ie, different key values that 'map' to the same address. IMS handles this by chaining the synonyms together with PHYSICAL TWIN POINTERS starting at the specified ANCHOR POINT. The reason for having multiple ANCHOR POINTS is to reduce the length of the synonym chains. As no randomizing routine can completely smoothe the irregular distribution of the key values, 'bunching' of SEGMENTS will occur. This results in some ROOT SEGMENTS not being stored in their HOME block, ie. in that block whose address was generated by the randomizing routine. Here, the length of the synonym chain can decisively affect performance. Fig. 2.3.2e shows the situation where multiple ROOT SEGMENT occurrences have randomized to the same Control Interval.

IMS space management always attempts to store synonyms as close to the home block as possible. After a series of deletes and inserts, it is possible for the situations represented in Fig. 2.3.2e (i) and (ii) to be reached, with the synonym

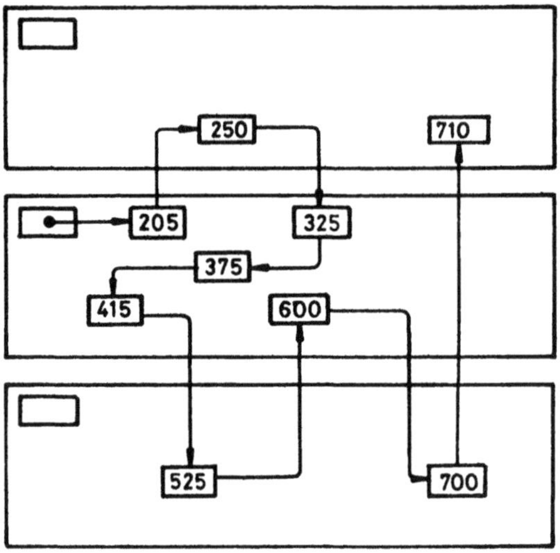

(i) Using only one ANCHOR POINT

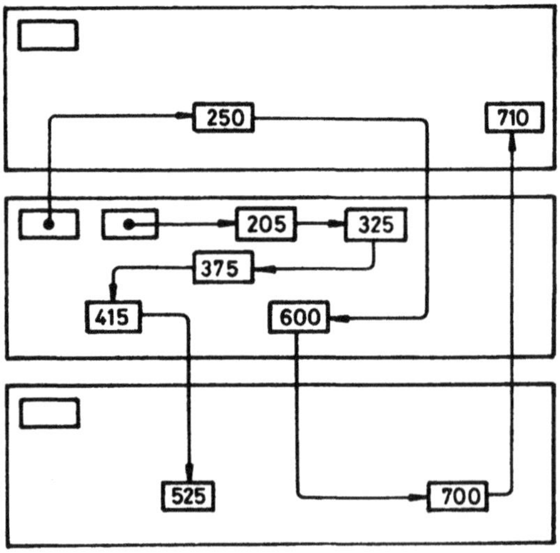

(ii) Using two ANCHOR POINTS

Fig. 2.3.2e: Synonym Handling

ROOT SEGMENTS being distributed over three control intervals. Using only one ANCHOR POINT (as in Fig. 2.3.2e (i)), more accesses are required to traverse all the synonyms than in Fig. 2.3.2e (ii), which has two ANCHOR POINTS. Naturally, a reorganisation can return most, if not all, of the synonyms to the home block.

When inserting dependent SEGMENTS, the space manager attempts to place them as close as possible to the control interval containing the parent SEGMENT (not necessarily the ROOT SEGMENT). If the parent of the dependent SEGMENTS to be added is in the ROOT ADDRESSABLE AREA (RAA), then the dependent SEGMENTS will be inserted into the same, or an adjacent, control interval – even if other dependent SEGMENTS have already been inserted into the OVERFLOW AREA.

These dependent SEGMENTS will, with consecutive INSERT commands, continue to be added to the RAA until the total number of bytes added (in this series of additions) exceeds the limit. All subsequent SEGMENTS for this database record which are added in this consecutive series of INSERT commands will then be accommodated in the OVERFLOW AREA.

This can lead to two unwanted conditions: the ROOT ADDRESSABLE AREA will be cluttered up with dependent SEGMENTS to the detriment of new ROOT SEGMENTS; and unacceptably long chains will be distributed over too many control intervals. Both problems can only be solved by reorganisation of the database as shown in Fig. 2.3.2f.

Deletion of a SEGMENT occurrence releases the space immediately for reuse by adding it to the space available chain. It is possible that the bit map has also to be updated (see section 2.8 on Space Management). The same procedure is also applied to any dependents of the deleted SEGMENT.

Performance of HDAM databases is heavily dependent on the size of the RAA. It can happen that ROOT SEGMENTS have to be stored in the OVERFLOW AREA because the RAA is full. This situation should be avoided at all costs!

4. HIDAM (Hierarchical Indexed Direct Access Method). A HIDAM database consists of two databases: an index database organised in HISAM and a database for the data based on an ESDS (similar to HDAM).

Each logical record at the lowest level of the index database (Primary HIDAM Index Database) consists of the unique key (SEQUENCE field) of a ROOT SEGMENT occurrence together with a direct pointer to it in the ESDS. Above this is the normal inverted file hierarchy of key value/ logical record pointers. The SEGMENTS of each database record stored in the ESDS are linked together with PHYSICAL CHILD and PHYSICAL TWIN pointers (see Fig. 2.3.1a).

Both HDAM and HIDAM use similar methods to store the database records, but their methods of accessing ROOT SEGMENTS are different. HDAM requires fewer accesses since the address is generated directly by the randomizing routine – although more than one access might be required to retrieve the desired ROOT SEGMENT because of synonyms. HIDAM has to process typically three or four levels of the index hierarchy before retrieving the address of the desired ROOT SEGMENT.

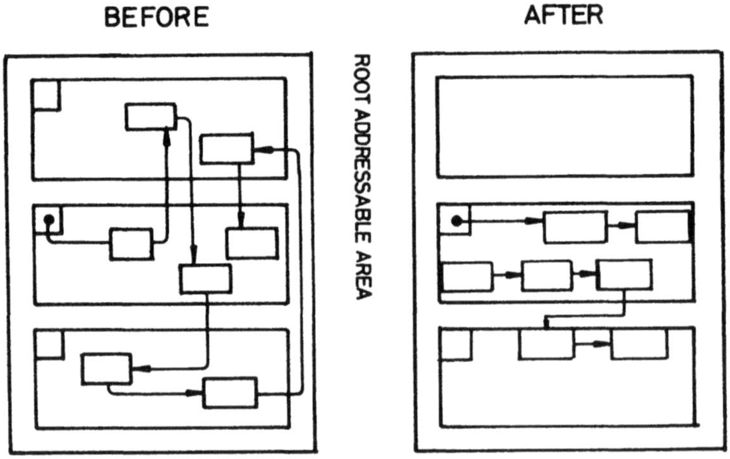

(i) Reorganisation of Synonyms

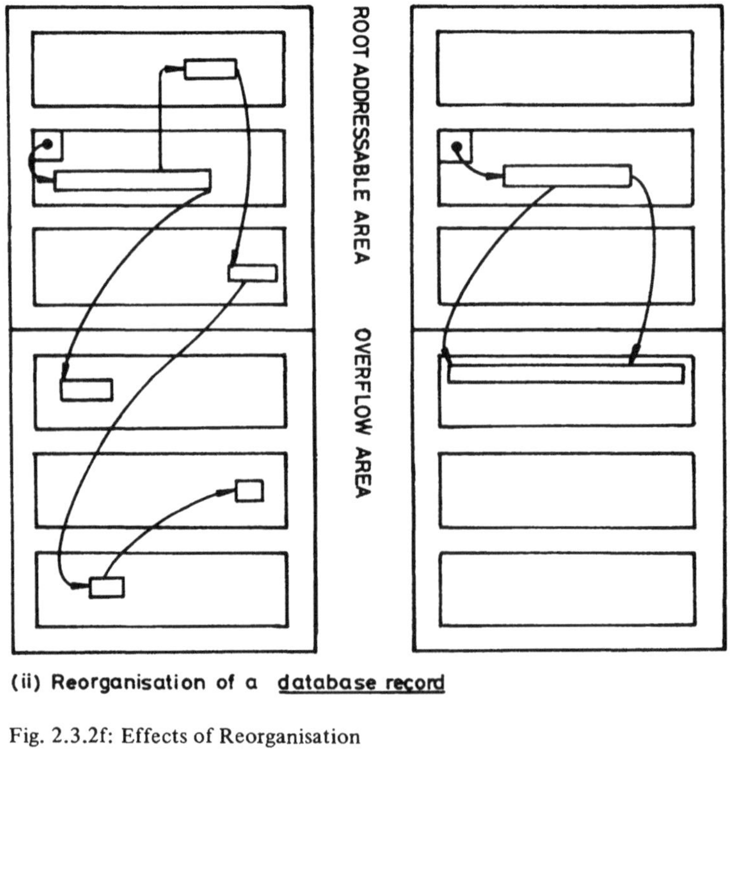

(ii) Reorganisation of a database record

Fig. 2.3.2f: Effects of Reorganisation

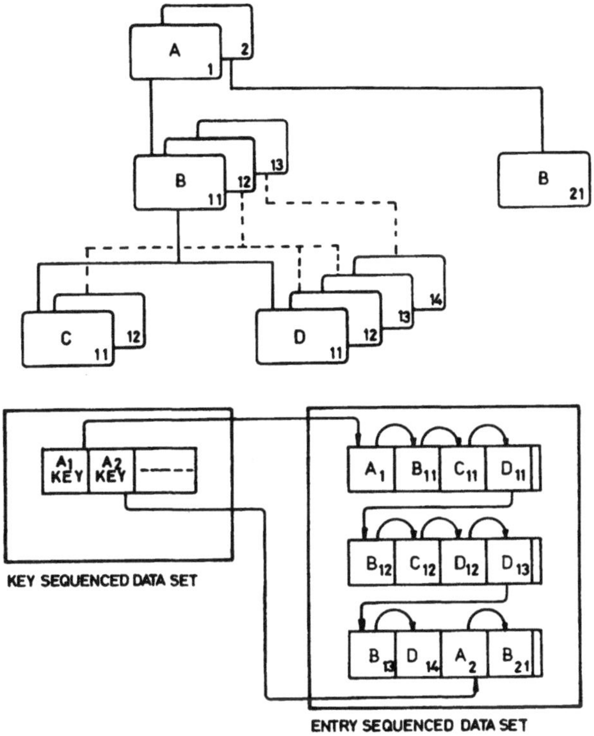

Fig. 2.3.2c: HIDAM Database

The relative inefficiency of HIDAM in this respect is compensated for by its superior sequential processing ability. The DL/1 'Get Next' command at the ROOT SEGMENT level functions logically for HIDAM and physically for HDAM. This means that the next ROOT SEGMENT, physically, will be retrieved using the command with HDAM. Using HIDAM, the ROOT SEGMENT with the next highest key value will be retrieved.

The sequential processing ability of HIDAM at ROOT SEGMENT level can be further enhanced by defining both forward and backward PHYSICAL TWIN (or HIERARCHICAL) pointers for the ROOT SEGMENT type, so that the index need only be referenced for the access to the first ROOT SEGMENT of a sequential series (see Fig. 2.3.2g).

2.3.3 Logical Relationships

The four storage organisations just described in section 2.3.2 are the basic building blocks of any IMS structure. The database so formed is called a PHYSI-

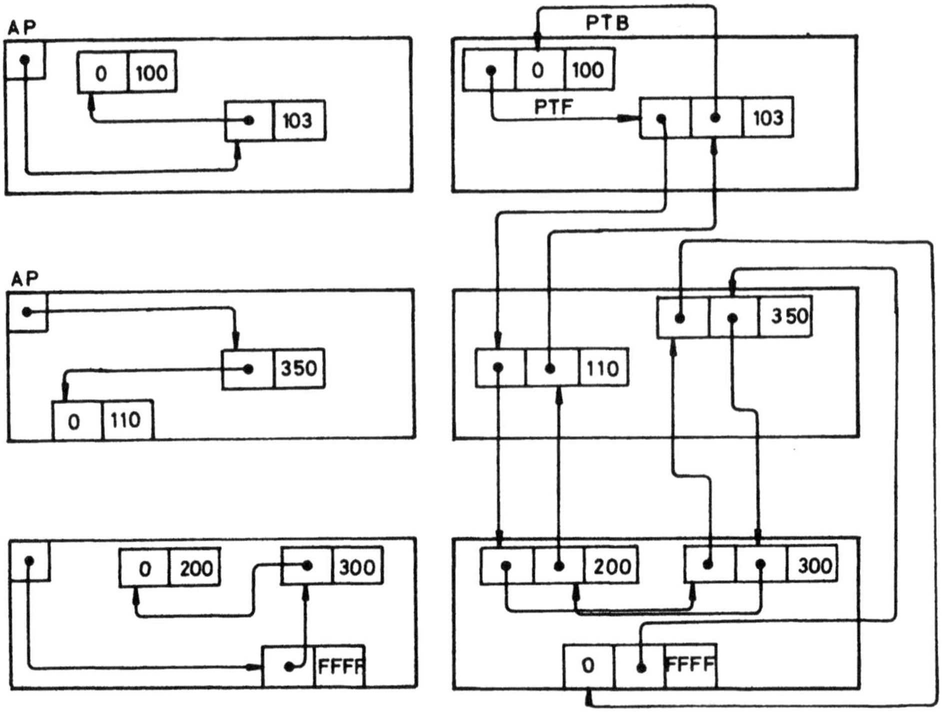

(i) Forward pointers only

one Anchor Point per CI starting a PHYSICAL TWIN FORWARD pointer chain with all the ROOTS in the CI in LIFO order.

(ii) Forward and backward pointers

no Anchor Point per CI. Instead two chains (PHYSICAL FORWARD and BACKWARD pointers) linking all ROOTS of the database in key sequence.

Fig. 2.3.2g: The Use of the PTB Pointer (Linking ROOT SEGMENTS) in a HIDAM Database

CAL DATABASE. Its greatest limitation is that it can only represent hierarchical structures. Logical relationships can extend the PHYSICAL DATABASE by linking the SEGMENTS in one or more databases to form more complex structures. Such databases are called PHYSICAL DATABASES with LOGICAL RELATIONSHIPS.

A LOGICAL DATABASE is a hierarchical subset of the PHYSICAL DATABASE; therefore, a series of LOGICAL DATABASES is necessary to represent a network structure. Another term for LOGICAL DATABASE is Logical or User View. Logical relationships are generated using Logical pointers in HISAM, HIDAM or

HDAM PHYSICAL DATABASES. Logical relationships cannot exist independently of PHYSICAL DATABASES.

Hierarchical relationships are limited to expressing 1:M relationships, eg. with FARMER as PARENT SEGMENT type and ANIMALS–OWNED as CHILD SEGMENT type. The general fault with this sort of construction is the data redundancy. Many different FARMERS have the same ANIMALS. Data redundancy would be multiplied if a further PHYSICAL DATABASE had to be constructed to answer the question, which FARMERS keep a particular ANIMAL, with ANIMALS–OWNED as PARENT SEGMENT and FARMER as CHILD SEGMENT.

The IMS solution to this problem is to have separate FARMER and ANIMAL PHYSICAL DATABASES, and to link the two databases with Logical pointers, the exact nature of which would depend upon the processing requirements.

One problem with an M:M relationships is INTERSECTION DATA. This is data applying to a particular FARMER–ANIMAL relationship occurrence, eg. how many ANIMALS of a particular type are owned by a particular FARMER. This data cannot be stored with the FARMER SEGMENT because he has many different sorts of animals; nor can it be stored with the ANIMAL SEGMENT for a similar reason.

Fig. 2.3.3a shows the IMS solution to this problem; namely a SEGMENT type as CHILD of both the two PARENT SEGMENT types. The Logical View is a hierarchy with either the FARMER or the ANIMAL SEGMENT concatenated with the INTERSECTION DATA as a Dependent SEGMENT of the other PARENT SEGMENT. Logical relationships are only an extension of PHYSICAL DATABASES, so that this CHILD SEGMENT type holding the INTERSECTION DATA must already exist as the PHYSICAL CHILD SEGMENT type of one or other of the two PARENT SEGMENT types, and will contain, in addition to the INTERSECTION DATA, a pointer to the other PARENT SEGMENT type.

This is called a UNIDIRECTIONAL LOGICAL RELATIONSHIP because the pointers only allow access via one particular PARENT SEGMENT type, that is via the PHYSICAL PARENT SEGMENT type, so named because both it and the CHILD SEGMENT type are in the same PHYSICAL DATABASE. The CHILD SEGMENT type is also a LOGICAL CHILD SEGMENT of the other PARENT, the LOGICAL PARENT SEGMENT type. The pointer stored in the LOGICAL (PHYSICAL) CHILD SEGMENT type is called a LOGICAL PARENT pointer.

There is only one Logical View, as shown in Fig. 2.3.3b (i). In order to be able to access the M:M Logical Relationship through the SEGMENT type known as the LOGICAL PARENT in the above described UNIDIRECTIONAL LOGICAL RELATIONSHIP, it is necessary to construct a second UNIDIRECTIONAL LOGICAL RELATIONSHIP in the 'opposite direction', ie. with the SEGMENT

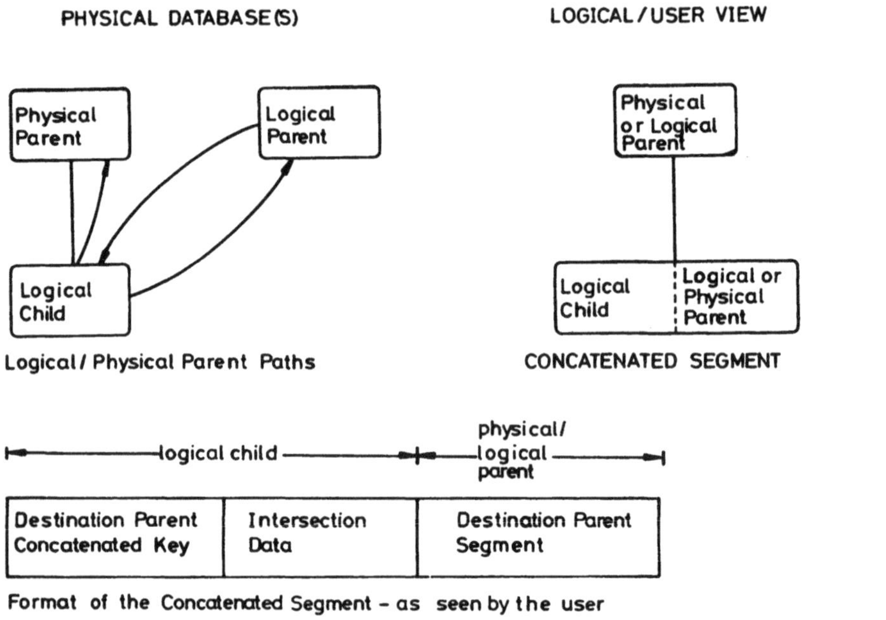

Fig. 2.3.3a: Logical Relationships 1

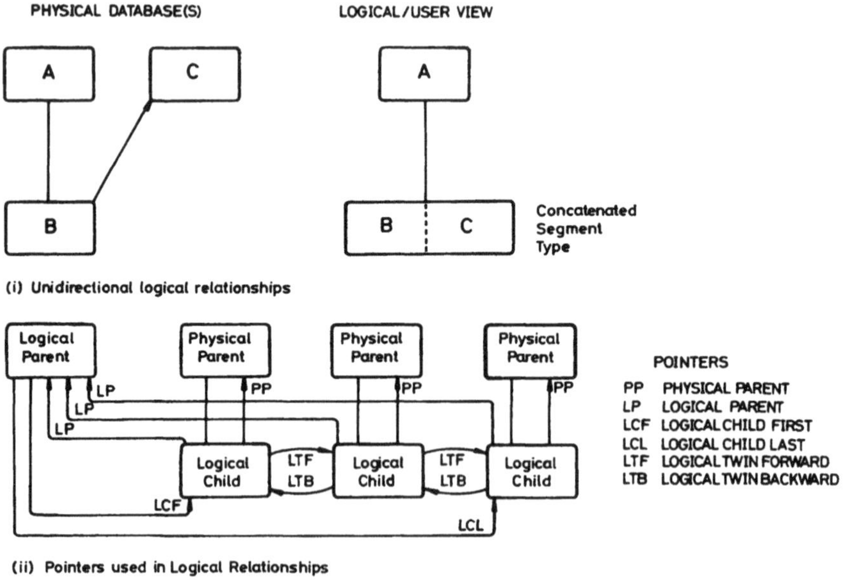

Fig. 2.3.3b: Locigal Relationships 2

type 'C' as the PHYSICAL PARENT etc. A new LOGICAL (PHYSICAL) CHILD SEGMENT type must be created to carry the new LOGICAL PARENT pointers.

The INTERSECTION DATA is the same in both LOGICAL CHILD SEGMENT types, and IMS must ensure that when one side is modified, the other is also modified. This is shown in Fig. 2.3.3c (iii), together with the two possible LOGICAL VIEWS. This is known as a BIDIRECTIONAL LOGICAL RELATIONSHIP. The DESTINATION PARENT CONCATENATED KEY will vary in the CONCATENATED SEGMENT, depending upon the access path.

The term DESTINATION PARENT is assigned to that PARENT SEGMENT which has not been accessed to reach the LOGICAL CHILD. In this case, the CONCATENATED SEGMENT contains the LOGICAL CHILD SEGMENT together with the DESTINATION PARENT SEGMENT as shown in Fig. 2.3.3a.

Three types of logical relationship can be defined:

1. UNIDIRECTIONAL LOGICAL RELATIONSHIP. This, as its name implies, is used to relate two SEGMENT types in one direction. Fig. 2.3.3b shows schematically how the two SEGMENT types are related – it is irrelevant whether they are in the same or different databases. The user view is also shown.

Within the database containing the PHYSICAL PARENT SEGMENT type, a LOGICAL CHILD SEGMENT type is defined as a PHYSICAL CHILD SEGMENT

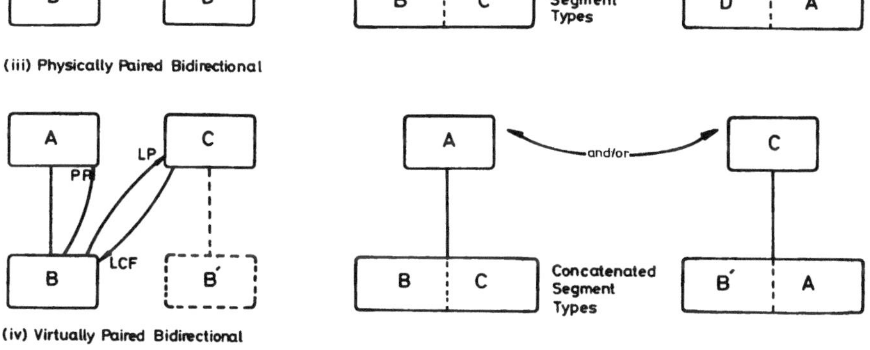

Fig. 2.3.3c: Logical Relationships 3

type. This SEGMENT will contain a LOGICAL PARENT pointer to the associated SEGMENT type. This pointer can be either DIRECT or SYMBOLIC. The name of this SEGMENT type is LOGICAL PARENT.

2. PHYSICALLY PAIRED BIDIRECTIONAL LOGICAL RELATIONHIPS. This type of logical relationship links two SEGMENT types in both directions and maintains identical intersection data in each direction. In this latter respect, it differs from a 'double' UNIDIRECTIONAL LOGICAL RELATIONSHIP, where the user would carry the responsibilitiy of maintaining the two sets of intersection data.

Fig. 2.3.3c shows schematically the relationship between the SEGMENT types and also the two possible user views.

In a way similar to that used in the UNIDIRECTIONAL LOGICAL RELATIONSHIP, a LOGICAL CHILD SEGMENT type is defined as a PHYSICAL CHILD of each of the SEGMENT types being related, and a LOGICAL PARENT pointer, (either DIRECT or SYMBOLIC) is specified in each LOGICAL CHILD SEGMENT type. Each LOGICAL CHILD SEGMENT type will create a PHYSICAL to LOGICAL PARENT path between occurrences of the two SEGMENT types in each direction. Each of the two LOGICAL CHILD SEGMENT types must be defined as being paired to the other one. This enables IMS to maintain identical data in each of the two associated LOGICAL CHILD SEGMENT occurrences. Each of the paired LOGICAL CHILD SEGMENT occurrences must be loaded initially with identical intersection data.

3. VIRTUALLY PAIRED BIDIRECTIONAL LOGICAL REALTIONSHIP. The difference between these and the PHYSICALLY PAIRED BIDIRECTIONAL LOGICAL RELATIONSHIPS is purely internal; the user views are exactly the same. In the latter case, the two LOGICAL CHILD SEGMENTS contain the same data, namely INTERSECTION DATA. An update to one LOGICAL CHILD SEGMENT automatically causes the opposite one to be updated as well.

This data redundancy and extra processing can be avoided by using VIRTUALLY PAIRED BIDIRECTIONAL LOGICAL RELATIONSHIPS. They should be used only when the relationship is not entered equally from each LOGICAL PARENT type, but when the majority of processing enters the relationship via one of the two LOGICAL PARENT types. This parent type should have the single LOGICAL CHILD SEGMENT type as (one of) its PHYSICAL CHILD SEGMENT type(s).

To differentiate between the two LOGICAL CHILD SEGMENT types, the one that is stored physically is called the REAL LOGICAL CHILD SEGMENT type (see SEGMENT type C in Fig. 2.3.3c); the other, which exists only theoretically is called the VIRTUAL LOGICAL CHILD SEGMENT type (see SEGMENT type D in Fig. 2.3.3c).

The VIRTUAL LOGICAL CHILD SEGMENT type cannot hold pointers, therefore the REAL LOGICAL CHILD must hold all the extra pointers necessary to express the relationship as before. The LP pointer from the suppressed (VIRTUAL) LOGICAL CHILD SEGMENT type is replaced by a PHYSICAL PARENT pointer. The PHYSICAL PARENT of the VIRTUAL LOGICAL CHILD no longer needs the PHYSICAL CHILD FIRST (and optionally LAST) pointer(s) to the PHYSICAL CHILD SEGMENT containing the INTERSECTION DATA, since this has been suppressed. In their place, a new pair of pointer types is introduced: LOGICAL CHILD FIRST (and optionally LAST).

The PHYSICAL TWIN FORWARD (and optionally BACKWARD) pointers from the suppressed (VIRTUAL) LOGICAL CHILD SEGMENT type are replaced by LOGICAL TWIN FORWARD (and optional BACKWARD) in the REAL LOGICAL CHILD SEGMENT type. In Fig. 2.3.3c, the extra pointers are included in the schematic representation. The PHYSICAL PARENT pointers are generated by IMS, but all other pointers must be manually specified.

The user has control over the sequence of the REAL LOGICAL CHILD SEGMENT occurrences for the PHYSICAL to LOGICAL PARENT direction, either by specifying a SEQUENCE field for the REAL LOGICAL CHILD SEGMENT type, or by specifying insert rules. For the LOGICAL to PHYSICAL PARENT direction, exactly the same possibilities are available. They are defined for the VIRTUAL LOGICAL CHILD SEGMENT type, but as this SEGMENT type is not held on storage, a series of LOGICAL TWIN pointers is held in the PREFIX of the REAL LOGICAL CHILD SEGMENT occurrences. The REAL LOGICAL CHILD SEGMENT occurrences can therefore have two TWIN chains linking different occurrences – the PHYSICAL TWIN chain and the LOGICAL TWIN chain.

The former is far more efficient to process because the SEGMENT occurrences will tend to be physically close to each other, whereas the LOGICAL TWIN chain may require a separate physical retrieval for each SEGMENT occurrence. This can also be a criterion for deciding which LOGICAL CHILD SEGMENT type should be suppressed. It is recommended that VIRTUAL PAIRING is only used where the VIRTUAL LOGICAL CHILD SEGMENTS occur singly. In this way, LOGICAL TWIN CHAINS are avoided completely.

Fig. 2.3.3b shows an example of a logical relationship using all the logical pointers. In both UNIDIRECTIONAL and PHYSICALLY PAIRED BIDIRECTIONAL RELATIONSHIPS, only LOGICAL PARENT pointers are necessary because each LOGICAL CHILD SEGMENT type is used to describe a logical relationship in a single direction. As these LOGICAL PARENT SEGMENT types do not contain LOGICAL CHILD pointers, there is no way of determining how many LOGICAL CHILD SEGMENTS point to a particular LOGICAL PARENT occur-

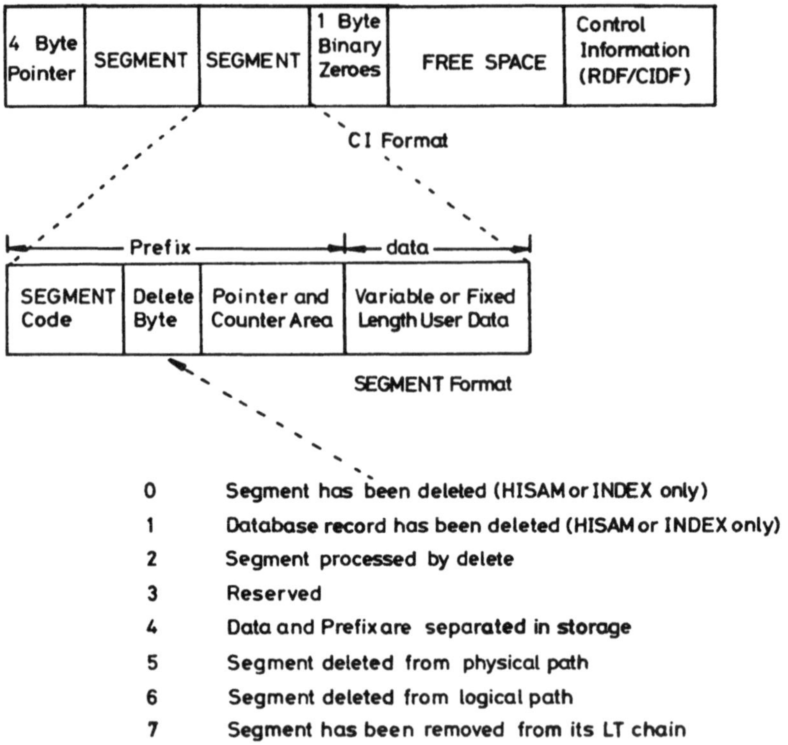

Fig. 2.3.3d: SEGMENT and C.I. Formats

rence. This lack is compensated by a four byte Counter field placed automatically in the Prefix of any LOGICAL PARENT SEGMENT type not containing a LOGICAL CHILD pointer. (see Fig 2.3.3d)

Direct and Symbolic Pointers

There are two types of pointer available within IMS: DIRECT and SYMBOLIC. The choice of which type to use is dictated sometimes by the type of file organisation employed, but mostly by the application.

SYMBOLIC pointers must be used when referencing SEGMENT occurrences in a HISAM database. For HIDAM and HDAM databases, both pointer types may be used.

DIRECT pointers are obviously more efficient because they point directly to the SEGMENT occurrence of interest, whereas a SYMBOLIC pointer contains the Concatenated Key and therefore if the SEGMENT of interest is not a ROOT SEGMENT, then a second I/O operation – if not more – would quite possibly be necessary to retrieve the SEGMENT of interest. Moreover, the DIRECT pointer occupies only four bytes in the SEGMENT Prefix and a CONCATENATED KEY will normally consist of many more than four bytes.

What then are the advantages of using SYMBOLIC pointers in a HIDAM or HDAM database? The answer is all too simple: if two or more databases are linked with DIRECT pointers and they have to be reorganised frequently, then DIRECT pointers increase the reorganisation run time dramatically. Even if only one of the two databases really needs reorganising, with DIRECT pointers, both must be reorganised together.

DIRECT pointers should only be used when the logical relationships are limited to one database, when the single database must be reorganised as a unit. A second possible application for DIRECT pointers would be where response time is critical and the LOGICAL PARENT SEGMENT type is deep in the hierarchy ie. below the fourth level.

The SYMBOLIC key, the full CONCATENATED KEY of the LOGICAL PARENT, is held as the first data field in the LOGICAL CHILD SEGMENT type.

2.3.4 Variable Length SEGMENTS

A SEGMENT consists of two parts: the data part and the Prefix. The Prefix contains a SEGMENT Code, Delete Byte and pointers which define the inter-SEGMENT relationships. The Prefix is managed by IMS and is never seen by the user. The data part consists of a series of fields, each of which is fixed in length, although the data part itself may be of either fixed length or variable length.

The variable length SEGMENT option is implemented by specifying the maximum ('Maxbytes') and minimum ('Minbytes') size of the SEGMENT type. Fig. 2.3.4a shows the user view of a 'normal' SEGMENT and of a CONCATENATED SEGMENT using the variable lengths feature.

The use of variable length SEGMENTS poses an extra problem for the programmer: the Size Field, which reflects the current length of a particular SEGMENT occurrence being processed, must be maintained by the user. This Size Field is two bytes in length.

Variable length SEGMENTS can be used in HISAM, HDAM and HIDAM databases. Fig. 2.3.4b (i) shows the format of a variable length SEGMENT. When initially loaded, a SEGMENT occupies that length specified by the Size Field. If however the Size Field is smaller than the 'Minbytes' parameter, the SEGMENT occurrence will be padded with blanks and stored in the 'Minbytes' length. This free space is available solely for this SEGMENT occurrence as it increases in size.

If, as a result of update activity, a SEGMENT returned to the database is too large for the space available for it, then space must be made available. The

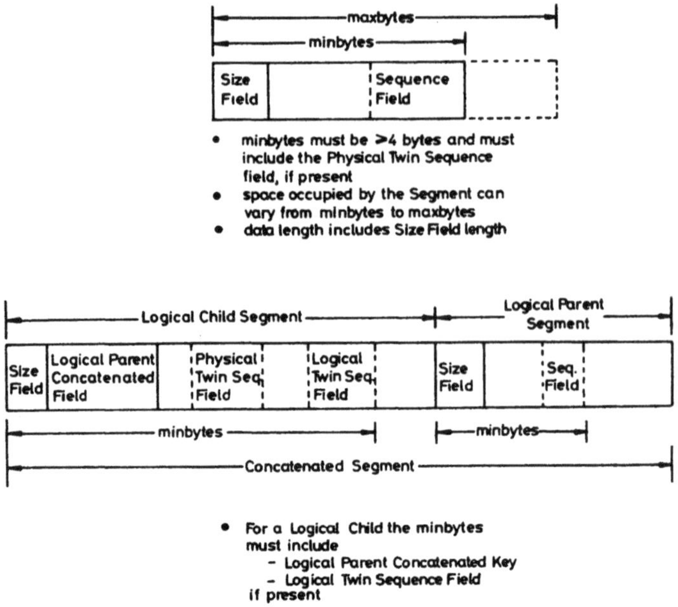

Fig. 2.3.4a: Variable Length SEGMENTS 1

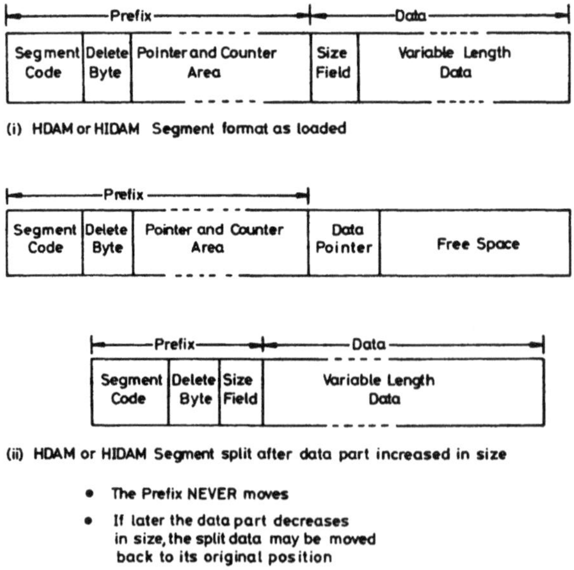

Fig. 2.3.4b: Variable Length SEGMENTS 2

method used depends upon the storage method. HISAM tries to make space within the CI, and, if this is not successful, the displaced SEGMENTS will be stored in an ESDS (overflow) CI and linked by a pointer to the 'home' CI. With HDAM and HIDAM databases, the Prefix and data portions of the SEGMENT are separated as shown in Fig. 2.3.4b (ii). A pointer is placed in the first four bytes of the space following the Prefix which is never moved. Should the data portion ever be reduced in size so that it would fit into its original space, it is returned to this place. The space originally occupied by the data portion is never made available for use by any other SEGMENT occurrence, so that the idea of saving space by using IMS's variable length feature is questionable, and more accesses are required to retrieve the split SEGMENTS than would otherwise be necessary.

Replacing data that is shorter in length than that retrieved has no effect on performance.

IMS offers a 'user-exit' for a compression/expansion routine but this would in many cases cause even more fragmentation. The variable length SEGMENT feature should only be used when SEGMENT occurrences can assume a range of values, but a SEGMENT never changes its length during the course of processing. In this case, SEGMENT splitting will not occur.

When field length sensitivity is used with variable length SEGMENT types, the user view is of a fixed length SEGMENT type – without the two byte Size Field. Fields which do not exist in a particular SEGMENT occurrence at retrieval time will appear in the users I/O area, filled with the default value based on the type of field. If such a field is returned to the database with an actual value, the system increases the Size Field to the minimum size required to hold the modified field.

2.3.5 Secondary Indexing

As already discussed, access to the ROOT SEGMENTS of HISAM and HIDAM databases is supported by means of an index based on the contents of the ROOT SEGMENT SEQUENCE FIELDS. This is referred to as the Primary Index; it may be viewed as the primary key. As the key specifies the order in which the ROOT SEGMENTS will be stored, ie. on ascending value of the SEQUENCE FIELD, this may be referred to as the Primary Processing Sequence.

IMS offers the user the possibility of processing the database in another sequence by building an index based on the contents of some other field in the database record. The index is called a SECONDARY INDEX and the processing sequence is called the Secondary Processing Sequence. This Secondary Indexing is available for any HDAM or HIDAM database and for any single data set HISAM database.

One of the main differences between primary and secondary indexing is that the latter does not have to be based on unique key values. It is, however, usual with

IMS to force uniqueness onto each key to improve performance, and this is explained in more detail later in this section.

The SECONDARY INDEX can consist of up to five fields from any SEGMENT type. These fields are known as the SEARCH field in the SECONDARY INDEX database. The SEGMENT type from which they were taken is known as the SOURCE SEGMENT type.

The pointer in each SECONDARY INDEX database SEGMENT need not necessarily point to the SOURCE SEGMENT upon which it is based. The index can alternatively point to any ancestor of the SOURCE SEGMENT. The SEGMENT pointed to is called the TARGET SEGMENT. It is recommended that the TARGET SEGMENT should be the ROOT SEGMENT (see Fig. 2.3.5a). The reason for this is somewhat complicated. The TARGET SEGMENT is always the ROOT SEGMENT of the logical view required to process via the SECONDARY INDEX. If it is not the ROOT SEGMENT in the physical database, then the Logical View presented will differ structurally from the physical database structures. This is shown in Fig. 2.3.5b(ii), where the primary database has SEGMENT type G defined as both SOURCE and TARGET SEGMENT type. This results in a logical view with SEGMENT type G as a ROOT SEGMENT type. This could cause the programmer particular difficulty especially if both structures were used in one program. A further difficulty with this Secondary Logical View is that not all SEGMENT types can be accessed – this can lead to further unnecessary processing and unwanted complication.

A SECONDARY INDEX database is composed of a VSAM KSDS only if all the keys are unique; if not, then all duplicate keys are stored in an ESDS with a pointer from the KSDS logical record, (see Fig. 2.3.5b (i)). Within each data set, one logical record is used to store each INDEX POINTER SEGMENT.

An INDEX POINTER SEGMENT is of fixed length and contains Prefix and data portions. The Prefix contains a one byte delete flag, followed by a four byte DIRECT pointer to the INDEX TARGET SEGMENT. This can only be used for HDAM and HIDAM primary databases. If SYMBOLIC pointing has been selected, instead of DIRECT pointing, IMS automatically places the CONCATENATED KEY into the INDEX POINTER SEGMENT as shown in Fig. 2.3.5b (ii). Alternatively, the CONCATENATED KEY can be defined as a SYSTEM-RELATED field, and the user can define its position within the data portion of the INDEX POINTER SEGMENT.

The data part of the SEGMENT contains in general four classes of system-maintained data: CONSTANT, SEARCH, SUBSEQUENCE, DUPLICATE DATA. Of these, only SEARCH data is mandatory.

1. CONSTANT FIELD. This one byte constant field must, when specified, occupy the first position in the data portion of the SEGMENT. It is only neces-

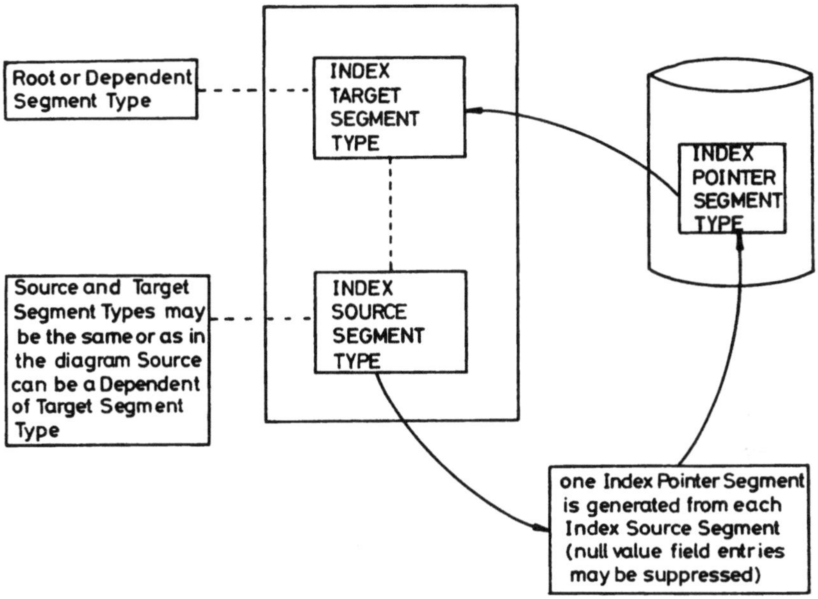

Fig. 2.3.5a: Secondary Indexing 1

sary when multiple SECONDARY INDEXES are stored within the same INDEX database, then all SEGMENTS belonging to a particular SECONDARY INDEX are given the same constant. This field is transparent to the user of the SECONDARY INDEX.

2. SEARCH FIELD. This is the data upon which the index key is based. It is the data extracted from the one to five SOURCE SEGMENT fields and upon which all retrievals are based.

3. SUBSEQUENCE FIELD. This field contains data extracted from the associated SOURCE SEGMENT. Its purpose is to make the key of the SOURCE SEGMENT unique. This is recommended because otherwise the duplicates of this value will have to be stored in an ESDS, which can seriously degrade performance. The contents of the SUBSEQUENCE FIELD are transparent to the user. It can also be used to order a series of non-unique SEARCH fields.

4. DUPLICATE DATA FIELD. Again, this data consists of one to five fields from the associated SOURCE SEGMENT. Its only purpose is for when the SECONDARY INDEX database is processed as a primary database.

All the above fields are maintained by the system ie. any change in the associated SOURCE SEGMENT will cause a change in the corresponding SECONDARY

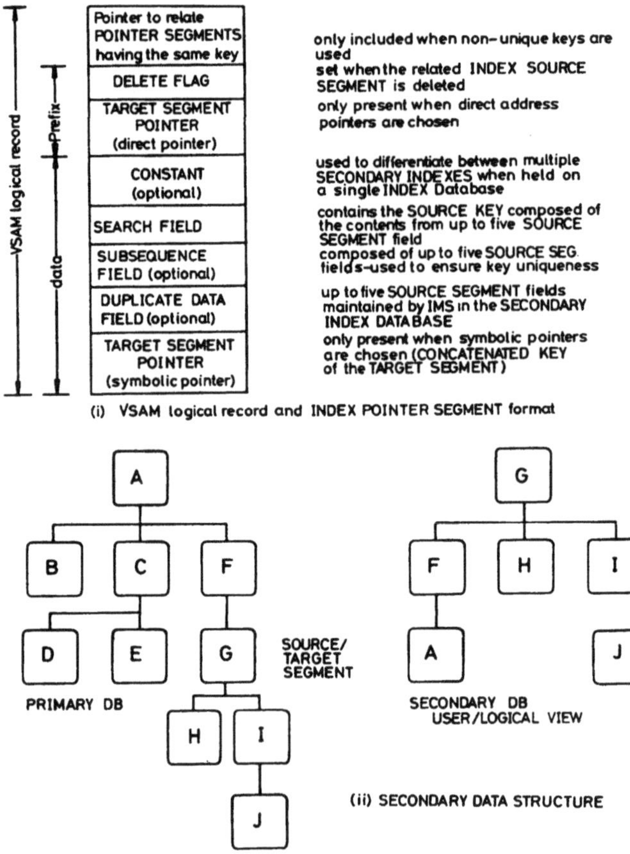

Fig. 2.3.5b: Secondary Indexing 2

INDEX SEGMENT. Here is another advantage of the secondary over the primary key ie. the key value may be changed.

Further data can be stored in a SECONDARY INDEX SEGMENT. This data is under user control, and will be lost during a reorganisation of the SECONDARY INDEX database.

2.4 Data Manipulation

2.4.1 The Parameters of the Data Manipulation Command

IMS was developed as a host language system and does not have a self-contained language interface. It is invoked from the host language (COBOL, PL/1 or

Assembler) via normal subroutine CALLS. An example of the format of a CALL statement (using COBOL) is shown in Fig. 2.4a (i). The 'PCB Name' parameter mentioned in the CALL is the communication area between IMS and the program. An example of the 'PCB Communication Area' is shown in Fig. 2.4a (ii).

One PCB (Program Control Block) is required for each database that is accessed by a program. All PCBs required by a particular program are defined together in a PSB (Program Specification Block). The first parameter of each PCB indentifies the (logical) database to be used. This (logical) database defines which SEGMENTS the program is sensitive to, ie. which it may access. The PCB only shows a hierarchical view of the data. Another of the parameters specifies which data manipulation commands may be used on this database. These points will be discussed in more detail in Section 2.5, Data Independence.

The 'work area' parameter indicates an area in storage where a SEGMENT or SEGMENTS are moved into or stored from. The final parameter of the CALL statement is optional, but, when present, consists of one or more Segment Search Arguments. An SSA is required by IMS for each level of the hierarchy down to the level of the SEGMENT of interest. If SSAs are not supplied by the program, they will be generated by IMS. A CALL statement without an SSA is termed 'unqualified'. Basically, an SSA allows the program to limit, qualify or modify the action of the CALL statement in the following ways:

- to limit the field of search to a particular SEGMENT type or SEGMENT occurrence,
- to modify the traversal procedure for this CALL or the currency for future CALLS,
- to qualify the processing to one SEGMENT or a path of SEGMENTS, either type or occurrence.

Since a database can contain a maximum of 15 levels, so a CALL can contain from 0–15 SSAs.

An SSA consists of one to three main elements (see Fig. 2.4a (iii)). If an SSA is specified, it must consist of a least a SEGMENT name, thereafter the command code, and a series of qualification statements may follow. The command code modifies the function of the IMS DML command. Basically, the qualification statement consists of three parts: a field name, a relational operator and a value, of the form:

FIELDA > 121

The field does not have to be a key (SEARCH or SEQUENCE) field, but of course searching on non-key fields is very inefficient. The possible relational operators are listed in Fig. 2.4a (iii). The value relates to the contents of the associated field.

```
CALL 'CBLTDLI' USING   dml      pcb   work   segment search argument . . . .
                     command,  name,  area,
```

(i) COBOL DL/1 CALL format.

```
LINKAGE SECTION.

Ø1 PCB-NAME.
     Ø3  DBD-NAME            PIC X(8).            database name
     Ø3  SEG-LEVEL-NR        PIC XX.              segment level indicator
     Ø3  STATUS-CODE         PIC XX.              results of latest access
     Ø3  PROC-OPTS           PIC X(4).            access permission
     Ø3  FILLER              PIC S9(5) COMP.      reserved for DL/1
     Ø3  SEG-NAME-FDB        PIC X(8).            segment name feedback area
     Ø3  KEY-LENGTH-FDB      PIC S9(5) COMP.      length of key delivered into
                                                  the key feedback area
     Ø3  NR-SENS-SEGS        PIC S9(5) COMP.      no. of segments to which
                                                  the program is sensitive
     Ø3  KEY-FDB-AREA.
         Ø5  KEY-A           PIC . . . . .        key feedback area
         Ø5  KEY-B           . . .
              .
              .
              .
              .
```

(ii) PCB MASK (programm communication area)

```
segment name [command code(s)] [(field name RO value
      [BO field name RO value . . . . . . . . . . ])]
                                             [ ] = optional entries
```

Relational Operators (RO)	Boolean Operators (BO)
EQ–equal to	& – logical (dependent) AND
GE–greater than or equal to	+ – logical OR
LE–less than or equal to	# – independent AND
GT–greater than	
LT–less than	
NE–not equal to	

(iii) SSA format

Fig. 2.4a: Data Manipulation

If required, a number of qualification statements can be specified for a particular SSA. They must be linked by one of the three Boolean operators:

- the dependent 'and'
- the 'or'
- the independent 'and'.

The first two have their normal logical meaning. The independent 'and' is used with Secondary Indexing in, for example, the search for a person who owns a blue car and a red car, where the information about each car is held on a separate SEGMENT occurrence.

Command Codes

The different Command Codes are examined here, although their exact function when used with particular DML commands will be examined within the description of the command itself.

1. 'F' (First). Start with the first occurrence of this SEGMENT type under current Parentage. This Command Code enables the user to travel hierarchically backwards within a database record.

2. 'L' (Last). This Command Code allows the user to establish currency at the end of a TWIN chain without having to traverse the chain.

3. 'D' (Path Call). This allows the user to retrieve and store a series of SEGMENTS (which constitute a hierarchical path) with one CALL statement. SEGMENTS from intermediate levels with SSAs not containing the 'D' Command Code will not be moved to the user I/O area with retrieval commands. On retrieval, when the lowest level(s) are not found, those SEGMENTS on the hierarchical path which are available are delivered into the program I/O area. For an INSERT command, only the highest level SSA must contain a 'D' Command Code.

4. 'N'. When a REPLACE Call follows a Path Retrieval, those SEGMENTS which have not been changed need not be returned to the database. This is indicated to IMS with the 'N' Command Code.

5. 'Q' (Queue). This is an extension of the 'Hold' logic. If a ROOT SEGMENT is retrieved with the 'Q' Command Code, no other user can access this complete database record. If the SEGMENT is a dependent, then this SEGMENT alone is enqueued, and 'read-only' access is permitted. One of the following actions will dequeue the SEGMENTS:

- a DEQ command being issued
- a SYNCHRONISATION POINT (Sync Point) being reached.

A Sync Point is reached when one of the following occurs:

- a CHKP (checkpoint) is issued
- the application program terminates

– the next new message is retrieved from the message queue (with a GU command).

6. 'C' (Concatenated Key). This Command Code enables the user to quote the full CONCATENATED KEY of the object SEGMENT immediately following the Command Code. This saves the work involved using a series of SSAs.

7. 'P' (Parentage). This Command Code sets Parentage or Currency.

8. 'U'. This Command Code sets 'temporary Parentage' at some level. This Parentage only applies for the duration of this command. This Command Code is particularly useful when processing dependent SEGMENTS without unique SEQUENCE fields.

9. 'V'. This functions in a similar manner to 'U', except that 'temporary Parentage' is automatically set at all higher levels.

2.4.2 Positioning (CURRENCY or PARENTAGE)

Position is established by the following commands:

– GET NEXT
– GET UNIQUE
– INSERT

Currency is maintained for each PCB used by a program. The default position is the start of the database. This default applies both after the end of the database has been reached and before any position has been established.

The only command which takes advantage of the positioning is the GET NEXT command.

The only difficulty with IMS positioning is after an unsuccessful retrieval operation; when IMS positions itself on the last SEGMENT that was successfully accessed on the hierarchical path to the object record. This information is normally of very little interest to the programmer. It would be of far greater use if Positioning remained unchanged after an unsuccessful Retrieval operation.

2.4.3 Retrieval Calls

There are three basic CALLS to retrieve SEGMENTS:

– GET UNIQUE (GU)
– GET NEXT (GN)
– GET NEXT WITHIN PARENT (GNP)

If the object SEGMENT is to be modified, (using the DELETE, REPLACE or INSERT commands) it must be retrieved with a 'lock' that prevents any other user from accessing it. These CALLS are:

– GET HOLD UNIQUE (GHU)
– GET HOLD NEXT (GHN)
– GET HOLD NEXT WITHIN PARENT (GHNP)

The GET UNIQUE command is used to retrieve a SEGMENT or path of SEGMENTS independently of the current database position and establishes a new database position. The command proceeds by finding the first ROOT in the database which satisfies the SSA and then seeks dependents of this ROOT which satisfy their respective SSAs. If SSAs above the lowest level are not specified, IMS will supply default values – normally with an unqualified SSA, ie. the first occurrence of this SEGMENT type satisfying the condition. If the ROOT LEVEL is unqualified, IMS starts scanning at the beginning of the database.

The GET NEXT command is used to retrieve a SEGMENT or a path of SEGMENTS based on the current position within the database. When the CALL is unqualified, ie. without SSA, the next occurrence of any SEGMENT type after the current position is retrieved. If the SSA is unqualified, ie. specifying a SEGMENT type but no field value, the first (next) occurrence of this SEGMENT type after the current position will be retrieved. With a qualifield SSA, the next SEGMENT of the specified type that contains the required value in a specified field will be retrieved.

With the GU and GN commands the retrieved record does not have to be a dependent of the SEGMENT upon which position has been established.

The GET NEXT WITHIN PARENT command functions in exactly the same way as the GET NEXT command, except that the scope of search is limited to one database record or less, depending on where Parentage has been set. (The GET NEXT has a scope of search from the current position forward to the end of the database.)

The following Command Codes can be used with the retrieval commands: C, D, F, L, P, Q, U, and V.

2.4.4 Insert Command

The INSERT Command adds new SEGMENT occurrences to HISAM, HDAM and HIDAM databases. A Dependent SEGMENT may only be added if its Parent SEGMENT or SEGMENTS are present; this applies equally to PHYSICAL and LOGICAL CHILD SEGMENTS. It is possible to order TWIN SEGMENTS without unique SEQUENCE fields, using the HERE, FIRST and LAST INSERT options.

The Command Codes used with this command are: C, D, F, L, U and V. The F and L Command Codes are particularly useful when the INSERT option specifies

HERE, and they can be used to add a new occurrence at the beginning or end of the TWIN chain.

2.4.5 Delete Command

With all network based systems, removing a SEGMENT can cause unexpected – and often unwanted – results. With IMS this is because a SEGMENT can have two Parents, one LOGICAL and one PHYSICAL, and thus cannot be removed physically from the database until it has been deleted from both paths.

The DELETE command causes the object SEGMENT and all its dependents to be no longer accessible via the path from which the object SEGMENT was retrieved prior to the DELETE command being issued.

No Command Codes are used with this command. If a series of SEGMENTS has been retrieved with a Path Call and the DELETE command does not contain an SSA, then the whole path will be deleted.

2.4.6 Replace Command

This command will return a SEGMENT to the database after it has been retrieved by a GET HOLD type command. All fields except the SEQUENCE field may be modified. Only the 'N' Command Code may be used with this command.

2.4.7 System Service Commands

These commands are used to control the IMS environment and not to transfer user data.

1. The Checkpoint Command. This command is used when a point is reached in the processing where a program restart could be made. IMS can optionally invoke an OS/VS checkpoint. IMS 'flushes' all the buffers of all modified SEGMENTS for databases used by the program that issued the Checkpoint Command. A log record is also created containing the identifier passed with the CALL. With the Extended Checkpoint, user information may also be included in the log message.

If the command is issued from a BMP or MPP region, the following actions are also undertaken:

– all DB resources enqueued for this application are freed
– for all TP applications, all output messages are enqueued for their final destination and the next input message (if one is available) is automatically returned to the application.

2. The Restart Command. This is only valid for a batch or BMP region. It causes IMS to restore the checkpointed user areas by activating the IMS/VS batch restart routine which reads the log tape until the requested checkpoint identifier is found. The application has to reposition itself from information supplied from IMS. The IMS log file has to be used as input to this job, therefore it is necessary to allocate a new log file to the IMS control region.

3. The Dequeue Command. This releases those SEGMENTS queued by a program by the use of the 'Q' Command Code. If, however, SEGMENTS have been modified, then they will not be released until a Sync Point is reached.

4. The Rollback Command. This is issued when a logical error arises during the processing of a transaction. It causes the elimination of all database changes and queued output messages since the last Sync Point.

It can also be used for non-transaction driven programs in a BMP region. No abnormal termination condition results from the issuing of this command and processing continues after the rollback has been successful.

5. The Log Command. This causes the system to write user-supplied information on the log tape. It is, however, only possible to read this information in a batch or BMP application program.

6. The GET SCD Command. This retrieves the addresses of the IMS/VS System Contents Directory and the Partition Specification Table.

7. The Statistics Command. With this command, the user can retrieve a wide range of statistics from IMS.

8. The Snap Command. This is used during the debugging phase. It can be used to dump DL/1 blocks for CALLS that execute correctly as well as incorrect ones.

9. The Purge Command. This command and the next one are strictly DC commands and have been included merely for the sake of comprehensiveness.

Except when the EXPRESS = YES option (in an alternative PCB) is in operation, the output message SEGMENTS are held on the output message queue until the program terminates correctly, or until it issues a 'GU' command to the input message queue. (The input and output message queues are addressed via the IO–PCB). Upon receiving the Purge Command, the IMS nucleus transmits the message SEGMENTS to their final destination immediately.

10. The Change Command. This can be issued by a program to reroute a message to a terminal other than the one that initiated the conversation. It can also be issued to activate another program. Both are effected via an alternative PCB.

2.5 Data Indepedence

IMS offers the user a high degree of data independence. Each application program can be limited to a subset of the physical database, which is known as a LOGICAL DATABASE (User View). The only limitation is that if a particular SEGMENT type is to be made available to a program, its parent SEGMENT type must also be available to the program, even if the PARENT SEGMENT type is not required by the program. For security reasons, access to the unwanted SEGMENT type can be limited to the key field.

The new release of IMS/VS (1.1.5) has taken Data Independence one step further. It is now possible to limit a user to only those fields within a SEGMENT type which are required for processing.

Field level sensitivity naturally imposes a small performance penalty. However, it does not allow the user views (as expressed in the PCB) to have a different format from that expressed in the DB definition. Thus the added Data Independence is much less than might appear after a superficial examination.

The DBA defines the total User View in a PSB (PROGRAM SPECIFICATION BLOCK) which consists of one or more PCBs (PROGRAM CONTROL BLOCKS), each of which describes a hierarchical User View of a particular database. A program is limited to a maximum of 255 User Views. They can be different views of a very complex database, or views of a series of different databases. A PCB can only represent a hierarchical structure, therefore any database of greater structural complexity requires more than one PCB to describe the structure for the user.

A PCB contains the following information:

- the Database name
- the access restrictions (cf. 2.7)
- the maximum key length associated with any hierarchical path. If this length is not specified, IMS takes 255 bytes per level as a default value.
- whether SINGLE or MULTIPLE POSITIONING is to be available. The latter offers the user the chance to maintain CURRENCY in each hierarchical path accessed, thus allowing different SEGMENT types under one Parent to be accessed in parallel.
- the name of a SECONDARY INDEX DATABASE should one be required for processing
- specification of the SEGMENT types to be processed and of the fields. If Field Level Sensitivity is selected then only those fields required are included. The order of the fields need not be as in the DBD. Processing options can also be specified at the SEGMENT level, if the specific SEGMENT requirement deviates from the global requirement specified for the PCB as a whole.

Even when the logical database structure is the same as that of the physical database, a logical DBD should be generated and used via the PCB. This will protect the current application from future changes, thus achieving the wanted data independence. The one rather weak feature of Field Sensitivity is that the fields' characteristics must remain the same in the user view as in the physical database. There is one situation where the application program can affect a SEGMENT type to which it is not sensitive and that is with the DELETE command. Here a non-sensitive dependent of a deleted SEGMENT is also deleted.

There is one further aspect to data independence in an IMS environment: an application program should be totally unaffected by a change in storage organisation, eg. from HISAM to HIDAM. This, in general, is achieved. Unfortunately, a change to HDAM will require a change of processing logic if a series of ROOTS are processed with GET NEXT type commands.

2.6 Concurrent Usage

IMS is available in two versions, either a database-only version, or a version offering integrated DB and DC functions. The database-only version executes in the same region as the user program, and there is no protection from concurrent updating by programs in other regions other than exclusive allocation of the database. Nor are automatic recovery features available. Using the integrated DB/DC version, each user-program resides in its own region and only one copy of the IMS (DB/DC) code is used. This is in the IMS control region which contains:

- a telecommunications facility
- a DML facility
- a message scheduling facility
- checkpoint/restart and automatic rollback facilities
- facilities for identifying and resolving deadlock.

This control region is responsible for scheduling all applications, TP or otherwise. Communication between the control region and the application programs running in all other regions is via two special SVCs.

IMS provides facilities for conversational programs. The first message in a conversation contains the transaction code, thereafter only data being entered from the terminal. Until the end of the conversation, the terminal remains 'connected' to the application program via the IMS Control Region.

Conversational programs do not remain in main memory throughout the conversation, but the status of the conversation is written onto a 'scratchpad' area of memory which is inserted onto the output queue after the output message. The program is now able to handle another input message or another program can be scheduled. When the answer to the output message is retrieved by the program, the 'scratchpad area' is also retrieved.

The rather limited transaction-oriented processing offered by IMS is known as PROGRAM ISOLATION. This limitation is due to the fact that a transaction is defined as the processing between two Sync Points ie. the retrieving of new messages from the input message queue with GU commands. The user has no control over this process. It means that one conversation consisting of a number of information exchanges between terminal and user programs cannot be defined as a single transaction. This can have the unfortunate consequence that a logical transaction viewed by the terminal user may not be completely backed out if something goes wrong either with the program or with IMS. IMS guarantees only the physical integrity of the database and not its logical integrity when conversational programs are being used.

Deadlock resolution is detected by an IMS program called Exclusive Control Enqueue/Dequeue. The program causing the deadlock situation is abnormally terminated with a special abnormal termination code. This results in the offending program being backed out to the last Sync Point (not necessarily the start of the logical transaction). All its held resources are freed. This program will not be aborted, but simply rescheduled. Neither the user program nor the terminal operator is involved in or aware of this process. The last terminal input is returned to the program message input queue for rescheduling.

All database updates are written initially to a Dynamic Log file held on disc. Only after the Sync Point has been reached are the changes committed permanently to the database log and hence to the database itself. This 'temporary' log is necessary to be able to back-out aborted transactions.

2.7 Security Controls and Recovery

IMS offers a fairly sophisticated level of security. Data can be protected by allowing each program to access only those SEGMENTS actually required and by limiting this access to only those fields within these SEGMENTS needed by the program (cf. 2.5 Data Independence).

The type of processing for the sensitive SEGMENTS can be specified either for the PCB as a whole, or for each sensitive SEGMENT individually. The processing options are:

G – GET
I – INSERT
R – REPLACE
D – DELETE
A – ALL (ie. G, I, R and D)
P – Path Call (cf. Command Code = D)
O – read only

E – enables exclusive use (for G, I, R, D and A)
L – for database loading (not HIDAM)
GS – GET SEGMENTS in ascending sequence only (HISAM)
LS – LOAD SEGMENTS in ascending sequence only (HIDAM/HDAM)
K – Key Sensitivity only; the SEGMENT is not moved into the user's I/O area

The last processing option is used primarily where a particular SEGMENT is not of interest to a program but its dependents are. In order to reach a particular dependent SEGMENT, it is necessary to read all its ancestors. This would reduce the effectiveness of the security feature; hence, key sensitivity is offered.

IMS offers comprehensive utilities to aid the recovery from the effects of data corruption caused by hardware or software failure. HSAM databases cannot however be recovered. The cornerstone of the IMS recovery utilities is the log tape. All BEFORE and AFTER IMAGES of each updated SEGMENT are automatically written to the central log tape. Each batch program not executing in a BMP region will have its own log file. The Rollforward Recovery facility consists of three utilities:

1. Database IMAGE COPY. This copies the data sets to tape (or disc).

2. Database CHANGE ACCUMULATION. This sorts all the changes on the log files and merges them with the previous CHANGE ACCUMULATION file in the order required by the RECOVERY utility. During this process, all changes to a SEGMENT that have been superceded by a later change are eliminated, thus reducing the time needed for a recovery run.

3. Database RECOVERY. This restores the database using the IMAGE COPY and applying the accumulated changes from the IMS log file.

In the event of an operating system or hardware failure, it is necessary to run a further utility to close the IMS log tape correctly, before the other utilities can usc thc log file.

There is a fourth utility, namely a program Rollback utility, which is also used when Emergency restart is not successful. This removes the changes made by a specific program and will return a database to the last checkpoint. It produces a log tape which contains a record of all the changes made, and this tape must be included in any future Rollforward RECOVERY attempts, although not in future Rollback attempts.

One problem facing the DBA is that the VSAM data sets used by IMS to hold the databases are only secure when used via IMS. There is no IMS security when they are used as pure VSAM data sets. This problem can be partially overcome by specifying that a password within the database definition parameters should be used. This results in the database name being used by VSAM as the password, to be specified before the data sets can be accessed.

2.8 Reorganisation and Space Management

The necessity to reorganise IMS databases is, to a large extent, the result of the Space Management strategy used by IMS. There is, however, a fundamental difference between the Space Management techniques used by the Sequential and the Direct access methods. In general, the latter provide faster access to lower level SEGMENTS and reuse of space after SEGMENT deletion, but with no movement of SEGMENTS once stored. The sequential access methods are characterised by better utilisation of space; deleted SEGMENT space is not reused however. Both access methods therefore require fairly frequent reorganisation when the database is subject to any degree of change. The need for reorganisation is increased by the use of variable length SEGMENTS with a Direct access method, and the length of the reorganisation run is adversely affected by the use of DIRECT POINTERS in Logical Relationships linking more than one PHYSICAL DATABASE.

2.8.1 Sequential Access Methods

There is no Space Management requirement with HSAM databases, since an insert requires the whole database to be read and re-written.

The ROOT SEGMENT occurrences in a HISAM database must always be maintained in ascending key sequence. This means that space is made available for a new occurrence in the Control Interval, by moving those database records with higher keys to the 'right' to accommodate it. If insufficient space is available, a Control Interval split occurs, ie. half the contents of the full Control Interval is moved to an empty one, thus generating adequate space for the new occurrence.

In HISAM databases, dependent SEGMENTS rely upon physical adjacency to define their hierarchical position and the hierarchical sequence must be maintained when a new dependent SEGMENT is inserted. If there is sufficient space within the logical record to accommodate it, all the hierarchically inferior SEGMENTS are moved to the 'right' to make space. If not, all the hierarchically inferior SEGMENTS are moved to an empty logical record in ESDS and the new dependent SEGMENT is accommodated in the available space in the first logical record. This SEGMENT will also contain a 4 byte DIRECT POINTER to the ESDS logical record. If the dependent SEGMENT is too large for the first logical record despite the relocation of the hierarchically inferior SEGMENTS, then it too will be accommodated in an ESDS logical record.First an attempt is made to accommodate this SEGMENT at the front of the same ESDS logical records as the relocated hierarchically inferior SEGMENTS. If this fails, a new empty ESDS logical record will be made available for this SEGMENT. The three logical records would then be chained together with 4 byte DIRECT POINTERS to reflect their hierarchical sequence.

When a dependent SEGMENT is deleted, the delete-byte is set in the SEGMENT prefix. When a ROOT SEGMENT is deleted, then it too only has the delete byte set, except in the following case. When executing in exclusive batch mode, where neither the ROOT nor its dependents are involved in an active logical relationship, an actual removal of the deleted database record will occur. All SEGMENTS with the delete-byte set (two for logical relationships) will be physically removed from the database by a reorganisation run.

2.8.2 Direct Access Methods

The direct access methods use bit maps to indicate in which Control Intervals space is available. Within each Control Interval, there is a free space chain linking the fragmented free space areas. Fragmentation occurs because no attempt is made to 'shift' all the SEGMENTS together so as to create one large free space area at the end of each CI. This is because the SEGMENTS are linked by DIRECT POINTERS, and any movement within a CI would have to be reflected in all these pointers.

The bit map can only indicate whether or not there is one free space area in the CI concerned capable of accommodating the largest SEGMENT type. This has the great disadvantage that CIs which contain sufficient space for the smaller SEGMENT types will not have this fact reflected in the bit map. Therefore, to use space reasonably efficiently, volatile databases have to be reorganised frequently.

ROOT ANCHOR POINTS in the ROOT ADDRESSABLE AREA of HDAM databases offer the possibility of keeping synonym chains short. They act as a 'fine control' on the randomizing algorithm and, used well, will help considerably towards optimal response times. They have the effect of reducing the home block size.

The techniques for inserting and deleting SEGMENTS are the same for both HDAM and HIDAM databases. These techniques use the bit maps and the space-available chain to find available space to insert a SEGMENT, and record the increase in free space following a deletion of a SEGMENT.

When inserting a SEGMENT, IMS tries to place it as close to its parent as possible, or, in the case of a HDAM ROOT, as close as possible to its ANCHOR POINT. The ideal situation is when space is available in the same CI. Should this space not be available, IMS tries to satisfy the request within CIs in the buffer from the same track, and then from the same cylinder. For this, no reference is made to the bit map, and so SEGMENTS smaller than the largest SEGMENT type will be inserted into CIs where, according to the bit map, no space is available.

Should these attempts fail to find space, then IMS uses the bit map (which reflects space available for the largest SEGMENT) to search for space with the following priorities:

- any block on the same track
- any block on the same cylinder.

When generating the database using a Direct access method, one parameter that must be specified is how many CIs on each side of the home CI may be scanned to find space for an insertion, before inserting the SEGMENT somewhere towards the end of the data set (in the overflow area). The priorities are as follows:

- any CI currently in the buffer pool from within the specified CI-scan-limits
- any CI from within the CI-scan-limits based on the bit map
- any CI in the buffer pool from the end of the data set
- any CI from the end of the data set, based on the bit map
- any CI from anywhere in the data set, based on the bit map.

IMS will always endeavour to use space within a CI so that the bit map is not changed, ie. IMS tries to find a free space element that is as nearly as possible the same size as the SEGMENT to be inserted.

In order to minimise the impact of insertions on performance, free space should be scattered throughout the file, when the database is loaded and also after reorganisation. Two parameters are involved: how much free space should be reserved per CI, and that every n^{th} CI should be held completely free. Deletion of a SEGMENT is a trivial matter. The pointers are updated to reflect the absence of the deleted SEGMENT and the free space element chain (within the block) is updated to reflect the consequent increase in free space. Contiguous free space elements are automatically combined.

2.8.3 Reorganisation

Reorganising a database will be necessary normally because performance has degraded because of framentation or because there is a lack of free space. This is known as physical reorganisation in IMS terminology. A further situation which leads to reorganisation being necessary is a change in structural design, and this is known as logical reorganisation.

1. Physical Reorganisation. As database records become fragmented over a number of CIs, more I/Os are required to achieve the same result. One symptom of this is an increase in CI and CA splits. A lack of free space can be seen from the VSAM catalogue, as can the number of CI/CA splits.

For HDAM, an increase in the number of I/Os per transaction would immediately suggest that the RAA (Root Addressable Area) is too small, and newly inserted ROOTS have been stored in overflow.

There are three major steps in any reorganisation:

- Unloading the database(s)
- Deleting the old files and redefining them; optionally altering the DBD or VSAM parameters
- Reloading the database(s)

An alternative to deleting an old database would be to rename it, thereby making it unnecessary to take an Image Copy prior to unloading, as is recommended. After the database(s) have been reloaded, a new Image Copy must be taken, prior to executing any application programs which alter the database.

2. Logical Reorganisation. Structural changes cannot normally be handled using the reorganisation utilities, except when very limited changes to the structure are to be made, as follows:

- a SEGMENT type may be removed from the structure provided no occurrences of this SEGMENT type are on the unload file
- a new SEGMENT type may be added, provided neither the hierarchical relationship between existing SEGMENT types nor the concatenated keys of LOGICALLY related SEGMENTS are changed
- existing SEGMENT lengths can be increased or decreased. When they are increased, the user is responsible for adding the new data via an update program
- access methods may be changed. HDAM may be changed to HISAM or HIDAM, but these may only be changed to HDAM if the randomising routine maintains ROOT key sequence, and this is most unusual.

In all other cases, a program must be written to unload and reload the database.

2.9 Performance

Because of its complexity, it is inconceivable that one person would be able to have detailed overall knowledge of all facets of IMS. This fact alone makes for performance inefficiency due to the normal problems of communication.

The major factors affecting the performance of IMS are:

- real memory available for the message queues
- real memory available for the I/O buffers
- choice of the storage organisation and database structure
- the type of pointers used in LOGICAL relationships
- the way the database is accessed and manipulated.

The first two of these tasks are normally the responsibility of the system programming group; the next two, that of the DBA; the last, that of the application programming. The job of co-ordinating all these functions tends to be the responsibility of the DBA. In general, the skill level required by the IMS programmer is seriously underestimated. DL/1 has some extremely powerful commands which can deliver the expected results despite inefficient programming techniques. When this happens, all the fine tuning of the DBA and system programming group will have been wasted. It is therefore also necessary to make the DBA responsible for the quality of the programmers' work.

IMS offers a very wide range of utilities to help the user with the various tasks related to database design, performance, monitoring and maintenance. Almost all of the performance monitoring and design aids are separately priced items.

1. DB SURVEYOR is a new utility which scans direct organised databases and reports on the condition of the database. It can be run as a batch message processing (BMP) program against on-line databases. Its main use is to help the DBA decide when a (partial) reorganisation is necessary.

2. The DB MONITOR REPORT PRINT program is a batch utility which collates and prints perfomance-related data which DB MONITOR collected during the normal processing of the IMS system. The reports produced include:

- DB buffer pools and VSAM buffer subpools statistics
- program I/O traffic
- DL/1 call summary
- VSAM statistics
- Distribution appendix

3. DB PROTOTYPE is used to compare the performance of various IMS structures and buffer sizes for a predefined sequence of DL/1 commands.

4. DB ANALYSER. This utility analyses HD-organised databases and the Direct Pointers of HISAM to HD databases. The databases need not reside on disc, but can also be analysed in their Image Copy form on either disc or tape.

DB ANALYSER serves two distinct purposes:

- reports in the state of disorganisation of a database
- checks the validity of the database pointers and identifies inaccessible SEGMENTS.

In the former function, statistics are collected on:

- free space
- number and location of pointers
- how many database records are contained in one CI.

In the latter function, the utility lists all 'bad' pointers. When these have been corrected, the utility creates a new corrected Image Copy.

5. DC MONITOR analyses a production system and produces reports on task scheduling, queuing and time spent in the wait state.

Although the database statistics are extremely good, certain information of interest to the DBA is missing, namely:

- twin chain count (maximum, minimum and distribution)
- DB record lengths (maximum, minimum and distribution)
- how a DB record is distributed physically across a number of CIs.

2.10 Conclusion

IMS is certainly the largest (in terms of total code), and the most complex of the six DBMSs examined. The interdependence of the DB and DC parts is such that it is not possible to consider them as separate products. IMS–DC has rarely, if ever, been installed without IMS–DB (DL/1), although the DB part has been used with many different TP monitors. Often, users of smaller S370 computers implement TP applications before DB ones. This means that DL/1 – should it be chosen – has to be interfaced to the existing TP monitor, particularly in the case of CICS. DL/1 alone is not capable of controlling multiple updating applications accessing common databases simultaneously in batch mode. This is because each partition/region would have its own DL/1 nucleus, and without one centralised version co-ordinating all accessing, no locking of records is possible.

It should always be borne in mind that either VSAM or ISAM/OSAM must be used as the supporting access method for all stored data. This is particularly relevant when calculating the real memory that IMS would occupy.

The complexity of IMS means that the designer is confronted with a wide range of choices when creating a database structure. There are four basic storage organisations available: HSAM, HISAM, HDAM and HIDAM. The hierarchical structure is defined by the SEGMENTS' physical placement with the sequential storage organisations. The 'direct' storage organisations use pointers to relate SEGMENTS in the hierarchical structure.

HSAM can only be used for classical sequential processing, since there is no possibility of inserting a SEGMENT into an existing structure, except at the very end of the 'database'. This restriction is hardly acceptable in typical database environments.

HISAM offers standard, partially-inverted access, similar to VSAM – although VSAM's key compression is not available.

HDAM is a random storage organisation for which an excellent key randomizing algorithm is available (DFSHDC40).

HIDAM uses the partially inverted file structure of HISAM to point to an ESDS data space where the SEGMENTS are linked with pointers. HIDAM appears to suffer from the disadvantages of HISAM and HDAM. In order to access a particular SEGMENT, an index hierarchy has to be traversed to the ROOT SEGMENT, and then a number of pointers must be followed, often over a number of Control Intervals. HIDAM is superior to HISAM in a very volatile database environment, where the shifting of SEGMENTS will degrade performance dramatically. It is also superior to HDAM in sequential processing in root key sequence because HDAM distributes the ROOT SEGMENTS randomly.

This superiority extends to the sequential processing of all ROOT SEGMENTS because HDAM retrieves the records linked to each RAP; this chain can be distributed over more than one CI. It should however be borne in mind that the majority of the processing is seldom sequential retrieval on the primary key.

Nevertheless, it is the author's opinion that HISAM and HDAM should be considered initially, and only when they are found to be inadequate should HIDAM be brought into consideration.

When linking the hierarchical databases with LOGICAL PARENT/CHILD pointers, the designer is confronted with the choice between symbolic and direct pointers. The problem is quite straightforward: the use of symbolic pointers means that the reorganisation of two or more databases linked by LOGICAL pointers is significantly faster than with the use of direct pointers, although the space occupied by the key will be greater than the four bytes of the direct pointer, and with symbolic pointers databases may be reorganised separately.

A further consideration is that the LOGICAL PARENT can only be accessed via the physical ROOT SEGMENT using the symbolic (concatenated) key in the LOGICAL CHILD SEGMENT. This means that symbolic keys result in slower processing in comparison with direct pointers where the LOGICAL PARENT is not the ROOT SEGMENT in its own hierarchical database (for HDAM).

It is recommended that symbolic pointers be used when one or more of the following conditions apply:

- reorganisation runs take place regularly
- the LOGICAL PARENT is a ROOT SEGMENT
- processing often requires only the LOGICAL PARENT key value, so that the retrieval of the LOGICAL PARENT SEGMENT can be avoided.

Another feature of the design process which is probably too powerful and complex for the vast majority of users and applications, is the chameleon-like change in the structure when using secondary indexing. This becomes possible when the SEGMENT containing the field used in the secondary index is not the ROOT SEGMENT. A logical view is then generated, with the 'subject' SEGMENT as the ROOT SEGMENT. This unnecessary complication can be avoided by always defining the ROOT SEGMENT above the SOURCE SEGMENT as the TARGET SEGMENT, so as to preserve the original user view. Even this has the disadvantage that the SOURCE SEGMENT can only be accessed via the TARGET SEGMENT, thus adversely affecting performance. One further advantage of using the ROOT SEGMENT as TARGET SEGMENT is that the SECONDARY INDEX can use SYMBOLIC POINTERS efficiently. This would mean that the SECONDARY INDEX would be independent of a reorganisation of the main database.

A further general rule is that VIRTUAL LOGICAL CHILDREN should never be used when LOGICAL TWIN pointers are necessary to link these VIRTUAL TWINS. This is because of the performance penalty. The rule can be summarised as follows: only use VIRTUAL PAIRING when there can never be more than one occurrence of the VIRTUAL LOGICAL CHILD SEGMENT under its 'PHYSICAL' PARENT.

2.11 Advantages of IMS

- Integrated DB/DC.
- IBM main-line product.
- Data dictionary.
- Secondary indexing implemented via inverted file techniques. Its primary purpose is to provide alternative access paths to the data, (cf. DISADVANTAGES of IMS Secondary Indexing)
- The object SEGMENT of a secondary index does not have to be the SEGMENT containing the value held in the secondary index; any ANCESTOR may be the object SEGMENT.
- Generic key searches are possible (except with HDAM).
- Reasonable on-line and batch interrogation of an IMS DB using GIS (Generalized Information System) for batch and IQF (Interactive Query Facility).
- Good access control features in PCB.
- 'Path Call' feature enables a complete Hierarchical path to be retrieved with one IMS CALL (not necessarily one I/O).
- Dual logging is a standard feature.
- Very comprehensive, if somewhat cumbersome, utilities.
- Huge user base.
- Interfaces (see Appendix III).
- The programmer can write messages to the system log. Unfortunately they cannot be retrieved by a program during on-line processing (except for Checkpoint/Restart).
- IMS offers four different access methods – although in practice only HISAM and HDAM, and sometimes HIDAM, are sensible choices.
- Direct access for fast response real-time applications and the user can write his own randomizer.
- Field level sensitivity but it is somewhat primitive – the field characteristics may not differ from those for the original record.

- Automatic warm restart.
- Searching can take place on non-key fields – this can sometimes be advantageous although it can require a sequential pass of the file. It can however sensibly be used in conjunction with a secondary index search (cf. Disadvantages of IMS Secondary Indexing)
- BTS (Batch Terminal Simulator), a superb tool for testing ca. 90% of an application program.
- The PRIMARY key of a HDAM DB need not be unique. If used it excludes the possibility of a change of IMS access method.
- IMS commands are easy to learn (except for some of the COMMAND CODES). Nevertheless a high degree of skill is required to traverse the database hierarchy efficiently.

2.12 Disadvantages of IMS

- The version 1.1.6 manuals are a great improvement over the previous editions; nevertheless all restrictions are still not adequately described and they still suffer from the complicated and sometimes unclear terminology.
- The previously established position (CURRENCY) is not necessarily maintained after an unsuccessful retrieval operation. Position is, in this case, established on the last SEGMENT in the Hierarchical Path 'retrieved' prior to establishing that the required SEGMENT was not present.
- DELETE removes DEPENDENT SEGMENTs not seen in the user-view.
- Using LOGICAL relationships can cause the user-view to change dramatically; a PARENT SEGMENT type can appear as the DEPENDENT of one of its CHILD SEGMENT types. This can lead to a program containing two apparently 'conflicting' user-views: a very confusing situation for a programmer, at least initially.
- The user-view (PCB) of the SEGMENT structure can only be hierarchical. It is therefore necessary to have multiple user views to process any structure more complicated than a simple hierarchy. Database position must be established anew when moving from one user-view to the next.
- A separate user-view is necessary for each secondary index.
- Retrieval requests involving multiple secondary index databases should not be used because IMS will only use the first secondary index and then retrieve the records one by one, checking for the other specified values in the retrieved records. This can be tremendously inefficient and demonstrates that IMS secondary indexing was not conceived to resolve complex queries but simply to make an alternative access path available.
- Secondary indexes created after the initial loading of the primary database requires that the primary database be reorganised: a resource consuming process particularly when the reorganisation itself is not necessary.

- Non-unique secondary indexes are handled in a less that optimal manner – using overflow areas and hence extra I/O traffic. IBM recommends that the user make the index unique by adding one or more user fields to the key or defining that IMS should automatically add the address (RBA) of the SOURCE SEGMENT to the secondary index value. This wastes space.
- Free space is controlled by a Bit Map reflecting space available only for the largest SEGMENT type. This leads to wasted space and/or bad organisation – both requiring more frequent reorganisation runs.
- No format checks are made on the data either during loading or updating.
- The knowledge of VSAM should not be underestimated (eg. HISAM free space can only be allocated via VSAM)
- With the Direct Access Methods no effort is made to restructure the blocks to have all free space together. This can only be done off-line during a reorganisation run. Thus often sufficient space is available in the block but because it is fragmented it cannot be used.
- TWIN CHAINs may not be sequenced in descending order on the contents of a particular field.
- TWIN CHAINs may not be traversed in a 'Backward' direction – even when TWIN BACKWARD pointers are being used. It is possible, however, to retrieve the last TWIN in a chain directly when CHILD LAST pointers are being used (from the PARENT SEGMENT type). TWIN BACKWARD pointers are only to improve DELETE performance.
- A LOGICAL CHILD SEGMENT cannot have a LOGICAL CHILD SEGMENT as its PHYSICAL CHILD. This restricts the networking capabilities of IMS.
- Generating the IMS control region is a time and resource consuming activity and must be done for almost every change.
- Data compression is only available via a user exit.
- Variable length records that continually expand cause IMS great performance problems because of fragmentation (with the DIRECT ACCESS METHODS).
- two separate sorts of 'HOLD' logic.
- IMS–DC main memory requirements tend to be high.
- DL/1 is single-threading without a TP Monitor. If two batch applications access a database simultaneously, no data protection would be in operation unless DL/1 was running in a BMP region with CONTROL REGION holding IMS/DC. Even if no actual DC operations are needed IMS/DC is required to guarantee data integrity.
- It is often claimed that a change of access method has no effect on program logic. In the following two cases a change to HDAM would cause a change in the SEGMENT retrieved:
  - GET NEXT 'ROOT–SEGMENT–NAME'
    HDAM retrieves the physically next ROOT SEGMENT
    HISAM/HIDAM retrieve the logically next ROOT SEGMENT

- GET NEXT 'ROOT–SEGMENT–NAME' > 'value'
  HDAM retrieves the next ROOT SEGMENT scanning through the DB in a physical sense which satisfies the condition.
  HISAM/HIDAM retrieve the next ROOT SEGMENT scanning through the index which logically satisfies the condition.
  HDAM retrieves the first higher value found scanning through the database in a physical sense – this can be any higher value. HISAM/HIDAM retrieve the logical next higher value.
- The contents of the SEQUENCE field may not be changed with an update command.
- Many of the worthwhile utilities cost extra.
- IMS only runs on S370 and S30XX hardware (and copies)
- The transaction oriented processing is inflexible. The program has no control over what should constitute a transaction. Every GU Call to the message queue automatically causes a transaction to end. Thus all positioning information is lost and integrity problems can arise if a transaction from the user point-of-view extends over more than one IMS transaction.
- Backing store requirements are ca. 70MB for IMS–DB/DC and ca. 30MB for DL/1.
- It is recommended that a utility be run periodically to check that all pointers are correct.
- If two PHYSICAL DATABASES are LOGICALLY linked using DIRECT pointers then they must be reorganised together.
- If two PHYSICAL DATABASES are LOGICALLY linked using SYMBOLIC POINTERS, then the full concatenated key of the LOGICAL PARENT must be stored in the LOGICAL CHILD SEGMENT type. This is a waste of space but it avoids the problem of having to reorganise both databases together. A futher disadvantage with SYMBOLIC pointers is that the LOGICAL PARENT can only accessed via its ROOT SEGMENT. This can cause processing inefficiency if the LP SEGMENT type is low down in the hierarchy.
- The user must write his own load programs.
- HISAM ROOT SEGMENTS that are deleted are not physically removed from the database until it is reorganised (except with VSAM in batch mode or in exclusive use with an MPP, and where no LOGICAL RELATIONSHIPS are involved). This presents not only a waste of space but it also slows down processing. The index hierarchy also contains this record's keys so that the fact that this record has been deleted can only be ascertained by checking the delete byte.
- In an IMS DB/DC environment each record retrieved, even with a 'GU' or 'GN' command is enqueued until a Sync Point is reached, thus increasing the chance of a deadlock situation arising.

One way of avoiding this is the use of the 'read only' option in the PCB (there is also a simple 'read' option!) The 'read only' option should only be used if no parallel deletion of SEGMENTS is being made.
This 'encourages' the user to strictly limit the number of programs updating the databases.

2.13 IMS Glossary

ACCESS METHOD: This term defines a storage organisation as well as an ACCESS METHOD.
1. The basic ACCESS METHOD is either VSAM or ISAM/OSAM which supports the DATABASE ACCESS METHOD. It is transparent to the user. If SECONDARY INDEXING or variable length SEGMENTS are to be used then VSAM must be used.
2. The DATABASE ACCESS METHOD specifies how the DATABASE storage is to be organised. Four possibilities are available HSAM, HISAM, HDAM and HIDAM although in practice only HISAM, and HDAM are used.

ANCHOR POINT See ROOT ANCHOR POINT.

BACKOUT: The process of removing all changes made to a database by a program which terminates abnormally. (cf. DYNAMIC BACKOUT)

BATCH MESSAGE PROCESSING (BMP): An IMS/VS batch processing program which executes under the control of the Control Region and thus has access to the message queue and on-line databases. BMP programs can also process OS/VS files. Like batch programs they are started via JCL.

CHILD SEGMENT: Within a hierarchical structure, each DEPENDENT SEGMENT is the CHILD SEGMENT of the SEGMENTS immediately above it in the structure (cf. SIBLING and TWIN SEGMENTS).

COMMAND CODES: These are extensions to the normal DML (DL/1) commands which can both extend and limit the power of basic commands. A number of COMMAND CODES are associated with each basic command.

CONCATENATED KEY: This is a key composed of the PRIMARY KEY in the ROOT SEGMENT together with the SEQUENCE FIELDS in the DEPENDENT SEGMENTS on the hierarchical path to the object SEGMENT.

CONTROL AREA (CA): The logical equivalent in VSAM to an ISAM cylinder. It contains a number of CIs.

CONTROL INTERVAL (CI): The logical equivalent in VSAM to an ISAM track. This is the unit of transfer between secondary storage and main memory as the result of one EXCP. FREE SPACE can be specified for each CI.

CONTROL REGION: The MVS region that contains the IMS/VS control program.

DATABASE: See PHYSICAL and LOGICAL DATABASES.

DATABASE RECORD: A DATABASE RECORD consists of an occurrence of a ROOT SEGMENT and all its DEPENDENT SEGMENTS.

DEPENDENT SEGMENT: This is a SEGMENT occurrence at any level in the hierarchy except at the ROOT SEGMENT level.

DESTINATION PARENT: In Bi-directional LOGICAL RELATIONSHIPS using VIRTUAL PAIRING, the LOGICAL CHILD SEGMENT may be accessed from either PARENT. That PARENT SEGMENT not used to access the LOGICAL CHILD is called the DESTINATION PARENT SEGMENT.

DIRECT POINTER: It consists of a four byte relative address (RBA) pointing directly to the location of the object record.

DL/1 (DATA LANGUAGE 1): The data manipulation language of the IMS/VS system. It can be used independently of IMS/VS-DC.

ESDS (ENTRY SEQUENCED DATA SET): See VSAM.

FIELD LEVEL SENSITIVITY: A feature which limits a program to accessing only those fields of a SEGMENT that are necessary.

GSAM (GENERALIZED SEQUENTIAL ACCESS METHOD): This ACCESS METHOD allows a standard OS/VS sequential data set to be processed in batch or in a BMP region as if it were a SHSAM DATABASE. Its main advantage is in its automatic repositioning in Checkpoint/Restart processing.

HDAM (HIERARCHICAL DIRECT ACCESS METHOD): A HDAM DATABASE consists of only an OSAM or ESDS – split into two areas: the Root Addressable Area (RAA) and the Overflow Area. A hashing routine assigns an address to a ROOT SEGMENT. This address is a block/CONTROL INTERVAL in the RAA and also a ROOT ANCHOR POINT. The ROOT SEGMENT and its DEPENDENT SEGMENTS should be stored here. If there is no space available either in the Home Block or in the neighbouring blocks then the SEGMENT will be stored in the Overflow Area.
DIRECT POINTERS link the SEGMENTS within a DATABASE RECORD in hierarchical sequence.

HIDAM (HIERARCHICAL INDEXED DIRECT ACCESS METHOD): The ROOT SEGMENTS are stored in PRIMARY KEY sequence in an ISAM/KSDS together with an Index Structure based on the PRIMARY KEY. The SEGMENTS are stored sequentially in an OSAM/ESDS.
DIRECT POINTERS link the SEGMENTS within a DATABASE RECORD.

HIERARCHICAL POINTERS: These are the pointers that link the SEGMENTS of a DATABASE RECORD in hierarchical sequence ie. top-to-bottom, front-to-back and left-to-right. Either HIERARCHICAL or PHYSICAL PARENT and PHYSICAL TWIN pointers may be selected to link the SEGMENTS of a DATABASE RECORD.

HISAM (HIERARCHICAL INDEXED SEQUENTIAL ACCESS METHOD): The ROOT SEGMENT and a specified number of DEPENDENT SEGMENTS are stored in an ISAM/KSDS together with an Index based on the PRIMARY KEY. The other DEPENDENT SEGMENTS are stored in an OSAM/ESDS. The relationship between SEGMENTS is defined by their physical adjacency.
VSAM can process ROOT-only HISAM (SHISAM) DATABASES.

HSAM (HIERARCHICAL SEQUENTIAL ACCESS METHOD): A HSAM DATABASE may only be processed sequentially; records may not be updated nor may records be inserted. It may be held on tape or disc. The records are stored in fixed length blocks.

ISAM INDEXED SEQUENTIAL ACCESS METHOD.

INDEX DATABASE: The DATABASE containing the SECONDARY INDEX – it can also be processed as a normal DATABASE.

INDEX POINTER SEGMENT: The SEGMENT in the INDEX DATABASE containing the data from the SOURCE SEGMENT and the pointer to the TARGET SEGMENT.

INDEX SOURCE SEGMENT: See SOURCE SEGMENT.

INDEX TARGET SEGMENT: See TARGET SEGMENT.

INDEXED SEGMENT: See TARGET SEGMENT.

INDEXING SEGMENT: See SOURCE SEGMENT.

KSDS (KEY SEQUENCED DATA SET): See VSAM.

KEY FIELD: The field in a SEGMENT type that determines the sequence of the TWIN SEGMENT OCCURRENCES (see SEQUENCE FIELD).

LOGICAL CHILD POINTER: The pointers are necessary in Bi-directional Logical Relationships using VIRTUAL LOGICAL CHILD SEGMENT types. They replace the PHYSICAL CHILD POINTERS that are lost because one of the CHILD SEGMENT types (the VIRTUAL CHILD) no longer physically exists. LOGICAL CHILD FIRST and optionally LAST POINTERS are available.

LOGICAL CHILD SEGMENT: This SEGMENT type has two PARENTS, one PHYSICAL and one LOGICAL. This SEGMENT is strictly the PHYSICAL CHILD of its PHYSICAL PARENT and the LOGICAL CHILD of its LOGICAL PARENT. The purpose of this construction is to link two separate PHYSICAL DATABASES or to extend the structure of a single PHYSICAL DATABASE beyond a simple hierarchy.

LOGICAL DATABASE: This is the User View. It may be exactly the same as a PHYSICAL DATABASE or it may show a hierarchical subset of a more complicated structure generated with LOGICAL POINTERS.

LOGICAL PARENT POINTER: This is a DIRECT or SYMBOLIC POINTER stored in the LOGICAL CHILD SEGMENT. It is necessary for the formation of LOGICAL RELATIONSHIPS.

LOGICAL PARENT SEGMENT: This is the SEGMENT pointed to by the LOGICAL PARENT POINTER in the LOGICAL (PHYSICAL) CHILD SEGMENT.

LOGICAL RELATIONSHIPS: IMS PHYSICAL DATABASES are strictly hierarchical in structure. More complicated structures can be generated using LOGICAL RELATIONSHIPS. They are implemented using LOGICAL CHILD, LOGICAL PARENT and LOGICAL TWIN POINTERS.

LOGICAL TWIN POINTERS: These are directly analogous to PHYSICAL TWIN POINTERS; they link LOGICAL TWIN SEGMENTS under a LOGICAL PARENT.

LOGICAL VIEW: See LOGICAL DATABASE.

OVERFLOW SEQUENTIAL ACCESS METHOD (OSAM): This is an IMS/VS access method used by some of the online pool management routines. It can also be used as an alternative to VSAM for HDAM DATABASES. It can also be used in conjunction with ISAM.

PCB (PROGRAM CONTROL BLOCK): This supplies the program with a LOGICAL VIEW of the DATABASE. Processing restrictions may also be specified. As the LOGICAL VIEW can only be hierarchical, it may be necessary to have more than one when processing more complicated structures than hierarchies.

PHYSICAL CHILD SEGMENT: This is a DEPENDENT SEGMENT in a PHYSICAL DATABASE. The PHYSICAL PARENT SEGMENT has a PHYSICAL CHILD FIRST (and optionally a PHYSICAL CHILD LAST) POINTER to the first (and optionally the last) occurrence of each type of PHYSICAL CHILD SEGMENT dependent on it.

PHYSICAL DATABASE: This consists of up to 255 SEGMENT types arranged in a hierarchical structure of not more than 15 levels.
The SEGMENTS are linked by HIERARCHICAL or PHYSICAL CHILD and PHYSICAL TWIN POINTERS.

PHYSICAL PARENT POINTER: This pointer is introduced automatically by IMS when VIRTUAL PAIRING is used. It is to replace the LOGICAL PARENT POINTER that is no longer available because the VIRTUAL LOGICAL CHILD does not exist physically.

PHYSICAL TWIN POINTERS: These pointers link the PHYSICAL CHILD SEGMENTS of the same type, dependent on one PARENT SEGMENT occurrence. They are always linked in a hierarchically forward direction using PHYSICAL TWIN FORWARD POINTERS and may be linked in the reverse direction using PHYSICAL TWIN BACKWARD POINTERS.

PSB (PROGRAM SPECIFICATION BLOCK): Each program has one PSB containing one or more PCBs.

RBA (RELATIVE BYTE ADDRESS): This is the byte address relative to the beginning of the file where a SEGMENT occurrence is stored. There is no Address Converter either explicit or implicit. The RBA is four bytes long; thus a file is limited to ca. 4.3 gigabytes.

REAL: This adjective describes entities that are physically stored in the database eg. REAL LOGICAL CHILD (cf. VIRTUAL).

RECORD: See DATABASE RECORD.

RELATIVE BLOCK NUMBER (RBN): Home Block.

ROOT ANCHOR POINT (RAP): The HDAM hashing routine produces an address consisting of an RBN and an RAP. Its purpose is to reduce the length of the synonym chains. Each ROOT SEGMENT is allocated to an ANCHOR POINT. This makes the blocks appear smaller thus providing a finer degree of tuning.

ROOT SEGMENT: This must occur once and may not occur more than once per DATABASE RECORD.

SEARCH FIELD: This is a field which forms the key for the SECONDARY INDEX. Up to five fields or parts of fields from a SEGMENT type may be used to form the SECONDARY INDEX.

SECONDARY INDEX: This provides an alternative processing sequence. (see INDEX DATABASE).

SEQUENCE FIELD: 1. The unique KEY FIELD in the ROOT SEGMENT used for the primary access path (nb. the ROOT SEGMENT KEY FIELD of a HDAM DATABASE need not contain unique values). 2. The KEY FIELD in DEPENDENT SEGMENT types used to order the TWIN chain occurrences. It may be unique but need not be.

SHISAM (SIMPLE HIERARCHICAL SEQUENTIAL ACCESS METHOD): This is a HISAM database consisting only of ROOT SEGMENTS, thus it does not require a SEGMENT PREFIX, which normally consists of SEGMENT type and delete bytes. Such a database structure is identical to a VSAM KSDS and can be processed as such.

SIBLINGS: These are occurrences of SEGMENTS of different types under one PARENT SEGMENT occurrence (at the same hierarchical level).

SSA (SEGMENT SEARCH ARGUMENT): This is part of the DML command; an SSA must be present (explicitly or implicitly) for each level of the hierarchy. It is used to:
- identify a particular SEGMENT type
- retrieve a SEGMENT dependent upon the value in one or more of its fields
- modify the function of certain DML commands via COMMAND CODES.

SOURCE SEGMENT: A concept used in SECONDARY INDEXING. This is the SEGMENT from which the field(s) are taken to construct the SECONDARY INDEX.

STORAGE ORGANISATION: See ACCESS METHOD.

SUBSEQUENCE DATA: Data used to make non-unique SECONDARY INDEX keys (cf. SEARCH FIELD) unique, or to provide a sequence for non-unique SECONDARY INDEX keys, eg. the department code is a SECONDARY INDEX key. In order to retrieve all persons in a department in alphabetical order on their family name, the family name is used as SUBSEQUENCE DATA.

SYMBOLIC POINTER: It consists of a concatenation of the keys in the hierarchical path to the object SEGMENT.

TARGET SEGMENT: A concept used in SECONDARY INDEXING. This is the SEGMENT that is retrieved via the SECONDARY INDEX; it may be any SEGMENT between the ROOT and SOURCE SEGMENT (inclusive).

TWIN: CHILD SEGMENT occurrences of the same type under a single occurrence of the PARENT SEGMENT.

USER VIEW: See LOGICAL DATABASE.

VIRTUAL: This adjective describes entities that are not physically stored in the database and have to be constructed from available data. The user sees VIRTUAL data as REAL data in the USER VIEW.

VSAM (VIRTUAL SEQUENTAL ACCESS METHOD): This Access Method supports the file organisations:
- KSDS records in key sequence.
- ESDS records in chronological sequence.
- RRDS records are stored and retrieved dependent on a user allocated Relative Record number.

Only the first two file organisations are used with IMS. Access to an ESDS record is only possible via the RBA. Access to a KSDS record is possible via the RBA and also using a key value via an INDEX.

The RRDS file organisation is used by some other DBMSs.

3. DATACOM/DB

The vendor's aim in developing DATACOM/DB was to produce a complementary package for their TP monitor GMT, which was renamed DATACOM/DC upon the release of DATACOM/DB in 1974.

The two products together are simply called DATACOM. They are, however, marketed separately with interfaces to other TP and DBMS products. Nevertheless it should be emphasised that the two products were designed by the same group of people to be totally compatible and complementary in their functions.

A query language, DATAQUERY, is available for use by non-EDP personnel to interrogate a DATACOM/DB database. A data dictionary is also available.

3.1 Classification

COBOL, FORTRAN, PL/1, RPG–II or Assembler, in fact any programming language containing a CALL verb, may be the host language for a DATACOM/DB application.

DATACOM/DB is based on inverted file structures with an index organisation which is unique. As it was designed to complement DATACOM/DC, it is strongly oriented towards providing fast response for multiple users in an on-line mode of operation. One of the consequences of this approach is that space management is kept to a minimum, which results in periodic reorganisation runs being necessary. Because the user data is maintained separately from the structure data, reorganisation is very simple – only those files which are disorganised need be reorganised.

One of the primary advantages of inverted file based systems over hierarchical/network based systems is the ability to resolve multiple key queries within the index structure, before accessing user data records. This has not yet been developed for the host language user of DATACOM/DB but is available for the DATAQUERY user.

The DBMS can operate under all current IBM/370 operating systems, DOS, OS and VS and also under EDOS (an independently-developed DOS replacement). DATACOM/DB can run on any IBM/360 or /370 hardware etc. The vendor claims that DATACOM/DB can run in as little as 25K bytes (excluding buffers). Even with data compression/expansion software and also the random and sequential access modules, the minimum main memory requirement is only 31K bytes.

3.2 Data Definition

DATACOM/DB is a pure inverted file DBMS. This means that there are no structure pointers embedded in the user data, nor is there an explicit data model. These factors make the definition of the database schema and the associated files and ELEMENTS relatively simple to understand and use. An ELEMENT consists of a number of contiguous data fields within a record. It can be as small as one field or as large as a record. ELEMENTS may overlap. It is viewed as the smallest logical piece of information capable of being processed by the application.

A database may contain up to 240 logical files. Each record type may contain up to a maximum of 15 keys, limited by a total of 255 keys per database. Each key can be composed of up to four fields with a limit of 180 bytes per key. An ELEMENT can consist of any number of contiguous fields. However, there is a maximum of 255 ELEMENT types allowed per file. A user program requests ELEMENTS from the database, not records. A maximum of 16 ELEMENT occurrences may be requested per access. One of the keys per record type must be defined as the NATIVE key. The value of this key's occurrences will determine the physical placement of the records.

Each file and its characteristics must be defined via three system macros. Also associated with each file is a DSECT, which describes the fields, their names and their characteristics within each record. The file itself is defined via the DB FILE macro and contains a series of parameters to specify:

- a unique name
- a numeric ID
- record length
- block size
- storage device
- whether or not data compression is to be applied
- with which DSECT it is associated
- whether the MASTER key may be changed via an update
- whether the MASTER key should be unique
- whether logging is required.

Each key is defined via the DB KEY macro. The following information is required:

- a unique name
- a numeric ID in the range 1–255. All similar key types within a database should be allocated the same numeric ID so that the unique index structure of DATACOM/DB can be used to full advantage.
- whether this key is the NATIVE key for the file. This would mean that the

logical and physical sequential order would be the same, thus making sequential processing on this key very efficient.
- those fields (from the DSECT) which constitute the key.

The final macro DBELMNT defines the ELEMENTS. The following information is necessary:

- an ELEMENT name (which is used in the application program)
- a one byte security code which the user program must supply before DATACOM/DB will deliver the ELEMENT to the user
- one or more field names from the DSECT. Choice of the composition of each ELEMENT can critically influence performance and data independence. ELEMENTS composed of too many fields could compromise data independence, while too many ELEMENTS containing one field might degrade performance without significantly enhancing data independence.

3.3 Data Storage Structures

A DATACOM/DB databank consists of the following secondary files:

- CONTROL FILE (CXX)
- HIGH LEVEL INDEX (IXX)
- DIRECT ACCESS INDEX (DXX).

The CONTROL FILE, as its name suggests, holds control information related to each database. The HIGH LEVEL INDEX is the link between the CONTROL FILE and the DIRECT INDEX. It is relatively small, containing two separate portions, the Higher Level (HLX) and the Lower Level (LLX). The DIRECT ACCESS INDEX holds all the key values and the pointers to their occurrences in the primary data. The relationship between the different files is shown in Fig. 3.3.

3.3.1 The Control File (CXX)

This file contains control information for all files and all databases within the DATACOM/DB system, together with information to resolve user requests. This file functions in a similar manner to a data directory.

The data directory of a database consists of one segment describing the database itself. This segment contains the following information:

- Master status of the database (eg. open, being loaded etc.)
- date and time when database was last processed
- number of files/record types in this database
- next index overflow pointer (into DXX)
- amount of index overflow

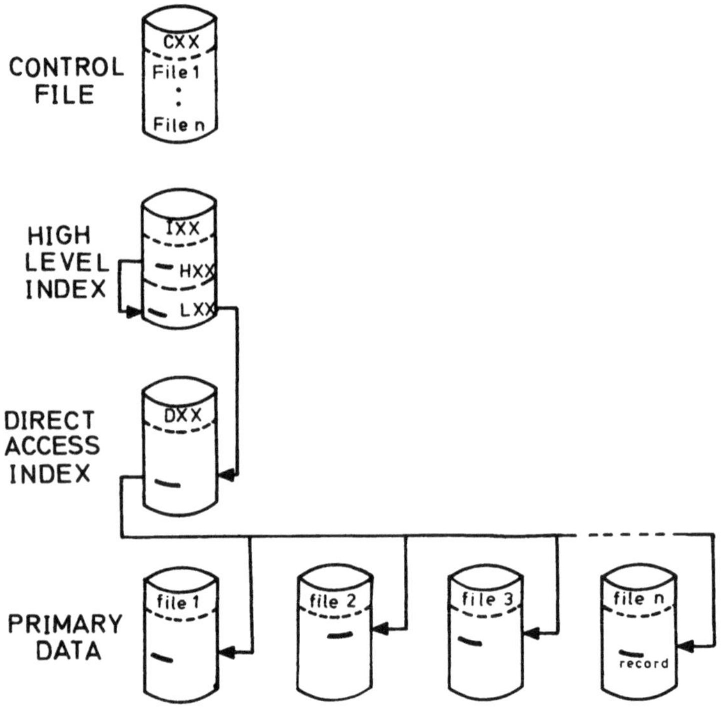

Fig. 3.3: Accessing a primary record

- maximum address for DXX (in TTR)
- DXX characteristics
- IXX characteristics.

Then follow a succession of segments, each describing one of the files within the database:

- file name
- file status
- file characteristics
- key information (name, location, length etc.)
- DATA ELEMENT information (name, location, security code, etc.)
- overflow information (start address and length).

3.3.2 The High Level Index (IXX)

This file is simply the two higher levels of index for the DXX. The essential difference between "normal" inverted file systems and DATACOM/DB is that the latter organises the keys on a database-wide basis. The HIGH LEVEL INDEX itself is split into two levels – the Higher Level (HLX) and the Lower Level (LLX).

For each block in the DXX there is one entry in the LLX. This entry is the highest key value from that block, together with its physical address (track and relative block number). The Higher Level Index is simply this same process repeated i.e. the highest key value in each track on the LLX.

The contents of the IXX cannot be changed after initial load. It is therefore incapable of reflecting any changes made to the DXX due to deletions, insertions etc. In order to have the IXX reflect the DXX after modifications, it is necessary to reorganise the IXX using DBIXUNLD and DBIXLOD. These two utilities cannot be run on anything but the complete database, and during their execution, no user can access the database.

3.3.3 The Direct Index (DXX)

This file, the lowest index level, is an unkeyed BDAM file containing the pointers to those records, in the various files, which contain the key value in question.

This index is also split into two separate portions; the Prime Area and the Overflow Area. The Prime Area is filled during the initial load, the Overflow Area for all subsequent modifications. This means that these modifications will cause no change to the IXX levels. The only alterations which can be made to the Prime Area are the insertion of pointers to the Overflow Area and the movement of compressed records from the Prime Area to the Overflow Area in uncompressed form after the first update to that particular record (when no space is present for the enlarged record in the original block).

Fig. 3.3.3 shows the format of the DXX entries. The "pointer count" field is not used when only one pointer is associated with a particular value.

3.3.4 Space Management

In the interest of fast response time, DATACOM/DB makes little attempt to use space efficiently. In the PRIMARY FILE neither space 'freed' by a delection nor space made available by compressed records being moved to the Overflow Area can be used for new record insertions. However, this space is used to accommodate enlarged compressed records, (see 3.5). If a compressed record is too large to fit its old block, due to update activity, then it is moved to an Overflow Area where it is stored in its uncompressed length. All insertions after initial load are also placed in the Overflow Area. No attempt is made to maintain NATIVE key sequence.

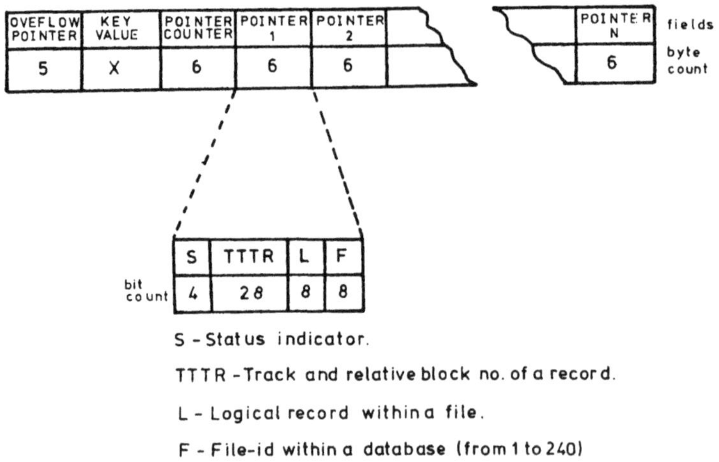

Fig. 3.3.3: Format of a DXX entry.

The same approach is used in the index portion of the database. Here, however, the DBA has some control over allocation of space within the Overflow Area.

The DXX is the lowest level of the index. It contains the pointers to the data record occurrences. The DXX is split into a Prime Area and an Overflow Area. Initially, and also after a reorganisation, all key occurrences and the associated pointers are in the Prime Area. Thereafter, all new key occurrences are placed in the Overflow Area, with a pointer to it from the Prime Area. New synonym occurrences are also placed in the Overflow Area.

There are a number of parameters in the DB key macro which can slow down the degradation of the database. One option causes the system to try to group the synonyms together, so avoiding the time-consuming process of having to follow long synonym chains. Another option causes groups of key value occurrences to be grouped together in the Overflow Area physical blocks.

3.3.5 Compression

Record compression can result in very significant space saving – sometimes as much as 50%. Data compression is implemented as an optional feature in DATACOM/DB. Fig. 3.3.5 shows how a compressed block appears on secondary storage.

The first two bytes of the block contain the length of unused space, SLACK, within the block. This SLACK is normally simply that space left at load-time since the next record to be loaded was too large for the block. It is however

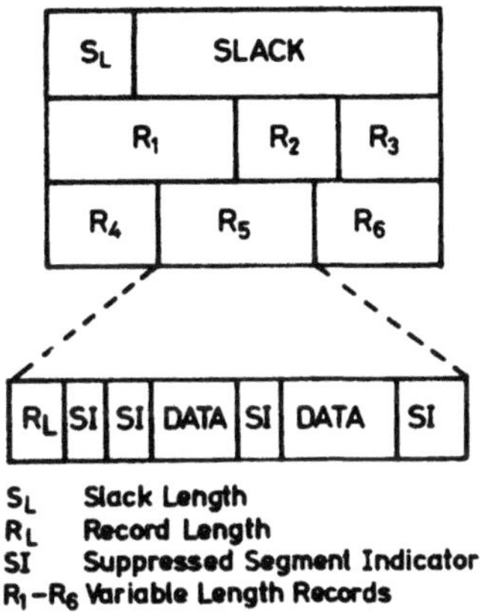

Fig. 3.3.5: A block Containing Compressed Records

possible to load the blocks with a particular value of SLACK. This SLACK is used to accommodate enlarged logical records resulting from update activity.

The compression algorithm operates on complete logical records – it ignores all field and ELEMENT boundaries. The only characters compressed are three or more occurrences of:

- space
- binary zero
- display zero

up to a maximum of 32 characters. Each compression is indicated by a SEGMENT INDICATOR (SI). Each group of uncompressed data (maximum length 128 bytes) is also preceded by a SEGMENT INDICATOR.

The only occasion when space is reused (either SLACK or deleted record space) is to accommodate compressed records which have been enlarged. This helps to preserve the NATIVE key sequence. If, however, the enlarged compressed record is too large for the original block, then the record is decompressed and stored in its full length in the Overflow Area. The original record in the Prime Area is flagged as deleted. In its uncompressed form, the record will never to be moved again. The reason for this is that movement costs processing time, all indexes having to be updated to reflect the new record location.

Data compression makes parameters such as block size difficult to calculate. Often it is necessary to change these parameters when the first reorganisation takes place in the light of performance analysis.

3.4 Data Manipulation

When examining and judging DATACOM/DB, it should be remembered that the primary design objective was to provide fast response for a large volume of on-line transactions. This approach has meant that all activities which can be are deferred. This can cause a gradual degrading of performance.

DATACOM/DB excels at direct access retrieval because the indexes contain pointers to each record containing the desired key value. The NATIVE key can be used for extremely efficient sequential processing.
No boolean functions are available to the host language user of DATACOM/DB. Complex queries must be resolved within the program. Therefore, the advantage of describing a field as a key is limited. The LOCKY and GSETL provide minor exceptions to this.

DATACOM/DB allows keys to be constructed from up to four fields. This, together with the generic key search capability, offers the competent system designer a high degree of flexibility. It can also compensate for the lack of conjunction of conditions.

The structure of the indexes is such that accesses may differentiate between:

- key type
- key value within key type
- file within key value.

This means that key value processing is possible without the record type being of any importance.

The DML can be divided into four basic types of command:

- LOCATE
- READ
- FILE MAINTENANCE
- BATCH SEQUENTIAL RETRIEVAL

3.4.1 LOCATE and READ Commands

The 15 LOCATE and READ commands are composite commands consisting of a three-character prefix and a two-character suffix. There are three prefixes:

LOC This retrieves meta-information eg. whether a certain key value occurrence exists and if so, in which file

RED This retrieves a record occurrence from the database and delivers data to the user according to the ELEMENT LIST

RDU This is a RED command together with a record occurrence lock, to prevent concurrent updating. This record must be unlocked by an UPDAT, DELET or RELES before another program can access it.

The seven suffixes act as qualifiers to the prefix and are:

KY random access
NE access the next occurrence with the same key value
NX access the next occurrence irrespective of key value
NK retrieve the value of the next higher key
LE retrieve an already LOCATED record
ID retrieve a record whose ID is known
PD identify the first entry in the previous index block.

Not all suffixes and prefixes may be combined (see Fig. 3.4.1).

The application programmer, using the host language, communicates with DATACOM/DB as follows:

CALL 'CBLDBMS' USING REQUESTAREA ELEMENTLIST.

The REQUESTAREA contains the following parameters:

COMMAND CODE	The actual command.
FILE–NAME	This parameter is optional in some commands, thus enabling the user to find desired data more easily.
KEY–NAME	The name of the key type.
RETURN–CODE	This field must be investigated after the CALL has been executed to ascertain the status of DATACOM/DB or the result of the CALL.
RECORD–ID	The record address is returned after some types of access.
DATABASE–ID	If a file name is used in more than one database, then the file can be uniquely identified using this parameter.

		prefix		
		LOC	RED	RDU
suffix	KY	LOCKY	REDKY	RDUKY
	NE	LOCNE	REDNE	RDUNE
	NX	LOCNX	REDNX	RDUNX
	NK	LOCNK		
	LE		REDLE	RDULE
	ID		REDID	RDUID
	PB	LOCPB		

Fig. 3.4.1: Valid LOCATE and READ Commands

RESERVED–AREA	An area reserved for use by DATACOM/DB.
WORK–AREA	This is the area used for transporting data between the program and DATACOM/DB. This can be the key and/or data.

The ELEMENT LIST contains up to 16 parameters. Each ELEMENT can have a SECURITY CODE associated with it. In this case, this must be present in the ELEMENT LIST.

LOCKY – LOCATE KEY

This command will identify the first record occurrence which contains a key value equal to, or greater than, the one in the WORK–AREA. It is possible to limit the search to a particular file.

LOCPB – LOCATE PREVIOUS KEY

This command delivers the first key occurrence of the previous index block. It is possible to specify a particular file, in which case, this file's first key occurrence will be returned.

LOCNE – LOCATE NEXT ENTRY

This command locates the next record occurrence which contains a particular key value. It is possible to limit the action of this command to a particular file.

LOCNX – LOCATE NEXT

This command differs from the LOCNE in that the next record is located irrespective of any key value. Nevertheless, a key name must be specified, otherwise 'next record' has no logical meaning.

LOCNK – LOCATE NEXT KEY

This command causes DATACOM/DB to return the address of that record occurrence which contains the next higher key value from the CURRENT position. This command can be limited to a particular file.

REDLE/RDULE – READ A PREVIOUSLY LOCATED ENTRY

These commands retrieve an ENTRY. It must have been preceded by one of the five LOCATE commands.

REDID/RDUID – READ AN ENTRY IDENTIFIED BY A RECORD–ID

These commands retrieve an ENTRY identified by the user specifying the RECORD–ID in the REQUEST–AREA. The RECORD–ID is the record address in the form of TTTRLF (see Fig. 3.3.3)

REDKY/RDUKY – READ ENTRY

These two commands do not need to be preceded by a LOCATE command. Both a key value and a file must be specified in the REQUEST AREA. If this key value is found within a record occurrence in the file specified, then the requested ELEMENTS will be retrieved.

REDNE/RDUNE – READ NEXT ENTRY WITHIN KEY AND FILE

These commands retrieve the next ENTRY within the key value and file specified in the REQUEST–AREA. A RDUNE command automatically releases the previously locked record.

REDNX/RDUNX – READ NEXT ENTRY WITHIN FILE

These commands retrieve the next ENTRY for the file specified, irrespective of key value. RDUNX automatically releases a previously locked record.

3.4.2 File Maintenance Commands

These are the commands which change (i.e. add, delete or update) records in the database. All these commands (except ADDIT) must be preceded by a successful ENTRY retrieval, under exclusive control.

ADDIT – ADD A RECORD

This command adds a new record to the specified file. Strictly, a series of ELEMENTS is added to the database. All key values are added to the indexes.

UPDAT – UPDATE A RECORD

This command causes a modified record occurrence to be returned to the database. Any ELEMENTS may be changed. DATACOM/DB checks whether or not key values have been changed and modifies the indexes accordingly. NB. The MASTER KEY may only be changed if it is so specified in the database file macro definition.

DELET – DELETE A RECORD

This command removes a record occurrence from the database, and all its associated index entries.

RELES – RELEASE A RECORD

This command removes the exclusive control over a record occurrence.

3.4.3 BATCH SEQUENTIAL RETRIEVAL Commands

When processing sequentially in a batch environment, two special commands are available. Although true sequential processing only occurs when the NATIVE key is specified, it is also possible to process on any other key. In the latter case, the records are retrieved randomly. The user program would notice no difference, but NATIVE key processing would be faster. In both cases, the processing is faster than using normal read commands. This speed is attributable to:

– multiple buffering
– chained channel commands
– a sophisticated look-ahead process.

Before using a series of GETIT commands to retrieve the records sequentially, the starting point and the direction (the key) of the subsequent processing must be defined by a GSETL command.

3.5 Data Independence

Total data independence can be achieved with DATACOM/DB because the application retrieves a logical record, which is composed of ELEMENTS. The order of these ELEMENTS does not need to correspond to the order in the physical record, and only those ELEMENTS needed by the application will be retrieved. It is therefore possible to add new fields or to delete fields to which the program is not sensitive without affecting the application. The disadvantage with this is that the number of ELEMENTS tends to be large, each field often being an ELEMENT, which of course reduces performance.

3.6 Concurrent Usage

The 'Multi-user Facility' enables one single copy of the DBMS to service multitasking application programs in a number of partitions concurrently. This offers the user distinct advantages:

– the economy of a single copy of the code
– the security that will protect the database from concurrent updating
– minimizing I/O traffic and maximizing available memory

3.7 Integrity Controls and Recovery

DATACOM/DB makes no check on the validity of data being stored, neither on its format nor value. All such validity checks are the responsibility of the application. Checks are carried out where the integrity of the system would be threatened eg. to ensure the uniqueness of a file MASTER key value occurrence (when so specified).

Integrity of the database itself is guaranteed by not allowing the user access to secondary data.

Recovery of a DATACOM/DB database is the responsibility of the user – no utilities are provided for this. An optional transaction logging feature is available, which logs both BEFORE and AFTER IMAGES. This information is sufficient for both FORWARD and BACKWARD recovery purposes. The DBUNLD utility provides a database copy typically used as input for a reorganisation. This may also be used to provide a back-up copy.

3.8 Security and Privacy Controls

Each ELEMENT may have a security code assigned to it. In order to access this ELEMENT, the user must supply the correct security code. A further level of security is provided through the FILE–TABLE. This can restrict the user to particular databases or files, or further restrict the user to read-only access. The FILE–TABLE also contains information about DATACOM/DB configuration and buffer sizes. It is defined using the DBFLTBL and DBUFSPAC macros.

3.9 Performance

DATACOM/DB is a relatively simple system to use. No special skill is required to define the REQUEST AREA or the ELEMENT LIST. The use of the commands is not particularly difficult, even when processing multiple files in parallel. Some knowledge of the DXX organisation is necessary to take advantage of DATACOM/BD's unique index structure. Nevertheless, the level of skill required is far less than that needed for navigation with a hierarchical- or network-based DBMS.

The performance of the system will normally degrade with time when updating activity occurs. The degree of degradation will be directly proportional to the volatility of the file. This is because all new record index occurrence in the DXX will be placed in an overflow area. Periodic reorganisation of the index will therefore be necessary. The primary-data area need not be reorganised so often, but here again, NATIVE sequence performance will degrade with time as new records are placed in the Overflow Area.

The buffer allocation within the FILE TABLE definition will have a critical effect on performance, but this can only be tuned by trial and error.

The DDL is simple to understand and use. This is true of all inverted file systems, since there are no pointer fields to be defined. However, the processing requirements can have a decided influence on the database design – although here, performance is gained at the expense of data independence. In general, DATACOM/DB requires fairly sophisticated skills to design efficient databases, but the requirements are not higher than those of the other DBMSs analysed here.

3.10 Conclusion

DATACOM/DB has profited by its late entry into the DBMS market by being able to analyse the strengths and weaknesses of the leading DBMSs – i.e. the other five DBMSs investigated in this book. The most outstanding feature of DATACOM/DB is its ability to search on a key that spans a number of files.

This system was developed for "speed", and many features were sacrificed to reach this goal eg. the approach to space management, which is more primitive than in most other systems, but which saves greatly on time. The consequence of this approach is that DATACOMB/DB tends to require frequent regorganisation.

DATACOM/DB does not yet offer all the features of a fully mature DBMS, for example recovery and also complex query resolution, which is normally amongst the strong points of a DBMS based on partially inverted file structures. This is most probably directly attributable to the newness of the system. Certainly the two hundred or so customers are generally more than just satisfied with the system. Since inverted file based systems need far less initial planning effort than network/hierarchical systems, the user can implement very quickly, creating almost instant respect and enthusiasm for the product.

Two other features of the system worth mentioning are the batch sequential processing facility and the data compression routine. The former makes use of sophisticated look-ahead techniques. The latter can often save up to 50% on data space and occasionally much more.

The system uses relatively little main memory. 31KB is adequate for the system, including the data compression/expansion routines, but excluding the buffers.

The system is easy to use, and should the user want a TP monitor, then DATACOM/DC, which has been developed by the same group, should be of great interest.

One of the problems with DATACOM/DB is to try to define the 'average' conditions of the database and to benchmark this situation. Normally benchmarks are taken on a freshly loaded database. In the case of DATACOM/DB this would give a completely false picture unless the database was to be used purely for retrieval purposes. All the records in a newly loaded (or reorganised) database are stored in compressed form and the records are stored in NATIVE KEY sequence. This optimal situation degrades almost from the first update because DATACOM/DB makes no effort to maintain order. All new records are placed uncompressed in an overflow area. As the location of data records is irrelevant for an inverted file system (except for logical sequential processing) this has little influence on performance. However the records being stored in their uncompressed length will influence the storage area (on average, records are compressed to less than half their original length) both in the buffer area and on secondary storage. This means that it is only half as likely that a required record is in the buffer – if the whole file were decompressed.

Far more serious from a performance point of view is the loss of physical order in the Inverted List (DXX). All additions to the file are noted in the overflow area and linked from the prime area with pointers. This takes place for all key values irrespective whether the value is already stored or not. Similarly updated key values are stored in overflow. This has the advantage that the addition or update is processed very rapidly but it has a far more serious disadvantage – all processing of these pointers will require more physical accesses. As these pointers are used more than once it is more efficient from a processing point of view to place them in the same block as their neighbours. This would of course mean that the initial storage of the values in the DXX would be slower due to shifting and block splits but that the far more frequent retrieval processing would have fewer physical accesses to perform.

The forgoing has been an attempt to place DATACOM/DB in pespective. The system shows promise but it cannot be compared with the leading Inverted File DBMSs for flexibility. It is certainly only a matter of time (and money) before DATACOM/DB takes its place as one of the leading DBMSs offering a full range of features and facilities. Certainly this system should be considered for the smaller user who expects to be able to 'grow' with the system or for the user who has simple processing and requires fast response time.

DATACOM/DB now offers complete transaction oriented processing. The log file can only be a preformatted disc file and logging is at the block level. Additions to the log file result from the execution of the following commands: OPEN (RUN–UNIT start), CLOSE (RUN–UNIT finish), ADDIT, UPDAT, DELET, LOGIT, LOGCP, and DEQUE commands.

The Recovery File is a sequential history file of the logged data records. It is updated periodically from the contents of the log file. Although forward recovery can be implemented from a tape or disc Recovery File, backward recovery can only be performed from a tape Recovery File. Thus in the latter case, when using a disc Recovery File, it must first be copied to tape before the backward recovery can be initiated. The transaction backout facility guarantees that all transactions that do not complete successfully will have all their modifications to the database(s) removed. Transactions may not complete successfully for one of the following reasons:

- hardware failure
- software failure in the operating system, DBMS or in the user program
- because of program logic.

The first two cases are under DBMS control (warm restart); the last case is activated using the LOGTB command.

The commands associated with the new transaction-oriented processing are:

LOGCP Writes a user checkpoint record to the log file, indicating the end of a sub–RUN–UNIT and the start of a new sub–RUN–UNIT.

LOGTB Requests transaction backout.

LOGIT Writes user information to the log file for later retrieval.

LOGLB Requests retrieval of a LOGIT record written by the same sub–RUN–UNIT. The last LOGIT record written will be retrieved first.

3.11 Advantages of DATACOM/DB

- Efficient and elegant solution to the problem of coupling key fields from different files.
- Simplicity of database design.
- Integrated DB/DC using DATACOM/DC.
- Data dictionary.
- Query language (DATAQUERY).
- Relatively cheap to buy.
- It performs well in a non-volatile environment.
- The records are initially stored in their compressed length. If an update causes the record to move block, then it is stored in its uncompressed length. However if it stays in its original block is stored in its compressed length; an illogical situation as data records are as at home in one block as another. The worst result is that the database will require regular reorganisation runs to keep the records compressed.
- A key may be designated as NATIVE KEY in which case the contents of this field will determine the sequence of the records when the file is being loaded. Unfortunately no effort is made to maintain this sequence thereafter.
- If a key field is known (and at least one other field) DATACOM/DB will retrieve a record and indicate which file it is from.
- Keys may be defined as unique, non-unique and/or non-changing as the design requirements dictate. All fields including key fields may be updated.

– User messages may be written to the log file.
– Database loading is via a utility.
– An encyphering facility (DATASECURE) is available. It is charged separately from the basic DATACOM/DB package.
– Transaction-oriented processing.

3.12 Disadvantages of DATACOM/DB

– Reorganisation is required frequently because no on-going reorganisation is carried out.
– No direct access method – using a hashing routine.
– The only operators available with the LOCATE command are '=' and '>'. No '<' is available.
– The compression routine treats the record as a string, thus on retrieval the whole string has to be expanded even when only one or two fields are required by the user. This is a great waste of CPU time.
– No facilities for variable length records.
– Space management is almost non-existent.
– No effort is made to maintain NATIVE KEY sequence.
– No complex queries can be formulated (this is very surprising as this is usually one of the strengths of an inverted file system; I am sure it will be implemented in the near future).
– It is not possible to retrieve a string of record addresses as a result of the LOCATE command.
– A new index can only be created by reloading the file.
– The contents of the ELEMENTS are never checked.
– A lack of certain utilities.
– The ELEMENTS requested in the ELEMENT LIST must have the same characteristics as in the database.

3.13 DATACOM/DB Glossary

COMMAND CODE: A DML command.

CONTROL FILE (CXX): This file contains the database definition and includes information about the files, keys and ELEMENTS in each database.

DATABASE: Those files which are managed as a unit, with a single DXX/IXX index pair.

DATA ELEMENT: One or more contiguous fields in a data record.

DIRECT ACCESS INDEX (DXX): This system file is the lowest level of the index hierarchy and contains all key values with pointers to the record occurrences containing these values.

ELEMENT: See DATA ELEMENT.

ELEMENT LIST: A storage area in all user programs specifying those ELEMENTS on which the COMMAND CODE should operate.

FILE TABLE: A series of parameters which regulate certain aspects of processing of a user program with DATACOM/DB. It includes buffer size, files which may be accessed, and system configuration.

HIGH LEVEL INDEX (IXX): This is the transitional index between the CXX file and the DXX file.

MASTER KEY: The first key specified for a database file. It is the only key for which system-supported uniqueness may be specified.

NATIVE KEY: This key defines the order in which the records are loaded into the database.

REQUEST (COMMUNICATIONS) AREA: The area within the user program for all communications with DATACOM/DB.

RETURN CODE: A two byte code returned by DATACOM/DB in the REQUEST AREA after each COMMAND CODE has been processed.

SECURITY CODE: A one byte code which may be optionally associated with each ELEMENT to restrict its accessibility.

SEGMENT INDICATOR (SI): A byte containing information data used only in compressed files.

SLACK SPACE: Space held at the start of blocks containing compressed records. It is used to accommodate the records from the block when they are enlarged.

4. TOTAL

This DBMS has most probably more installations than any other. This is due in part to the number of different versions of TOTAL available. It is available for the IBM System 360/370 etc. running under DOS, DOS/VS, OS, VS1, SVS and MVS; the RCA Spectra series; the UNIVAC 70 and 9000 series; the Honeywell Series 200/2000 under Mod 1 and OS/2000; the Honeywell Levels 62 and 66 under GCOS; the ICL 1900 and 2903 series; NCR Century and Criterion series; CDC 6000 and Cyber series; Burroughs medium-to-large-scale systems running under MCP; the VARIAN (UNIVAC) V70 series under VORTEX II; Harris minicomputers running under VULCAN; INTERDATA minicomputers under OS32; DEC PDP–11 series running under RSX and IAS and IBM System 3. This report is however only concerned with the IBM System 360/370 etc. versions.

TOTAL was developed by a group of people who left IBM after having participated in the development of DBOMP. The intention was to develop software tools to help clients implement management information systems. TOTAL was released in 1968 by the company this group founded – CINCOM Systems Inc.

TOTAL is now supported by several other software packages developed by CINCOM:

- a general-purpose TP monitor, ENVIRON/1
- a sophisticated report writer, SOCRATES
- a data dictionary
- a number of generalised application packages.

TOTAL together with ENVIRON/1 now offers a number of optional features:

- a multi-threading capability
- checkpoint restart
- point-of-failure restart
- a terminal-oriented version of COBOL called COBOL–XT.

The system is written completely in Assembler. The access method was originally BDAM but a new version with VSAM is now available.

CINCOM has recently announced TIS (Total Information System). This will be the successor system to TOTAL, but it is far more a new approach to data management, in which a data dictionary provides the only access path to the database nucleus. At present, the DBMS used in TIS is TOTAL. CINCOM has long-term plans to develop a successor system to TOTAL, but is awaiting the next hardware generation.

4.1 Classification

TOTAL can best be viewed as a limited network-oriented system with inverted lists distributed as address pointers within the records themselves. The database is accessed via a host language CALL statement. All relationships in TOTAL, both inter-record and inter-file, are implemented via physical pointers. This structural data is stored in the record prefix. It is maintained by the system and completely transparent to the user. This means that TOTAL is not oriented towards fast data retrieval.

All TOTAL modules are reentrant and one copy can support either single- or multi-partition working. Should the installation wish, a separate copy of the TOTAL code may be loaded in each partition. In this case, TOTAL will not allow multiple batch partitions to update the same file concurrently. It is possible for one partition to update a file while other partitions are reading it.

Each application program must be link-edited to an interface module (DATBAS). It occupies only 224 bytes and is consequently irrelevant from a space standpoint.

For on-line working, TOTAL offers a multi-programming version which allows multi-access facilities to be provided in conjunction with a teleprocessing monitor. TOTAL normally operates as a subtask of the TP monitor. When used with ENVIRON/1, TOTAL's option logging facility is not normally used, as ENVIRON/1's own logging facility provides both point-of-failure and checkpoint/restart.

TOTAL's system resource requirements are lower than most of the other systems examined only DATACOM/DB has comparable resource requirements. For the complete TOTAL package, excluding ENVIRON/1, maximum DOS/VS main memory requirments are ca. 22–23 KB, while with OS/VS, ca. 35–36 KB are required. Both theses figures exclude the buffering, as this is application dependent. ENVIRON/1 can operate with 30 KB – 60 KB real and 100–150 KB virtual. Further requirements are: direct access device/devices for the database; one tape drive.

The data dictionary requires 64 KB and the report writer, SOCRATES, 35 KB.

4.2 Data Definition

A TOTAL database consists of MASTER and VARIABLE ENTRY data sets. Each data set is subdivided into records and fields. The MASTER data set (SINGLE ENTRY file) can only consist of one single record type. VARIABLE ENTRY records are of fixed length, but may optionally be of variable format

(CODED RECORDS). There is no limit to the number of fields that can be defined in a record.

A MASTER data set record consists of a ROOT, a CONTROL KEY, a data portion and a series of LINKAGE PATH fields; dependent on the relationships. The ROOT field is used for linking synonyms. The VARIABLE ENTRY data set records contain CONTROL–KEY fields, a data portion and a series of LINKAGE PATH fields. The CODED RECORD option acts like a REDEFINES clause in COBOL. Up to a maximum of 32 different CODED RECORDS may be defined for any one VARIABLE ENTRY file.

A two byte field will be reserved to hold the RECORD CODE for each record type. The REDEFINE may contain CONTROL KEY, data and LINKAGE PATH fields. However, all records of a VARIAGLE ENTRY data set must be the same length.

The DBA defines each TOTAL database using the DBDL macro. The information is split into three parts:

- database information
- the MASTER data set definitions
- the VARIABLE ENTRY data set definitions.

4.2.1 Database Description

The database itself is very simple to describe, by naming the database and specifying which buffers can be shared between the files. The only restriction on this is that I/O areas, used by MASTER and VARIABLE ENTRY data sets, cannot be shared by each other.

4.2.2 MASTER Data Set Definition

Each MASTER data set description consists of:

- a unique four-character data set name
- an optional parameter which defines the I/O area
- a record description which describes the characteristics and layout of the MASTER record.

The first two fields of the record description are mandatory. They specify the ROOT field, used by TOTAL for synonym handling, and the CONTROL KEY. These two fields are followed by one or more control statements defining which relationships (LINKAGE PATHS) are to be generated. This is followed by a series of DATA ELEMENT descriptions. The remaining statements are concerned with mapping the records into physical storage.

4.2.3 VARIABLE ENTRY Data Set Definition

The VARIABLE ENTRY data set consists of fixed length records, but within this restriction, it is possible to define different record types, using the CODED RECORD facility.

The first two parameters have a similar meaning to those in the MASTER data set description. These are followed by at least one field description entry. The final statements are concerned with mapping the record type/types into physical storage.

The record description is a series of DATA ELEMENT entries describing the characteristics of the record type. Those fields which form the links with one or more MASTER data sets carry an extra parameter indicating the LINKAGE PATH with which it is to be associated. If a second record type is to be defined, this intention is indicated by the RECORD–CODE parameter followed by a number of DATA ELEMENTS used to form the LINKAGE PATHS and finally a series of user data fields.

4.3 Data Storage Structures

A TOTAL database consists of at least one MASTER data set, although typically, both MASTER and VARIABLE ENTRY data sets are present. VARIABLE ENTRY records can only be accessed via MASTER records.

All MASTER records are placed randomly in the available data space. The address is generated by a CINCOM-supplied randomizing routine, using the CONTROL KEY, which is composed of one field, or several concatenated fields. The precise nature of the randomizing routine has not been revealed by CINCOM, nor is it possible to replace it with a user-written algorithm. As with all radomizing algorithms, different keys 'map' to the same address. TOTAL places these synonyms as close as possible to the 'home' record and constructs a synonym chain using the ROOT field. When a MASTER record is inserted, and its 'home' space is occupied by a synonym from another chain, this synonym is moved. If a MASTER record is deleted, the last synonym of the chain would be moved to the 'home' position.

TOTAL attempts to store all records from a LINKAGE PATH set as physically close together as possible. When a record participates in more than one LINKAGE PATH, this is no longer possible, so TOTAL optimises the storage for the LINKAGE PATH which is used when inserting the record. This leaves the storage optimization as a reponsibility of the programmer and not under the control of the DBA.

When a data set become full, it must be unloaded, the space for it enlarged and then the file must be reloaded. In general, the space made available through a record being deleted is immediately available for reuse.

4.3.1 Inter-file and Inter-record Relationships

It is not possible to express relationships between MASTER records, but MASTER records can be linked to VARIABLE records with the related VARIABLE records linked to each other. All records carry both backward and forward pointers, which are transparent to the user. The MASTER record points to the first and last VARIABLE records with the same CONTROL KEY.

Complex structures can be represented because MASTER records may 'own' more than one VARIABLE record chain, with the latter located in one or more files. VARIABLE records may also participate in more than one relationship. There are five possible relationships between the MASTER and VARIABLE data sets:

- Stand-alone MASTER file. This is the simplest file structure within TOTAL, requiring only a CONTROL KEY and at least one data item. (This corresponds to a random file).
- Single MASTER file, single VARIABLE ENTRY file. This is represented in Fig. 4.3.1a. Each MASTER ENTRY contains one CONTROL–KEY. All records in the VARIABLE ENTRY file which contain the same value in their CONTROL KEY field are linked. The VARIABLE records are linked together with NEXT and PRIOR pointers. The MASTER record points to the FIRST and

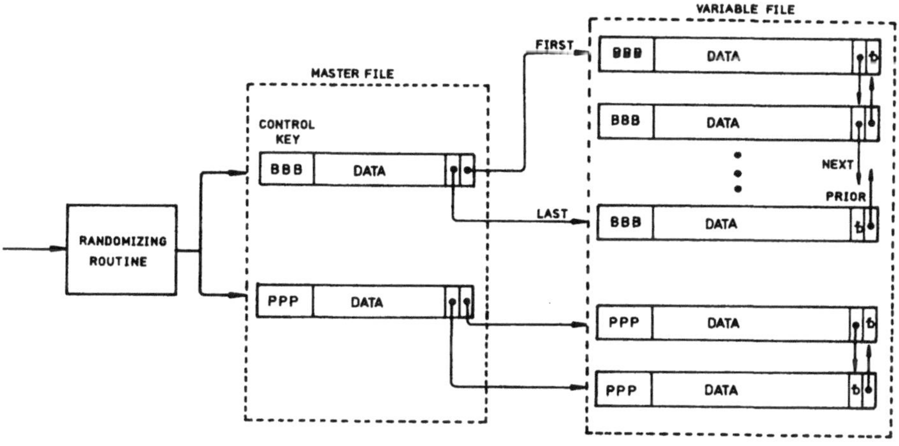

Fig. 4.3.1a: TOTAL Using a Single MASTER File and Single VARIABLE File

the LAST VARIABLE records in the linked sequence with the same CONTROL KEY value.

- Single MASTER file, multiple VARIABLE ENTRY files. This is represented in Fig. 4.3.1b. The records in either VARIABLE file are accessed through the MASTER record to which they are linked. Those VARIABLE records within a VARIABLE ENTRY file which are associated with a particular MASTER record, by the contents of a CONTROL KEY are linked together to form a chain (with both NEXT and PRIOR pointers). The FIRST and LAST records in the chain are linked from the MASTER record. Processing of the VARIABLE record chain can be in either logical direction.
- Multiple MASTER files, single VARIABLE file. This type of relationship is similar to the one described above with the extension that each VARIABLE record can be associated with more than one MASTER record, one for each MASTER file. Pointer space will be reserved for each possible linkage.
- Multiple MASTER files, multiple VARIABLE files. This is the most complicated relationship offered by TOTAL, allowing many-to-many relationships. This relationship combines the previous two relationships. See Fig. 4.3.1c. Even in this case MASTER records may not be directly linked to each other.

4.3.2 Inter-field Relationships

Both MASTER and VARIABLE records are defined in terms of DATA ELEMENTS (group items) which in turn may contain one or more DATA ITEMS (fields). There is no facility for defining repeating groups.

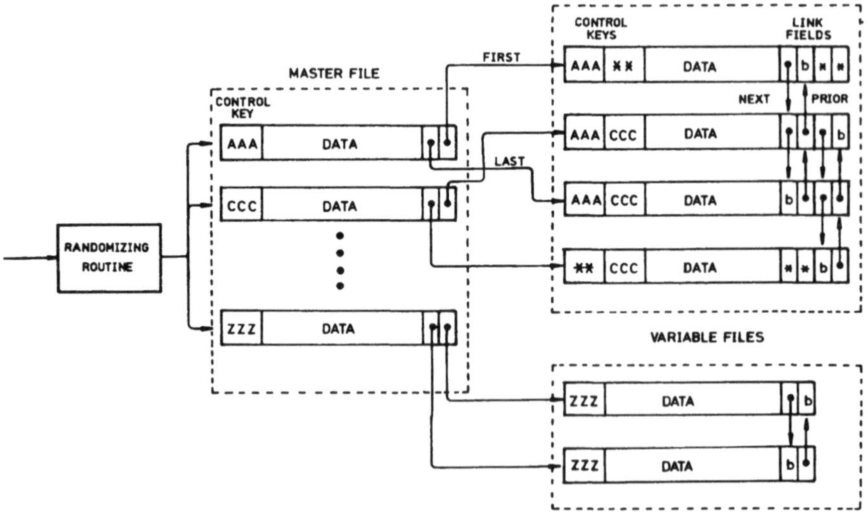

Fig. 4.3.1b: TOTAL Using a Single MASTER File and Multiple VARIABLE Files

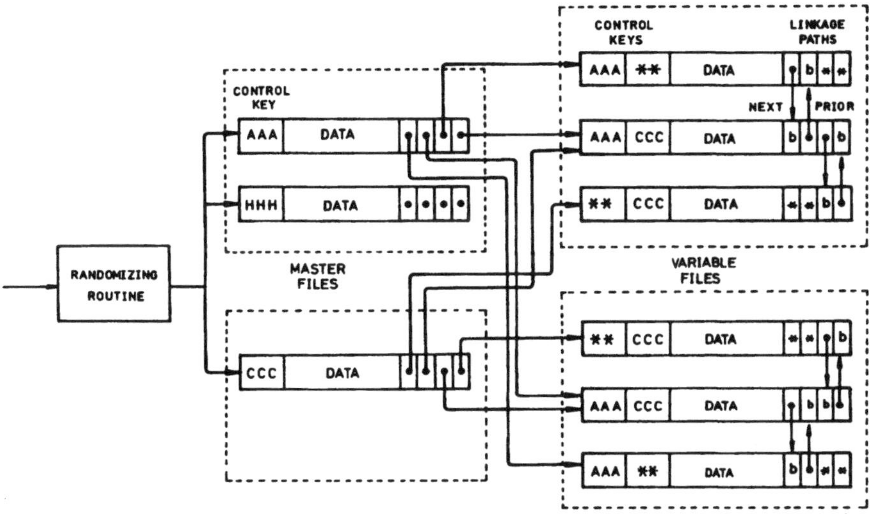

Fig. 4.3.1c: TOTAL Using Multiple MASTER and VARIABLE Files

4.4 Data Manipulation

Each DML command consists of a CALL statement followed by up to nine parameters. It is possible to access data logically, sequentially or randomly.

A COBOL application program request to TOTAL is formulated as follows:

CALL 'DATABAS' USING *function* ,*status* [,*file*] [,*reference*] [,*linkpath*] [,*control-key*] [,*realm*] [,*argument*] [,*qualifier*] [,*access*] [,*data-list*] [,*data-area*] [,*dbmod*] [,*task*] [,*options*] ,*end*.

Figure 4.4 shows the parameters required with each DML command. The parameters have the following meanings:

1. *function* parameter. This points to a user-defined field containing a five character code identifying the DML command to be executed.

2. *status* parameter. After each DML command has been executed, this field will contain a four character code indicating the successful execution, or otherwise, of the command.

3. *file* parameter. With this four-byte parameter, the user identifies the file to be operated on.

4. *reference* parameter. This parameter names a field which will contain the INTERNAL REFERENCE POINT within a VARIABLE ENTRY data set, or the last four characters of a LINKAGE PATH name. This allows the application to

name the starting point in a chain, from which the processing is to begin. When the LINKAGE PATH option is used, processing begins at the beginning of that LINKAGE PATH chain.

5. *link-path* parameter. This parameter allows the user to define the relationship, ie. chain, along which processing is to proceed.

6. *control-key* parameter. This parameter points to a variable length field which contains the key of a MASTER record.

7. *qualifier* parameter. For control functions, this parameter indicates a variable length field containing the control function to be performed. For the RDNXT and FINDX commands, it indicates a field to be used to maintain the current position in the file being processed.

8. *data-list* parameter. This points to a list of DATA ELEMENT names (ROOT and LINKAGE fields excepted). The order of the DATA ELEMENT names need not correspond with the description in the DBD module. They will be retrieved in the order specified in the data-list.

9. *data-area* parameter. This indicates the data I/O area. The data must conform with the description of DATA ELEMENTS as defined in the data-list parameter.

10. *end* parameter. This points to a four character field which must contain 'END', if the retrieval record is to be placed in 'hold' status; otherwise 'RLSE'.

TOTAL offers the user only very simple CURRENCY positioning. A program has only one position per file, namely on the last record retrieved. The direct address of each record (the INTERNAL REFERENCE POINT) is placed in the REFERENCE field when a record is retrieved. This enables the programmer to store the CURRENCY information should it be needed for processing later in the program.

The DML commands can be split into a number of categories: control commands, data manipulation commands, modification commands and DBA commands.

4.4.1 CONTROL Commands

These are not concerned with transferring data between the user and the database, but with controlling the logical and physical connections between application program and the data sets.

1. CLOSX (Close Multiple Files). The file(s) specified are both logically and physically closed. The logical close includes flushing the I/O buffers and resetting the LOCK BYTE. The physical close involves issuing a CLOSE command to the operating system for each file involved. In a multitasking environment, logical and physical close commands are issued for all tasks using the files involved.

Commands	status	file	reference	linkage-path	control-key	realm	argument	qualifier	access	data-list	data-area	dbmod	task	options	end
ADD-M	X	X			X					X	X				X
ADDVA	X	X	X	X	X					X	X				X
ADDVB	X	X	X	X	X					X	X				X
ADDVC	X	X	X	X	X					X	X				X
CLOSX	X					X									X
DEL-M	X	X			X					X	X				X
DELVD	X	X	X	X	X					X	X				X
FINDX	X	X					X	X		X	X				X
OPENX	X					X									X
RDNXT	X	X						X		X	X				X
READD	X	X	X	X	X					X	X				X
READM	X	X			X					X	X				X
READR	X	X	X	X	X					X	X				X
READV	X	X	X	X	X					X	X				X
SINOF	X												X		X
SINON	X								X			X	X	X	X
WRITM	X	X			X					X	X				X
WRITV	X	X	X	X	X					X	X				X

Fig. 4.4: Parameters Associated With Each TOTAL Command

2. OPENX (Open Multiple Files). The file(s) specified are initialized for read only, shared update or exclusive update by executing logical, and, if necessary, physical open commands. One of the open activities is to check and set the LOCK BYTE in the control record. In a multitasking environment, the specified files are made available to all tasks.

3. SINOF (Sign off). This command performs the task termination activities.

4. SINON (Sign on). This command causes the TOTAL nucleus and the DATA-BASE DESCRIPTOR modules to be dynamically loaded; the LOGGING SUP-

PORT module will also be loaded if necessary. The type of logging may also be specified (see Section 4.7).

4.4.2 Data Manipulation Commands

1. FINDX (Find Records). This command retrieves data according to the search criteria specified via the *argument* parameter. The search criteria consist of a list of DATA ELEMENTS to be examined, a list of values against which the data elements are to be compared, and a single operator. It may be any one of the following: GREATER THAN, LESS THAN, EQUAL TO, NOT EQUAL TO, GREATER THAN OR EQUAL TO, LESS THAN OR EQUAL TO. The DATA ELEMENTS specified in the *argument* parameter should not be confused with the ELEMENTS to be retrieved, specified via the *data-list* parameter. The execution of the FINDX command is accomplished via the serial search feature of TOTAL.

2. RDNXT (Read Next). This command makes a number of serial retrieval options available. The options are specified via the *qualifier* parameter, and may be used to retrieve both MASTER and VARIABLE logical records. During serial processing, the field indicated by the *qualifier* parameter is used to hold the INTERNAL SEQUENCE NUMBER of the record just retrieved.

A MASTER file may be processed in physical sequence, either from the beginning of the file, from a particular key value, or from a specific record (identified by its INTERNAL REFERENCE POINT).

The VARIABLE ENTRY file can be read in physical or logical sequence, depending on the value specified via the *qualifier* parameter. The options are:

- processing in physical sequence from the beginning or from an INTERNAL REFERENCE POINT
- processing in a logical sequence along a LINKAGE PATH either from the beginning or from a particular INTERNAL REFERENCE POINT
- processing in a logical sequence along a particular LINKAGE PATH from a specified MASTER file value.

3. READD (Read Direct). This retrieves the logical record specified by the INTERNAL REFERENCE POINT from a VARIABLE ENTRY file. Processing may thereafter continue along any LINKAGE PATH valid for the retrieved record.

4. READM (Read MASTER). This command retrieves those ELEMENTS specified via the *data-list* parameter from that MASTER record whose key value is in the *control-key* field.

5. READR (Read Reverse). This allows the application to process a complete chain in a backward direction, by following the backward pointers. Only VARIABLE records can be read with this command.

6. READV (Read VARIABLE). This command enables the application to process a complete chain in a forward direction, by following the forward pointers. Only VARIABLE records can be read with this command.

7. RQLOC (Request Location). This takes the contents of the *control-key* field and, using the randomizing algorithm, returns the INTERNAL REFERENCE POINT of the MASTER record to the application. The MASTER record itself is not returned. This command can build up a table of the INTERNAL REFERENCE POINTS associated with each of the key values. Then, having sorted the INTERNAL REFERENCE POINTS, the user can retrieve the MASTER records with maximum efficiency.

4.4.3 Data Modification Commands

1. ADD–M (Add MASTER). This command inserts a new MASTER record into the MASTER file. The address, where the record will be stored, is generated by the randomizing algorithm operating on the contents of the *control-key* field.

2. ADDVA (Add VARIABLE After). This causes a VARIABLE record to be placed logically in the VARIABLE ENTRY file, directly after the record whose INTERNAL REFERENCE POINT is in the *reference* field and in the LINKAGE PATH specified via the *linkage-path* parameter. In all other LINKAGE PATHS, the record will be placed at the end of the chains.

3. ADDVB (Add VARIABLE Before). This is similar to the previous command, except that the record is placed before and not after the record identified in the *reference* field.

4. ADDVC (Add VARIABLE Continue). This command logically adds a record at the end of all the LINKAGE PATHS defined for the record by the *control-keys* specified in the *data-area*.

5. ADDVR (Add VARIABLE Replace). This command logically relinks an existing VARIABLE record into different chains, dependent on the contents of the *data-area*. The record retains its physical position, but is logically added at the end of the new chain(s). This is done by retrieving the record indicated by the INTERNAL REFERENCE POINT in the *reference* field, and comparing its *control-keys* with those in the *data-area*. This is the only command which may change CONTROL KEYS.

6. DEL–M (Delete MASTER). This command uses the contents of the *control-key* field together with the randomizing algorithm to identify a particular MASTER record. This record is deleted and the space made immediately available for reuse. Synonyms are not deleted. The MASTER record will not be deleted if VARIABLE ENTRY records are linked to it.

7. DELVD (Delete VARIABLE Direct). This command removes from the file that VARIABLE record which is identified by the INTERNAL REFERENCE POINT contained in the *reference* field. It is also removed from all relationships in which it participated. The space which results is immediately available for reuse. Upon successful completion of this command, TOTAL places the backward pointer from the deleted record in the *reference* field.

8. WRITM (Write MASTER). This command updates an already existing MASTER record. TOTAL retrieves that MASTER record identified by the contents of the *control-key*. The DATA–ELEMENTS in the *data-area* field are moved to the record, which is them returned to the MASTER file. NB. CONTROL KEYS cannot be changed with this command, cf. ADDVR.

9. WRITV (Write VARIABLE). This command updates that VARIABLE record identified by the INTERNAL REFERENCE POINT contained in the *reference* field only for those DATA–ELEMENTS in the *data-area* field. The CONTROL KEY may not be changed.

4.4.4 DBA Commands

These commands are coded and processed in a similar manner to the standard commands, but they are restricted to use by the Database Administrator because their misuse can violate the integrity of the database. They are used mainly to recover the database after a software or hardware system failure.

Although the format of these commands is similar to those already described, there is one extra parameter: ($_{**}$REST$_{**}$END), which may be used by the DBA with all commands. This parameter allows the DBA to retrieve records completely – including ROOT and LINKAGE PATH fields. These fields are necessary for the user-written restore programs, which must be named RESTORxx (where xx are valid alphanumeric characters) in order to bypass TOTAL's record-holding logic.

DBA commands are:

1. CNTRL (Control). This command removed module names from the list of active modules, thus allowing a task to execute in less main memory that would otherwise be required. Indiscriminate use of this command could lead to thrashing. The *qualifier* parameter must point to a field containing the word 'PURGE'. This command is functional only in a batch environment.

2. ENDLG (End Log). This causes the log file to be both physically and logically closed and then reopened. The I/O buffers will be flushed. It need not be the same physical unit which is closed and then opened.

3. ENDTO (End TOTAL). This command shuts down TOTAL, and this is the only method of doing so. The command functions differently in a multi-tasking

environment than for a single user in batch. In the former it is normal to have a separate task whose sole function is to issue this command. Thereafter, the TOTAL nucleus will not accept any further commands, and the commands already accepted are processed to completion. The I/O buffers will be flushed and the files will be closed. Then, and only then, will TOTAL terminate itself. In a batch environment, the DBMOD and TOTAL modules are simply deleted from the partition.

4. FREEX (Free Held Resources). This command frees the named (or all) files held by the task which issued the command. All records held by these files are also released. If this is not done, then all those records read for update and not yet updated are held until a total of 1000 requests for them have been executed from other tasks. This command functions only in a multi-tasking environment.

5. MARKL (Mark Log). This command allows the user to write user-oriented information to the log file, together with the task name and time. This command functions only in a multi-tasking environment and is used for checkpointing.

6. QMARK (Quiet-Mark Log). This combines the functions of the QUIET and the MARKL commands, necessitating the writing of only one record onto the log file.

7. QUIET (Quiescing the Database). This causes the TOTAL nucleus to stop accepting new commands. All accepted commands are processed to completion, then all I/O buffers are flushed. This synchronises the physical and logical databases by writing a checkpoint, and provides a point from which a restart can be made. This command applies only to a multi-tasking environment.

8. RSTAT (Read Statistics). This command provides the DBA with information about the internal activities and functioning of TOTAL. The information available is as follows:

- the time each task signed on and signed off
- a count of all the physical and logical I/O activities, which is used to judge the appropriateness of the current buffer sizes
- counts of the total number of records held, the maximum held at one time and the number of deadlock situations
- statistics accumulated on the number of log records and on the number of times that the writing of log records hindered some record writing activity
- statistics accumulated on the number of each type of command executed, and their concurrency.

9. WRITD (Write Direct). This command is only used in the writing of database recovery programs. It writes complete TOTAL records, ie. data plus the normally transparent record prefix to the database. These records are the BEFORE (or AFTER) Images recorded on the log file for this purpose. The recovery programs

must be named RESTORxx (where xx are any two valid alphanumeric characters) in order to bypass TOTAL's record-holding logic.

4.5 Data Independence

The way in which data is physically stored and structured is the responsibility of the DBA, and the programmer is involved only with his local view of the database as specified in the *data-list* parameter. This contains a list of the fields necessary to construct the required logical record. The field order need not be the same as that in the physical record.

The statment of data requirements (*data-list* parameter) is part of the CALL command and bound to the program at compile time. This means that the program receives data in the format and length as described in the DATABASE DESCRIPTOR MODULE (DBDM), which is a severe limitation of the DATA INDEPENDENCE as each change is field characteristics requires that all programs using this field have to be changed and recompiled. Processing is dependent upon LINKAGE PATHS, so that any removal of relationship will require compilation. Additional relationships may however be developed without changing existing programs.

4.6 Concurrent Usage

In a multi-tasking (multi-programming) environment, it is possible to have all tasks in one region, or to have multiple tasks operating in multiple regions. In either case, all database requests are serviced by a single copy of TOTAL.

In a batch environment, programs operate either in update or read mode. In a multi-tasking environment, all programs operate in an update mode. This means that each record retrieved is automatically locked from all other users. If the user does not want to update the record, this intention can be signalled to TOTAL with a parameter in the CALL command, so that the record remains available to other tasks (see *end* parameter).

As soon as a task opens a particular file, this file is reserved for the exclusive use of all tasks being serviced by the particular copy of TOTAL that opened the file. It is possible to use TOTAL on-line by interfacing it with a TP monitor. CINCOM markets a TP monitor, ENVIRON/1, which interfaces with TOTAL. Typically, both systems will run in the same partition with TOTAL executing as a subtask to ENVIRON/1.

4.7 Integrity Controls and Recovery

Structural data, held in each MASTER and VARIABLE ENTRY record in the LINKAGE fields, is never made available to the programmer, thus eliminating this possible source of corruption.

TOTAL does not carry out any format checks on the contents of the data fields but does carry out the following checks:

- the CONTROL KEY must not contain any blank characters
- the MASTER record CONTROL KEYS must be unique
- a MASTER record which is to be deleted may not be removed if VARIABLE records are dependent on it.

In general, the integrity checks carried out by TOTAL are those necessary to keep the DBMS functioning. This has the disadvantage that the programmer becomes responsible for the contents of the records and the DBA has no automatic control or check on this.

Three modes of operation are available to the programmer:

- update mode
- read only mode
- recovery mode.

The mode of operation desired is communicated to the DBMS in the SINON command. This command is also used to specify the type of logging required. The options available are:

- no logging
- logging of BEFORE Images
- logging of AFTER Images
- logging of both BEFORE and AFTER Images
- logging at the completion of specified TOTAL commands.

The log file may be either tape or disc, but no duplicate logging option is available.

Three commands are associated with the log file. The QMARK (QUIET MARK) command is issued by an application program and causes TOTAL to synchronise the file and log contents by stopping acceptance of further DML commands, processing those accepted to completion and then emptying the buffers of all blocks containing charges Additionally, the user may write information to the log file. These synchronisation points are used to identify points in processing which are used in ROLLBACK recovery. The MARKL (MARK LOGGING) command simply writes user information to the log file. The QUIET command simply flushes the buffers.

TOTAL does not offer a utility to dump TOTAL files. The standard OS/DOS utilities must be used to provide the necessary back-up database copies.

No warm restart facilities are available with TOTAL, nor is there any command available to backout a single program, but cold restart is available via a program called RECOVER. For VSAM users, the IDCAMS utility must be run prior to RECOVER.

The RECOVER program offers ROLLFORWARD or ROLLBACK recovery. A separate execution of RECOVER is necessary for each log file to be processed. This program should only be executed in batch mode. The options available are:

- ROLLFORWARD including all AFTER Images
- ROLLFORWARD to the last synchronisation point resulting from a QUIET or QMARK command
- ROLLBACK including all BEFORE Images
- ROLLBACK to the last synchronisation point from the end of the log file applying BEFORE Images.

Somewhat greater flexibility is offered in a TP environment. Using the facilities offered by TOTAL only the latest synchronisation point can be used for recovery purposes and ROLLBACK involves all tasks, not just that one which has ended in error.

4.8 Privacy Controls

TOTAL does not provide any access control features.

4.9 Performance

The DBA is not always able to tune a TOTAL database for optimal performance, simply because the options are not available or not under his control. An example of this is the lack of any facility for ordering a VARIABLE record chain on a field within the VARIABLE record: the only options available place a record either at the beginning or end of the chain or before or after the current position.

This means that placement of VARIABLE records and checks on possible duplication are dependent on the program logic not on the DBA's tuning of TOTAL.

A further example is the logical placement of VARIABLE records involved in multiple LINKAGE PATHS. Here again, the programmer and not the DBA is responsible for placement. The programmer must explicitly insert the new occurrence of a VARIABLE record into one relationship and TOTAL will automatically include it in all other necessary relationships, placing it logically at the end of the relevant chains. The DBA can only influence the placement indirectly by specifying the LINKAGE PATH to be explicitly used and checking that the programmer follows these instructions. This has a further disadvantage from the Data Independence point of view, namely that any new relationship added requiring a change in logical placement strategy will need program changes to be made.

Accessing a MASTER record will typically require one I/O operation, as the address of the home block can be generated directly from the randomizing routine. Nevertheless, synonyms will require more I/O operations, the number depending on the size of the MASTER records in relation to the block size, the number of synonyms and how densely the file is filled.

TOTAL optimises the storage of MASTER records by ensuring that records belonging in a particular location will displace synonyms overflowed from another location and by returning overflowed synonyms to the home block as soon as space is available. The last synonym in the chain is placed in the home block, which means that the synonyms are not chained in CONTROL KEY sequence. Thus searching a synonym chain for a record that is not present means processing the chain to the end each time – a time-consuming process, particularly if the chain extends over a number of blocks.

The VARIABLE records are normally retrieved via a MASTER record, although they can be retrieved directly when the INTERNAL REFERENCE POINT is known. Consequently VARIABLE records will normally require more accesses than MASTER records to be retrieved. The number of accesses is dependent upon the length of the chain the degree of fragmentation and also the block size. The fragmentation of VARIABLE record chains can be removed (for one of the multiple LINKAGE paths) using the LOADER/UNLOADER utility.

The design of the database structure involving many interlinked MASTER and VARIABLE datasets will need a high degree of skill to match the processing requirements to the structure. Similarly, the applications programmer must have an intimate knowledge of the structure and of TOTAL to develop efficiently executing programs. Because additions to a VARIABLE file can only be placed in one chain at any chosed position (in all other chains they will be placed at the end), it is very important to consider which chain will be used. This can have considerable impact on the system performance. The fact that in-depth knowledge of data frequency and the database structure is a prerequisite for developing efficient programs, means that a change in data frequency could result in dramatically slower processing.

4.10 Conclusion

This very small system has achieved unbelievable success, which is partly due to the rapid implementation possible as a result of TOTAL's simplicity, in as far as the choice of options is very limited. CINCOM recognises that a DBMS 'features count' will result in TOTAL coming last, but they believe that they offer what the majority of users need from a DBMS. The area in which TOTAL is most successful is the middle-to-small computer section where this argument might be relevant.

The *lack* of such features as:

- optional record compression
- variable length record handling
- full automatic warm restart
- encyphering routines
- complex query handling
- secondary keys supported by inverted files
- transaction oriented processing

certainly detract greatly form the system's attraction for the larger computer user.

Although TOTAL does not offer all the recorvery facilities that might be expected, CINCOM maintain that it is reasonably certain that at least one of the very large circle users will already have developed any required routine or interface if it is at all possible. However, the disadvantage with the approach of 'borrowing' software is that the borrowed software will be neither guaranteed nor supported by CINCOM.

No other system has been implement on such a wide range of computer hardware, and this has played no small part in TOTAL's success, making it the most 'portable' of all DBMSs. CODASYL-oriented systems do not run on as many different computer ranges as TOTAL, although the gap is narrowing. This could be the deciding factor for a large organisation with very mixed hardware.

If, however, the aim is to buy a DBMS which is capable of flexibly and efficiently supporting a wide range of application types, then a DBMS will almost certainly be needed containing features not available with TOTAL.

4.11 Advantages of TOTAL

- Simple to understand.
- Small memory requirements.
- Portable over a wide range of computer types.

- Data independence down to the field level.
- Interfaces (see Appendix III).
- Quite efficient for random single key processing on-line
- Large user base (even larger than IBM's)
- Limited networks may be generated
  - two MASTER records types may not be linked
  - two VARIABLE records types may not be linked directly.
- Intergrated DB/DC via ENVIRON/1.
- Report writer (SOCRATES).
- Data dictionary (CINCOM DD).
- On-line query language (T–ASK).
- LOGICAL and PHYSICAL sequential processing available.
- It is impossible to delete a MASTER record if it has VARIABLE records dependent on it.
- Multithreading nucleus.
- Checkpoints may be written from the program.
- Space from deleted records is available immediately for reuse.
- Log file may be disc or tape.

4.12 Disadvantages of TOTAL

- There is no Secondary Indexing based on inverted file techniques. Complex query resolution requires that the VARIABLE record chain be processed sequentially; an extremely time and resource consuming process.
- Limited flexibility in the phrasing of a complex query.
- No transaction oriented processing.
- No variable length record option.
  Even when multiple record types are used in one file they must all have the length of the longest record type.
- No data compression facilities.
- TOTAL is not oriented towards fast data retrieval, due to inflexible processing paths.
- VARIABLE ENTRY file organisation degrades with activity.
- Volatile environments are not handled at all well.
- No security at the DATA ITEM level.
- No password lock.
- No warm restart facilities.
- Weak program/data independence – changes in the database frequently affect existing programs.
- The order of the VARIABLE records in a chain is not controlled by TOTAL, except for placement at end of chain. Thus the programmer not the DBA can become responsible for record placement.

- VARIABLE records' physical placement is dependent on the LINKAGE PATH specified when inserting the record. Thus the programmer is responsible for the efficient placement of VARIABLE records not the DBA.
- It is impossible to place two records from the same file in 'HOLD' status simultaneously.
- DEADLY EMBRACE is resolved by allowing a user to retrieve a a 'held' record after requesting it a specified number of times, typically 1000 times.
- No dual logging facilities.
- Changes to the LINKAGE PATHS can affect existing programs, but new LINKAGE PATHS can be added without affecting them.
- Field formats are not checked on loading or updating.
- Use of the CINCOM supplied randomizing routine is mandatory.
- No facilities for copying a file for backup purposes.
- Primitive CURRENCY – only one position per RUN UNIT.
- No high-level self-contained DML.
- No command is available to delete a MASTER record and all its dependent VARIABLE records. They must be deleted singly. This is extremely inefficient.
- The ROLLBACK facilities are only capable of returning a whole database to a Checkpoint not a particular task. Only the last Checkpoint may be specified.
- The handing of synonyms in the MASTER file is weak. The synonym chain is not ordered on the CONTROL KEY values thus the whole chain must be followed in order to identify a duplicate key or determine that a key is not present. Further, the last synonym in the chain replaces any previous synonym that is deleted – this means that the whole synonym chain has to be retrieved.
- All VARIABLE records are automatically placed in all relationships (cf. AUTOMATIC and MANUAL rules for IDMS).

4.13 TOTAL Glossary

CONTROL KEY: This field identifies each record in a SINGLE ENTRY FILE.

DATABASE DESCRIPTOR MODULE: A machine-readable module containing a description of the database. It is generated by the Database Generation Program.

DATABASE DEFINITION LANGUAGE: This language is used to define the database. It forms the input to the Database Generation Program.

DATA ELEMENT: An identifiable DATA ITEM or group of DATA ITEMS. The DATA ITEMS of a DATA ELEMENT cannot be accessed individually.

DATA FIELD: see DATA ELEMENT.

DATA FILE: An organised, accessible group of data records processed as a logical unit.

DATA ITEM: The smallest unit of data having independent existence.

DML: (DATA MANAGEMENT LANGUAGE). A set of commands used to access and manipulate the contents of a database. These commands are embedded within a CALL statement of the host programming language.

INTERLOCK: See DEADLOCK in the General DB Glossary.

INTERNAL REFERENCE POINT: A record's relative address within the file.

KEY: A DATA ITEM which uniquely identifies the MASTER RECORD (see CONTROL KEY).

LINK: A logical interconnector between files.

LINKAGE PATH: A bidirectional chain which must be followed to access one or more specific records in a VARIABLE record chain.

LINKPATH SET: The MASTER record and its associated VARIABLE record chain.

MASTER FILE: A file consisting of MASTER records. A MASTER FILE can exist independently, or be linked to one or more VARIABLE files. It cannot be linked directly to other MASTER FILES.

MASTER RECORD: A record of a non-volatile nature.

RECORD CODE: A two-byte field used in VARIABLE records to identify the record's format.

SINGLE ENTRY FILE: see MASTER FILE.

VARIABLE ENTRY FILE: see VARIABLE FILE.

VARIABLE FILE: A file consisting of VARIABLE RECORDS. All VARIABLE RECORDS must be of the same physical length, but multiple records may exist for a particular key. Such records are chained together with a MASTER RECORD (containing the same key) as the entry to this chain. VARIABLE RECORDS may have multiple formats, with each record having multiple keys.

VARIABLE RECORD: A record in a VARIABLE FILE.

VARIABLE RECORD CHAIN: A number of VARIABLE RECORDS containing the same key value.

5. SYSTEM 2000

SYSTEM 2000 (S2000) is conceptually the most interesting of the six DBMSs examined because although it is based on inverted list structures, it offers the capability of processing hierarchically-structured databases. The origins of S2000 can be traced to a package called TDMS (Timeshared Data Management System). The CODASYL Systems Committee examined TDMS and the results were published in May 1971 in the 'Feature Analysis of Generalised Database Management Systems'. The vendors of S2000, MRI Systems Corp., acquired a copy of TDMS in 1967. The experience gained with this package enabled MRI to develop a completely new DBMS. The aim was to provide a generalised solution to the problem of database management for both batch and on-line environments. The first version was released early in 1970 for use on CDC 6000 series equipment. In 1971, the CDC version was completely rewritten and a UNIVAC 1100 version was released. By May 1972, an IBM System 360 version was available. This was a single-user system with only a COBOL host-language interface. In August 1972, Version 2.22 was released, containing a multi-user feature capable of handling 64 databases and 16 users. During 1973, versions 2.30 and 2.40 were released, both primarily concerned with "feature enhancement". The primary objective of Version 2.45, which was released in February 1975, was performance enhancement.

In August 1975, Version 2.60 was released. This was a major enhancement in terms of both performance and features, offering for example:

- a multi-thread monitor
- a fully rewritten Report Writer
- extensions to the host-language interface for FORTRAN and PL/1
- host-language networking capability for FORTRAN only.

The next version (2.70), released in April 1976, was designed to take advantage of the IBM virtual operating systems, with improvements centring around a new buffer manager. Other improvements included:

- extension of host-language interfaces (including the LINK command for COBOL and PL/1)
- query facilities for non-indexed fields.

Recovery features were consolidated in Version 2.80 released in December 1976.

The most recent version (2.90) was released in April 1979 and included:

- HLI record-level lockout
- an increase in the number of concurrent users

– VM/CMS compatibility at the source level
– HLI Multi-user concurrent MODIFY/REMOVE for non-key data.

Some 65% of S2000 coding is in FORTRAN, with the rest in Assembler. MRI is planning to rewrite S2000 in CPL/1 to increase its portability amongst hardware ranges. Although S2000 runs on CDC, UNIVAC and IBM hardware, this report is primarily concerned with the IBM version and any examples of the host-language interface will be in COBOL.

5.1 Classification

SYSTEM 2000 structures data logically in strict hierarchies but the linkage information is not stored with the user data. The records in this hierarchy are called REPEATING GROUPS, and consist of a fixed number of fields, any of which may be declared as a key. Access via inverted lists is provided for all key fields. The data manipulation facilities of S2000 are available both in a self-contained language called 'NATURAL LANGUAGE' or embedded in a host-language. Preprocessors, called HOST LANGUAGE INTERFACES are availabe for COBOL, FORTRAN, PL/1, and Assembler. NATURAL LANGUAGE provides two separate data manipulation options, either QUEUED ACCESS or IMMEDIATE ACCESS. The former is supplied as standard with the basic S2000 package, the latter is charged extra, but is far more flexible than the former. Both subsets of the S2000 Self Contained Language can be used interactively. S2000 requires ca. twenty-five 3330 cylinders including not only the S2000 executable load libraries and relocatable object code, but also validation and test libraries. User space requirements are dependent on application. No tape unit is required when operating under the Multi-User version, unless creating an archival copy of the database or when dumping the disc Update Log to tape for back-up purposes. Each database has its own independent disc log file, thus enabling each database to be backed-up without affecting other processing.

The minimum recommended core requirements are ca. 180KB for a Single-User version with a three level overlay structure. This would include the buffer space. In a VS environment 50KB–70KB would have to be 'real'. With a Multi-User environment, at least 275KB would be necessary, but the 'real' amount would, of course, be dependent on such factors as:

– the overlay structure
– number and size of the buffers
– number of threads (with the Multi-Thread feature).

Typically, a VS partition of 500KB would be necessary, of which ca. 100KB would have to be 'real'. VS paging is more efficient than overlay loading, so that within a VS environment, S2000 should be generated with fewer overlays than standard.

S2000 databases may reside on any mass-storage device supporting BDAM. The DBA is responsible for choosing the page size that will optimize storage on the particular device used; the type of processing (random/sequential) and the available buffer space.

The minimum mainframes are IBM S360/40 or S370/135 with the following operating systems: OS/MFT, OS/MVT, OS/VS1, OS/SVS, OS/MVS, VM/CMS, DOS/E and DOS/VS. The only incompatibility on upward migration within the IBM range occurs with a change from DOS to OS and then, only the S2000 code need be change – the databases themselves are compatible. When used in conjunction with a TP monitor, S2000 can run as a subtask to the TP monitor. Alternatively, it may run in a separate partition servicing both batch and TP programs.

5.1.1 The S2000 Overlay Structure

S2000 has a three-tier overlay structure (see Fig. 5.1.1) with the root module involved with management of the lower level modules, buffers and I/O. The second tier of the overlay structure contains three modules: the DEFINE module, the CONTROL module and the ACCESS module. Only the ACCESS module has dependent modules which are involved in executing the DML commands from the Host Language Interface (HLI) and the Self-Contained Language.

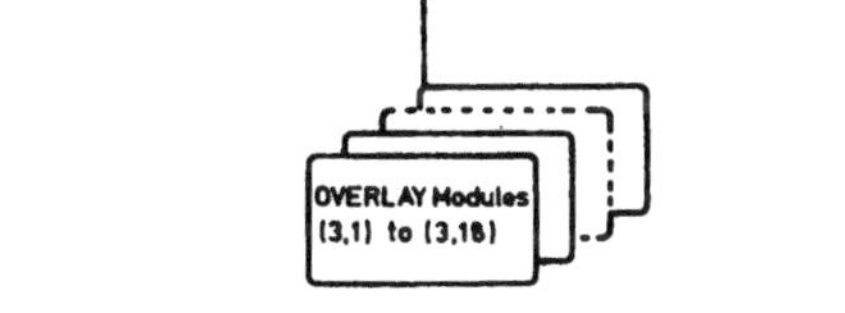

Fig. 5.1.1: S2000 Overlay Structure

5.2 Data Definition

A database is defined by a series of database definition statements called COMPONENTS. These COMPONENTS are processed mainly by the DEFINE module and to a lesser extent the CONTROL module. The first command is the assigning of a password. This is called the MASTER PASSWORD for the database as is normally only known to the DBA. This is followed by the allocation of a unique name to the database.

These two parameters are followed by a series of COMPONENTS describing the structure of the user data to be stored within the database. Each entry has the following format:

Component Number	System Separator	Component Name	(Component Description)

The Component Number must be in the range 1–4095, but no more than 1000 COMPONENTS are allowed per database. The System Separator is, as its name suggests, a separator between Component Number and Name, its default value being an asterisk. The Component Name can be up to 250 characters in length. The Component Description defines the type of entry and is of four types:

- REPEATING GROUP description
- USER DEFINED functions
- STRINGS
- field (ELEMENT) description

5.2.1 Repeating Group (SCHEMA RECORD is the new terminology)

This is a specification that indicates that the associated ELEMENT or group of ELEMENTS may occur a variable number of times under each PARENT REPEATING GROUP (see Fig. 5.2a). Up to 32 levels of nesting are permitted.

5.2.2 User Defined Functions

These only apply when the IMMEDIATE ACCESS mode is being used. It allows arithmetic expressions to be included in a COMPONENT specification.

5.2.3 String

This allows the user to develop NATURAL LANGUAGE routines which may be invoked later via QUEUE and IMMEDIATE ACCESS modes.

```
1*  ORGANISATION          (KEY NAME X(23)):
2*  COGNIZANT OFFICIAL    (NON–KEY NAME X(20)):
3*  ADDRESS               (NON–KEY NAME X(20)):
4*  CITY                  (NON–KEY NAME X(13)):
5*  STATE                 (NON–KEY NAME X(10)):
6*  ZIP CODE              (NON–KEY INTEGER NUMBER 9(5)):
7*  CURRENT DATE          (NON–KEY DATE):
8*  PORTFOLIOS            (RG):

     9*  PORTFOLIO NAME     (KEY NAME X(10) IN 8):
    10*  PORTFOLIO CODE     (NON–KEY NAME XX IN 8):
    11*  MANAGER            (NON–KEY NAME X(14) IN 8):
    12*  STOCKS             (RG IN 8):

        13*  NAME OF STOCK           (KEY NAME X(20) IN 12):
        14*  TICKER SYMBOL           (KEY NAME X(5) IN 12):
        15*  EXCHANGE                (KEY NAME X(4) IN 12):
        16*  INDUSTRY NAME           (KEY NAME X(19) IN 12):
        17*  INDUSTRY CODE           (NON–KEY INTEGER 9(4) IN 12):
        18*  SHARES OUTSTANDING      (NON–KEY INTEGER 9(9) IN 12):
        19*  LATEST EARNINGS         (NON–KEY MONEY 99.99 IN 12):
        20*  LATEST EARNINGS DATE (NON–KEY DATE IN 12):
        21*  ESTIMATED EARNINGS      (KEY MONEY 99.99 IN 12):
        22*  ESTIMATED EARNINGS DATE (NON–KEY DATE IN 12):
        23*  DIVIDEND                (KEY DECIMAL 99.9(3) IN 12):
        24*  CURRENT PRICE           (KEY DECIMAL 9(3).9(4) IN 12):
        25*  TRANSACTIONS            (RG IN 12):

             26* BLOCK NUMBER        (KEY INTEGER 9(8) IN 25):
             27* TRANSACTION TYPE (KEY NAME X(4) IN 25):
             28* DATE                (KEY DATE IN 25):
             29* SHARES              (NON–KEY INTEGER 9(5) IN 25):
             30* PRICE               (NON–KEYDECIMAL 9(3).9(4) IN 25):

    31*  BONDS                       (RG IN 8):
        32*  NAME OF ISSUER     (KEYNAME X(20) IN 31):
        33*  ASKED PRICE        (KEY  DECIMAL 9(5).9(4) IN 31):
        34*  PURCHASE PRICE     (NON–KEY DECIMAL 9(5).9(4) IN 31):
        35*  MATURITY DATE      (KEY DATE IN 31):
        36*  PURCHASE DATE      (NON–KEY DATE IN 31):
        37*  FACE AMOUNT        (NON–KEY MONEY 9(5).99 IN 31):
```

Fig. 5.2a: A Database Definition Example

5.2.4 Element

This entry describes a data field – the smallest logical unit within an S2000 database. Each field is automatically a key field unless the contrary is explicitly stated. Six different types of Data Description are supported:

1. Character. This consists of alphanumeric data with all leading, trailing and embedded consecutive blanks suppressed. Fields can be variable in length irrespective of the specified size. Up to 250 bytes will be accepted.

2. Text. This consists of alphanumeric data without blank character suppression. It also accepts fields of up to 250 bytes, irrespective of specified size. It supports one byte binary fields.

3. Date. Input and output can be in the format specified by the user. Internally, it is a four byte packed decimal field with an offset from October 15, 1582.

4. Decimal can be up to fifteen numeric digits with a maximum of ten to the left or right of a decimal point, and is stored in packed decimal format.

5. Money is the same as Decimal with a floating currency sign and 'CR' for negative qualities. It is accepted on input and printed on output under the Self-Contained Language.

6. Integer can be any numeric quantity up to a maximum of 15 significant digits and is stored in packed decimal format.

5.2.5 Key and Padding Parameters

These two parameters are needed to complete the data field specification.

1. KEY. Each data field is automatically assumed to be a KEY field even when the parameter KEY is not specified. This results in an index being maintained for this field. If this is not required, the parameter NON–KEY should be specified. NON–KEY data fields may be used in qualification criteria, but it is obviously inefficient.

2. The PADDING factor can be expressed as one of the following:

$$\text{WITH} \begin{bmatrix} \text{NO} \\ \text{FEW} \\ \text{SOME} \\ \text{MANY} \end{bmatrix} \text{FUTURE OCCURRENCES}$$

It is used to reserve contiguous space for later entries in the MULTIPLE OCCURRENCE TABLE whenever a new index page is created. Judicious use of the PADDING factor can reduce I/O requirements to process qualification criteria in update or retrieval commands. Only KEY fields may have PADDING. The default value is NO PADDING.

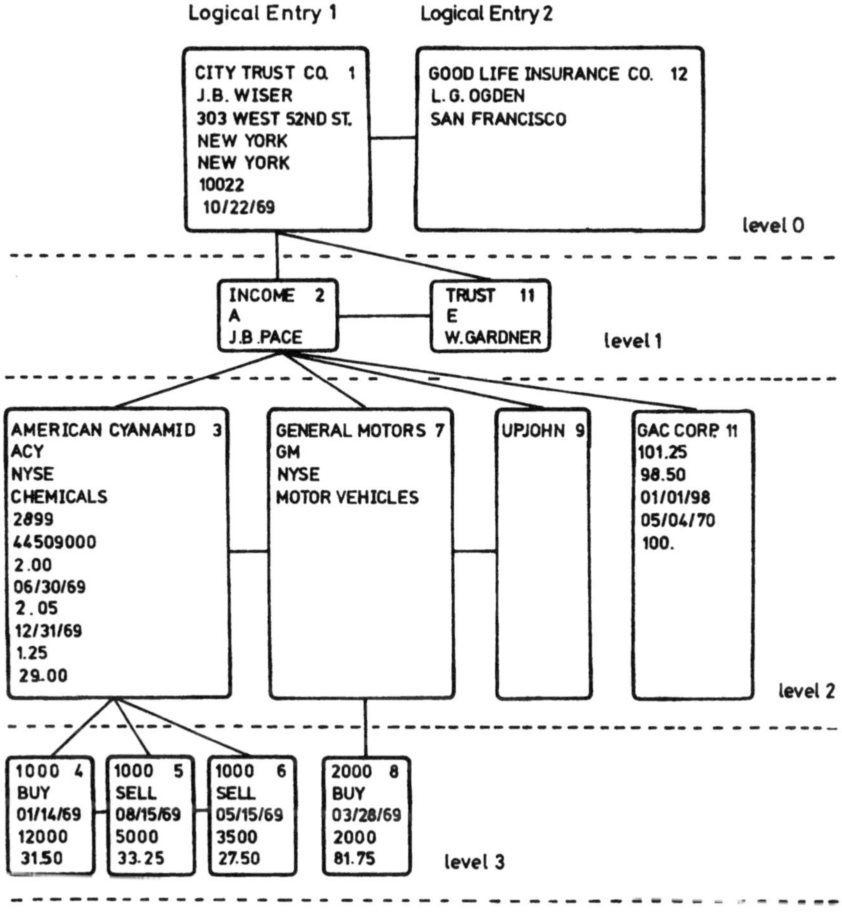

Fig. 5.2b: A Data Structure Example

5.3 Data Structures

S2000 designers have produced a very interesting solution which is a DBMS based on inverted file techniques operating on data which is structured hierarchically. Nevertheless, all pointer data is held in a separate file from the user data.

5.3.1 Physical Data Structures

Each S2000 database is a stand-alone entity consisting of six physical BDAM data sets (see Fig. 5.3.1a). It contains only relative pointers indicating the record or character number displacement from the start of the file (Table).

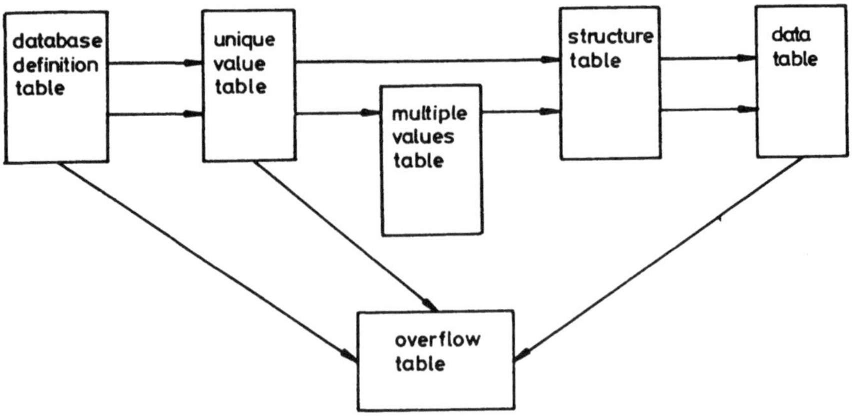

Fig. 5.3.1a: Database Tables

The DATA TABLE contains variable length records. Each record holds one REPEATING GROUP. All numeric data, (Integer, Decimal and Money) is stored as packed decimal. All data is stored in fixed length fields. These field lengths need not be the maximum possible field length for Text or character fields. Instead, the fields should be defined to accommodate 70–90% of the maximum data length. The remaining 10–30% of the field occurrences will contain data too large to fit into the field. This extra portion will be stored in the OVERFLOW TABLE. A four byte pointer in the original field occurrence will indicate the position of the extra portion in the OVERFLOW TABLE. The total length of the two portions of the field may not exceed 250 bytes.

The DB DEFINITION TABLE contains structural information and ELEMENT descriptions. The UNIQUE VALUE TABLE contains one entry for each unique value of a KEY ELEMENT in ascending order, with a pointer to the MULTIPLE VALUE TABLE or to the HIERARCHICAL LOCATION TABLE. The former is necessary if the KEY ELEMENT does not contain unique values. The UNIQUE VALUE TABLE contains a hierarchical index structure, thus enabling any given key to be accessed efficiently.

The MULTIPLE VALUES TABLE (also called the MULTIPLE OCCURRENCE TABLE) functions in a similar manner to the UNIQUE VALUE TABLE, but instead of having a single entry for each key value, there is a block of pointers for the synonyms. The size of these blocks is determined by S2000 at load time. The DBA can influence this with the PADDING parameter, (see section 5.2.4). When a block is full, an additional one is made available and chained to the original.

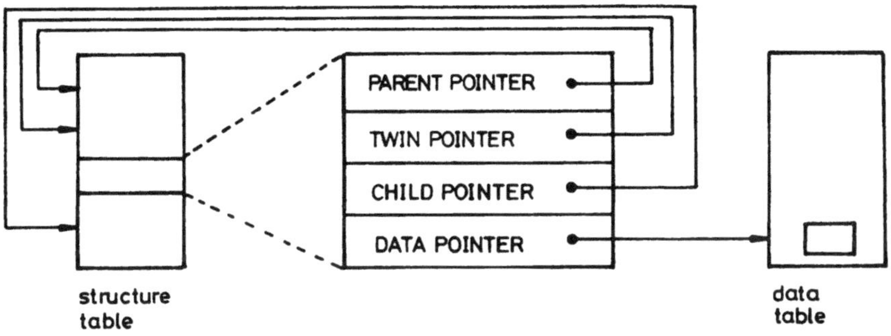

Fig. 5.3.1b: Structure Table Entry Format

The HIERARCHICAL TABLE (or STRUCTURE TABLE) contains four pointers associated with each REPEATING GROUP, (see Fig. 5.3.1b). Three pointers refer to other groups of pointers in the HIERARCHICAL LOCATION TABLE. These are the Parent, Child and Twin (or Sibling) pointers. The fourth pointer refers to a REPEATING GROUP occurrence in the DATA TABLE.

Each of these six data sets may be allocated to a different device and/or channel so as to optimize processing. Each data set may be allocated with primary and secondary extents on different devices. Different block sizes may be specified for each data set.

5.3.2 Logical Data Structures

A S2000 database can be considered to consist of a file containing one variable length record type (LOGICAL ENTRY), which consists of a number of REPEATING GROUPS related to each other hierarchically. Nevertheless, the LOGICAL ENTRY is not a particularly useful concept. It is better to consider a database simply as a collection of REPEATING GROUPS organised hierarchically, each consisting of ELEMENTS (see Fig. 5.3.2).

Although S2000 structures are pure hierarchies, the LINK command of the Host Language Interface (see section 5.4) allows inter-database relationships to be generated temporarily. This enables the HLI-user to generate limited network structures.

REPEATING GROUP occurrences are inter-related via Parent, Child and Twin (Sibling) pointers. This hierarchical structure may not contain more than 32 levels. It is possible to declare any ELEMENT at any level a KEY field. This can be used as an entry point into the hierarchy, making it unnecessary to access via the root.

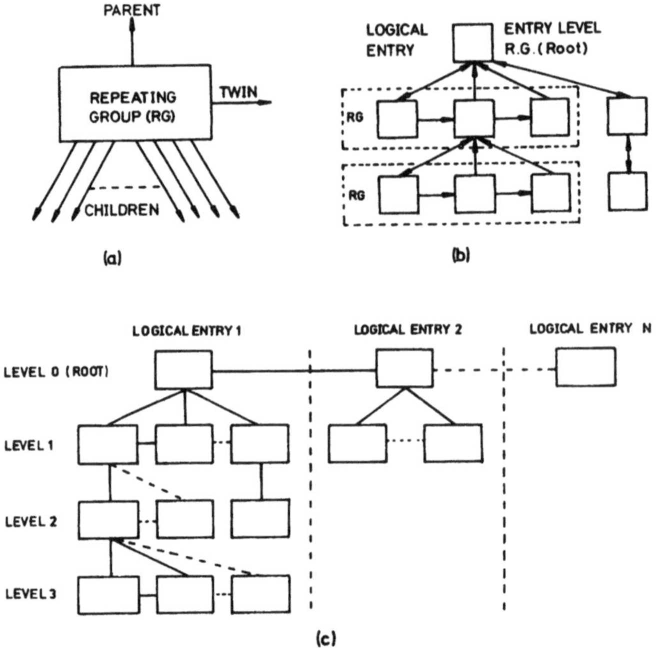

Fig. 5.3.2: S2000 Logical Data Structure and ist Terminology

5.3.3 Space Management

S2000 provides for the automatic re-use of space within the Database Tables via 'reusable space chains' held separately for each record type. Each space released through a deletion is 'added' to the front of this chain. Then for each insertion, S2000 scans through the chain looking for the first space that is at least large enough to accommodate the record.

These free space chains are maintained for the DATA TABLE (per REPEATING GROUP) for the parallel HIERARCHICAL LOCATION TABLE, for the MULTIPLE VALUE TABLE and also for the OVERFLOW TABLE.

The pointers in the HIERARCHICAL TABLE contain the character displacement of the record from the start of the DATA TABLE. This means that any movement of a REPEATING GROUP will result in the HIERARCHICAL TABLE pointer, which is associated with the REPEATING GROUP, having to be updated to reflect the new position.

When using LOAD mode, for either initial or incremented Load, a simplified method is used. The REPEATING GROUPS are placed in the free space after the last REPEATING GROUP occurrence in the DATA TABLE (instead of trying to reuse space available throughout the database). The entries for the other TABLES are written to scratch files and then sorted before being entered into the relevant tables.

5.4 Data Manipulation

There are two completely separate languages for manipulating S2000 databases: NATURAL LANGUAGE and the HOST LANGUAGE INTERFACE (HLI). The former is a stand-alone language, while the latter is embedded in a host language. There are preprocessors available for COBOL, PL/1, Assembler and FORTRAN. Any language supporting a CALL statement can use the HLI directly. Within NATURAL LANGUAGE, two distinct processing options are available, namely QUEUE ACCESS and IMMEDIATE ACCESS. The former is essentially for batch processing and the latter for on-line work, although IMMEDIATE ACCESS can be used in batch mode and can include QUEUED ACCESS commands.

The main difference between NATURAL LANGUAGE and HLI is in their respective approaches to data manipulation. HLI embodies the normal approach, whereby the system 'remembers' the results of the last command. These results are then available to future commands. This is particularly important with positioning information. NATURAL LANGUAGE, on the other hand, operates on a syntactic unit with the system 'remembering' nothing from any previous syntactic unit.

There are advantages and disadvantages to both approaches. The HLI user is better able to navigate through the database hierarchy. This results in a finer control over processing logic, but also requires more experience and more detailed knowledge of the database structure. The NATURAL LANGUAGE user does not need to be an experienced programmer; normally it will be used only by an end-user to answer ad hoc enquiries. Nevertheless, where processing efficiency is not of primary importance, NATURAL LANGUAGE can be used to good effect.

Both HLI and NATURAL LANGUAGE contain update, insert and delete commands.

5.4.1 Host Language Interface (HLI)

The HLI user has to define a communications area (COMMBLOCK) in the WORKING–STORAGE SECTION of his COBOL program for each database to be accessed. Special SCHEMA statements specify which REPEATING GROUPS are to be accessed by the program. The data manipulation commands are embedded in the program logic in the PROCEDURE DIVISION.

QUEUED ACCESS	IMMEDIATE ACCESS	HOST LANGUAGE	WHERE CLAUSE
SAVE DATA BASE RESTORE DATA BASE KEEP APPLY SUSPEND RELOAD REORGANISE PRINT (element,group or tree) REMOVE (") ADD (element or group) APPEND (") ASSIGN (") CHANGE (") IF-THEN-ELSE WHERE WHERE Operators EXISTS EQ NE GT GE LT LE [RG] HAS [condition]	1 Update ADD ASSIGN ASSIGN TREE CHANGE INSERT TREE REMOVE REMOVE TREE 2 Retrieval DESCRIBE LIST ORDER BY PRINT TALLY UNLOAD WHERE LOAD QUEUE STOP IF USER DATABASE IS	1 Control APPLY KEEP RELEASE LOAD RESTORE SAVE SUSPEND 2 Update INSERT MODIFY REMOVE REMOVE TREE 3 Retrieval GET GETA GETD GET1 LOCATE ORDER BY WHERE LINK 4 QUEUE TERMINATE	IMMEDIATE ACCESS 1 [element] [EXISTS / FAILS] 2 [element] [EQ / NE / LT / LE / GT / GE] [value] 3 [element] [EQ / SPANS / NE] [value] [system seperator] [value] 4 [repeating group] HAS [condition]

Fig. 5.4: The Commands Available in NATURAL LANGUAGE (IMMEDIATE and QUEUED ACCESS options) and HOST LANGUAGE INTERFACE

CURRENCY information is maintained by the system in a STACK which is created when the Database OPEN command is issued. Multiple STACKS will be maintained by the system if a subscript is attached to the relevant HLI commands. The contents of a STACK identify those REPEATING GROUPS at each level which were last accessed. There is always a PRIMARY POSITION in the STACK, and it may be at any level. The other positions are called SECONDARY POSITIONS. A PRIMARY POSITION can only be established by GET and GET1 commands. The establishment of a new PRIMARY POSITION deletes all other entries in the STACK.

The COMMBLOCK consists of 16 COBOL statements, and a separate COMMBLOCK is necessary for each database accessed.

COMMBLOCK OF DATA BASE name
01 DATA BASE name
    05 SCHEMA name
    05 return code
    05 filler
    05 last REPEATING GROUP occurrence
    05 password
    05 number of REPEATING GROUP
    05 REPEATING GROUP position

05 level
05 time
05 date
05 cycle
05 separator symbol
05 end terminator
05 status

The SCHEMA statements defines which ELEMENTS are to be retrieved for a particular REPEATING GROUP type. One SCHEMA must exist for each REPEATING GROUP type to be accessed. The format is as follows:

SCHEMA schema name OF data base name
01 schema name
05 component identifier PICTURE IS picture notation
.
.
.
.
.

The statement 'END SCHEMAS' informs the preprocessor that all SCHEMA definitions have been specified.

The PROCEDURE DIVISION commands can be grouped into three classes: control commands, retrieval commands and modification commands. Generic or global selection criteria are available for both retrieval and update commands, and are also available with both the Self-Contained Languages. The selection criteria may contain any combination of:

- the normal binary operators
- the ternary operators (SPANS, NE) to provide both inclusive and exclusive range checks
- the unary operators (EXISTS, FAILS) to verify the existence or otherwise of data occurrences
- the Boolean operators (AND, OR, NOT) for logically connecting the individual search criteria.

They may also be nested, using brackets, to control the order of the processing of the selection criteria. It is also possible, by the use of the LIMIT command, to control the number of DATA SETS to be selected.

5.4.1.1 Control Commands

1. Precompiler Control. There are only two precompiler control commands:

- START S2K(n)
- END PRODECURE

The subscript (n) can have a value in the range 0–15, and specifies the numer of scratch (LOCATE) files that are to be OPENED during the execution of the program.

2. OPEN. It is not necessary to issue a special command to OPEN a database – although it is good programming practice to do so, since the first DML command for a particular database will, providing the password is correct, automatically cause an internal OPEN command to be issued. A STATUS FLAG is returned in the COMMBLOCK, indicating whether or not the database may be used. A maximum of 16 databases may be OPEN simultaneously, although up to 64 may be declared in a program.

OPEN database identifier

3. CLOSE. This command is necessary only under one of the two following conditions, although, once again, it is good programming practice to issue this command.

- in place of the CLEAR command when the contents of a database have been modified
- more than 16 databases are to be processed by the one program.

Should a program not issue a CLOSE command in either of the above conditions, then the database will be flagged as damaged.

CLOSE database identifier

4. QUEUE ACCESS. This command signals to the pre-processor that QUEUE ACCESS commands follow. The reason for this is that a batch of updates can be performed more efficiently under QUEUE ACCESS. Retrieval may be from any number of databases, but only one may be updated. The QUEUE ACCESS commands are delimited by the two commands QUEUE and TERMINATE.

The philosophy behind QUEUE ACCESS is that all retrieval commands are executed immediately they are issued, but the updates are 'queued' awaiting a TERMINATE command. If a CANCEL QUEUE command is issued, all the 'queued' update commands are deleted and processing is allowed to continue normally.

5. CLEAR. As a general rule, buffers are not returned to the database until the space is required for other blocks (PAGES), or the job ends normally. The user has two commands at his disposal to influence I/O buffer management:

- CLEAR causes all buffers, containing modified REPEATING GROUPS, to be returned to their databases

- CLEAR AUTOMATICALLY results in PAGES being returned to their database immediately after the update command has been executed. This command can only be cancelled by issuing a CLEAR command.

6. APPLY. This command is used to reconstruct a database using an archival copy (see SAVE Command) and the updates recorded in internal form in a KEEPFILE (see KEEP Command). The reconstruction of the database can be effected to any cycle of recorded updates.

APPLY database identifier [ALL | THRU cycle-no.]

7. KEEP. This command causes processed updates to be noted on the KEEPFILE. For a single user environment, (Direct Mode), the program issues a KEEP command before issuing the first modification command, then the results of each modification command are recorded directly onto the KEEPFILE.

In a multi-user environment, modifications are held on an Update Log file (disc or tape) until a KEEP command is issued, when the Update Log records for the program issuing the KEEP command will be transferred to the KEEPFILE.

KEEP database identifier

8. RELEASE. This command deletes a database on secondary storage. The STACKS and LOCATE FILES are cancelled. Prior to issuing this command, the program should have gained exclusive control over the database and have placed the Master Password in the COMMBLOCK.

RELEASE database identifier

9. RESTORE. This command copies an archival copy of a database, the SAVEFILE, onto direct secondary storage. The KEEPFILE only needs to be mentioned if it was not activated by a previous SAVE, or if a change is required in the identifier or the Update Log mode.

RESTORE database FROM identifier [/KEEPFILE [/INDIRECT | /DIRECT]]

10. SUSPEND. This command causes the recording of database modifications on the Update Log to be suspended. This command can be issued during the execution of a program.

SUSPEND database identifier

11. ENABLE/DISABLE ROLLBACK. These commands specify that rollback processing is to be performed (or not) for a specific database if it is damaged. Rollback is the process of returning a database to an intact situation after it becomes damaged. A Rollback Log is used to achieve this. Only one Rollback file may be allocated per database – and may only be used by one program at a time. This means that two programs updating a database in parallel cannot use ROLLBACK simultaneously.

The ENABLE ROLLBACK command does not cause Rollback recovery to occur, but merely causes the Rollback Log to be written, (cf. FRAME and END-

FRAME commands). This request remains in force until a DISABLE command for the same database is issued. These commands are only available to the Master Password holders.

[ENABLE / DISABLE] ROLLBACK FOR database identifier

12. FRAME/END FRAME. These commands indicate the limits of a logical transaction. A maximum of 16 databases may be included in the synchronised checkpoint. These commands may only be used for databases with the Rollback option enabled.

Before any database modification command is executed, the Before Image of the PAGE containing the object record (or space for it) is copied to the Rollback Log. In the case of a Rollback, the contents of the KEEPFILE and, as necessary, the Update Log are adjusted to reflect the new situation.

An END FRAME or FRAME command causes the following to occur:

- termination of the current Frame
- flushing of the I/O buffers
- ending of all Global Holds secured through the previous FRAME command

FRAME [/IMMEDIATE/ / /CONDITIONAL/] database list

With the IMMEDIATE option, a FRAME command requests that the Global Holds obtained in the previous Frame be maintained in the next Frame. With the CONDITIONAL option, a FRAME command specifies that a non-zero return code should be issued if any of the requested databases are not available.

13. SAVE. This command copies a database onto secondary storage (either disc or tape). It can also activate or suspend the Update Log for the database.

SAVE database ON identifier [/KEEPFILE [/INDIRECT / /DIRECT]]

5.4.1.2 Retrieval Commands

1. LOCATE. This command enables the user to ascertain whether or not a REPEATING GROUP(S) satisfying specified criteria exists. No STACK information is changed as a result of this command. This command results in the addresses of qualified REPEATING GROUPS being stored in a LOCATE file. The number of REPEATING GROUPS located is passed to the user in the communications area.

LOCATE(n) schema name WHERE condition-1 [AND / OR / AND NOT / OR NOT] condition-2 . . .

The subscript 'n' if specified allows multiple LOCATE files to be used.

A CONDITION has the form:

ELEMENT relational operator field name

where the relational operator may be:

- equal (EQ)
- not equal (NE)
- less than (LT)
- greater than (GT)
- greater than or equal (GE)
- less than or equal (LE)
- the ELEMENT occurs (EXISTS)
- the ELEMENT does not occur (FAILS)
- Text search (CONTAINS)

The user must place the relevant value in the KEY ELEMENT field of the SCHEMA.

2. ORDERED BY. This is a further extension of LOCATE command, which enables the user to sort the REPEATING GROUPS found by a LOCATE command. Its format is:

ORDER BY [LOW / HIGH] item-1 [LOW / HIGH] item-2 . . .

If the ORDERED BY option is not used then the REPEATING GROUPS will be retrieved in the physical order that they occur in the HIERARCHICAL LOCATION TABLE.

3. GET. This command retrieves a REPEATING GROUP occurrence via the address held in the LOCATE file. The format is as follows:

GET schema name [FIRST / NEXT / LAST / S2KCOUNT / PRESENT / PREVIOUS]

The meaning of FIRST, NEXT, PREVIOUS and LAST options are self-evident. They all establish a new PRIMARY POSITION in the STACK. The PRESENT option reestablishes an old PRIMARY POSITION after a GET1 has established a new one. The S2KCOUNT option causes S2000 to reference a field in storage containing a numeric value which specifies a displacement from the current position for the next retrieval operation.

4. GET1. This command has two formats:

$$\text{GET1 schema name} \begin{bmatrix} \text{FIRST} \\ \text{LAST} \\ \text{NEXT} \\ \text{S2KCOUNT} \end{bmatrix}$$

$$\text{GET1} \quad \text{schema-name WHERE condition-1} \begin{bmatrix} \text{OR} \\ \text{AND NOT} \\ \text{OR NOT} \\ \text{AND} \end{bmatrix} \text{condition-2} \ldots$$

Both formats establish a PRIMARY POSITION. The first format allows the user to specify displacements from a previously established PRIMARY POSITION. GET1 is useful for direct navigation through a database. The 'FIRST' parameter is an exception to this; it is completely independent of positioning. The second format locates a REPEATING GROUP occurrence according to the criteria specified in the 'WHERE' clause. If more than one occurrence is found, only the first will be retrieved.

5. GETA. This command allows the user to retrieve the direct ancestor (parent) of the REPEATING GROUP occurrence on which the user is currently positioned. The format is:

GETA schema name

6. GETD. This command allows the user to retrieve any descendant of a REPEATING GROUP occurrence.

The format is:

$$\text{GETD schema name} \begin{bmatrix} \text{FIRST} \\ \text{LAST} \\ \text{NEXT} \\ \text{S2KCOUNT} \end{bmatrix}$$

Both the GETA and GETD commands establish SECONDARY POSITIONS in the STACK.

7. LINK. This most powerful feature allows the user to establish temporary logical relationships between REPEATING GROUPS in the same or different databases (and to cancel them). The retrieval of one REPEATING GROUP occurrence can trigger off multiple retrievals. S2000 automatically creates, modifies and deactivates these temporary relationships.

A series of LINK commands can be issued by the user, but they will not be executed until the first GET type command is issued. The format of the command is as follows:

LINK m (n) (source control) source schema TO (target control) target schema VIA association list.

The LINK subscript 'm' can assume the values 0–9 which uniquely identifies the LINK command and a maximum of 10 LINK commands may be active at any one time.

When operating with multiple LOCATE files, the subscript 'n' specifies that a separate STACK should be maintained for each LOCATE file.

The Source Control parameter may also contain either a plus or minus sign. The plus sign specifies that the LINK command may initiate a cascade of retrievals, but not continue the process. A minus sign has the opposite effect. The omission of this parameter allows both the initiation and concatenation of a cascade.

The Target Control parameter contains either a plus or minus sign. The plus sign specifies that the cascade of retrievals is to continue even when none of the criteria for retrieval are satisfied, provided that the Target Segment appears as a Source Segment (with Source Control parameter of minus) in another LINK command. The minus sign specifies that a cascade of retrievals cannot continue via this LINK command. The omission of this parameter will allow cascading of retrievals to continue only when the retrieval criteria are satisfied ie. if the return code is zero. An Association List can be composed of up to 2 logically-linked Associations, as follows:

association-1 AND association-2 . . .

with each Association composed of: – variable/item

variable: – a variable in the WORKING-STORAGE SECTION (of a COBOL program). It may be in a subschema REPEATING GROUP.

item: – the alias of a database schema ELEMENT declared in a subschema REPEATING GROUP. This ELEMENT must belong to the same database as the schema REPEATING GROUP corresponding to the Target subschema REPEATING GROUP.

The '/' character in the Association is equivalent to an 'EQUALS' operator.

The use of the LINK command will often result in a large number of REPEATING GROUP occurrences being identified which satisfy the selection criteria. The addresses of these REPEATING GROUP occurrences are stored in LOCATE files, which can then be retrieved with GET type commands. A LINK command may be disabled by either issuing another LINK command with the same subscript, or by issuing a dummy LINK command consisting of only the LINK command with the relevant subscript and no other parameters.

5.4.1.3 Modification Commands

1. INSERT. This command allows the user to add a new occurrence of a REPEATING GROUP to a database. Prior to this command being issued, the necessary position has to be established in the hierarchical structure by a GET type command, or even by a previous INSERT. The format is:

INSERT schema name [AFTER / BEFORE]

2. MODIFY. This command allows the user to change the contents of one or more ELEMENTS of a REPEATING GROUP. The format is:

MODIFY schema name component list

The 'component list' parameter is optional

If the 'component list' parameter is not used, the command applies to all ELEMENTS of the REPEATING GROUP. There is no restriction on the number or type of ELEMENTS that may be modified. Prior to issuing the MODIFY command, the REPEATING GROUP must have been retrieved with a GET type command.

3. REMOVE. This command allows the user to remove one or more ELEMENTS from a REPEATING GROUP occurrence which must have been retrieved by a GET type command before the REMOVE command is issued. The format is:

REMOVE schema name component list

The restrictions on the optional 'component list' parameter are the same as for the MODIFY command. Even after all ELEMENTS have been removed from a REPEATING GROUP, it retains its position in the hierarchy, ie. new ELEMENT occurrences are added to the REPEATING GROUP occurrence with MODIFY commands not INSERT commands.

4. REMOVE TREE. This command removes the REPEATING GROUP occurrence (and all its dependent REPEATING GROUP occurrences) from the database. No password protection is provided for the dependent REPEATING GROUP occurrences. The REPEATING GROUP must first have been retrieved by one of the GET commands. The format is:

REMOVE TREE schema name

5.4.2 Self-Contained-Language

NATURAL LANGUAGE provides a complete set of commands, not only for retrieving and updating REPEATING GROUPS, but also for definition, modification, security, backup and recovery, and performance monitoring. Additionally composition and generation of reports is accomplished through NATURAL LANGUAGE commands within the Report Writer.

There are two separate languages within NATURAL LANGUAGE: QUEUE ACCESS, which is part of basic S2000; and IMMEDIATE ACCESS, which is an optional extra. Both can be used in batch and on-line environments, but the former is oriented towards batch operations and the latter towards on-line.

5.4.2.1 QUEUE ACCESS

QUEUE ACCESS commands are processed in blocks. The QUEUE command identifies the start of a block and the TERMINATE command identifies the end of the block. Processing of the block of commands will not start until the TERMINATE command has been issued. The commands will not simply be processed in the order they were issued but in the following sequence:

- all WHERE clauses are processed in parallel
- PRINT TREE commands are executed
- REMOVE TREE commands are executed in the order that they occur
- all other commands are executed in the order that they were issued.

QUEUE ACCESS commands may also be issued from within a HLI program.

The QUEUE ACCESS processing commands are:

1. PRINT/PRINT TREE. ELEMENTS can be retrieved selectively from REPEATING GROUP occurrences with these commands.

2. REMOVE/REMOVE TREE. With these commands, ELEMENTS can be removed from REPEATING GROUP occurrences or REPEATING GROUP occurrences can be removed from databases.

3. APPEND TREE. This causes a DATA TREE to be added to a database.

4. ADD. This command introduces a value to an ELEMENT occurrence when the occurrence held none before.

5. ASSIGN. This command alters defined ELEMENT values unconditionally.

6. CHANGE. This command alters the ELEMENT occurrence value, provided that the ELEMENT occurrence held a value previously.

5.4.2.2 IMMEDIATE ACCESS

This provides full, nested, Boolean logic, and processes each retrieval or update command before processing any subsequent command. It allows heuristic browsing, arithmetic function processing, and immediate data modification. IMMEDIATE ACCESS is thus oriented toward interactive operation, but it can be used in batch mode just as effectively.

Complex selection criteria are available to the IMMEDIATE ACCESS user, and these operate on both Key and Non-key ELEMENTS.

There are six System Functions which make arithmetic statistics about the data values available to the user:

- AGV calculates the average value of an ELEMENT
- COUNT counts the number of occurrences of an ELEMENT
- MAX/MIN calculates the maximum/minimum value of an ELEMENT
- SIGMA calculates the standard deviation
- SUM adds up the numeric values

The IMMEDIATE ACCESS processing commands are:

1. TALLY. This command provides information about specified KEY ELEMENTS.

2. PRINT. This lists the values of a REPEATING GROUP one value per line with double spacing between groups.

3. LIST. This lists the values of named ELEMENTS. Page and column headings may be included.

4. UNLOAD. This command offers the possibility of unloading part of a database in Value String format suitable for loading into another database.

5. ASSIGN TREE. This command allows the user to replace DATA TREES.

6. INSERT TREE. This allows the user to insert DATA TREES.

7. ADD, ASSIGN, CHANGE, REMOVE and REMOVE TREE all have the same meaning as in QUEUE ACCESS processing.

5.5 Data Independence

Programs need only retrieve those fields required by the program logic. Data is retrieved by a HLI program via a SCHEMA, which is an area in the WORKING–STORAGE SECTION (for COBOL) which contains the names of those fields which the program requires. Each SCHEMA represents one REPEATING GROUP. The fields specified in the SCHEMA do not have to be in the same order, nor do they have to have the same length and format as in the original definition. Moreover, not all fields need be present in the SCHEMA. This means that a HLI program is not affected by changes to a database which are not directly referenced by the program. Even if the characteristics of referenced fields are changed, then they will only necessitate changes to the program if the new characteristics are incompatible with those of the SCHEMA. Adding a new REPEATING GROUP type at the end of the present hierarchy or adding a completely new hierarchy type to a database definition does not require any internal storage reorganisation. However, the introduction of a new REPEATING GROUP type into the hierarchical structure or the adding/deleting of a field will require a structural reorganisation. This is carried out automatically by S2000.

Changing non-key fields to key fields (and vice-versa) is done using CREATE (DELETE) INDEX. Multiple Secondary Indexes may be created in a single pass of the database. The INDEX command is a normal S2000 command – not a utility – and does not require exclusive use of the database.

5.6 Concurrent Usage

S2000 has two possible approaches to a multi-user environment – the Multi-User feature and the Multi-Thread feature. The former is supplied as a part of the basic system, and provides for concurrent access to the same or different databases (up to a maximum of 63 different databases), co-ordinated by a single copy of S200 code. Jobs can be both TP and batch, using either the Self-Contained Language or the Host Language Interface.

The main features of the Multi-User capability are:

1. Updating of a particular database may occur from different concurrently operating run-units with data protection guaranteed. However, each command is processed to completion before the next command is processed (cf. 5.7 Integrity Controls and Recovery).

2. On request, the system provides status information on user programs and database activity.

3. The occurrence of an ABEND in a program will be recognised by S2000 and the run-unit will be terminated in an orderly manner.

4. Deadlock is prevented by resource enqueuing logic.

The Multi-Thead (MT) capability is, in essence, a high performance extension of the Multi-User feature. It should be used in a high volume, complex transaction environment. Up to a maximum of 9 users (threads) can be serviced simultaneously. Servicing of the 9 threads is carried out on a non-priority basis, dependent on sharable resource contentions.

There are a number of limitations to concurrent usage. With QUEUE ACCESS, a Global Hold on a database is set when a REPEATING GROUP is retrieved for update. A Global Hold allows all other users to access the database, but not to modify it. QUEUE ACCESS cannot modify more than one database at any one time, thus a QUEUE ACCESS user cannot 'lock out' all other users from the databases.

A Hold issued by an IMMEDIATE ACCESS user normally results in a Local Hold. This is a Hold only on the object REPEATING GROUP, all other REPEATING GROUPS being available for update by the remaining users. Although a user can issue a Hold command for all available databases, only one Hold per database is allowed. If, however, an IMMEDIATE ACCESS user issues a FRAME command, the Local Holds are converted to Global Holds. This is necessary because each database has only one ROLLBACK file associated with it, which can only be used by one program at any one time. In this way, no other program may update a database already under the control of a FRAME command.

By definition, a program is in IMMEDIATE ACCESS mode if it has not issued the QUEUE command.

5.7 Integrity Controls and Recovery

Concurrent update protection is provided in both Multi-User and Multi-Thread environments via a Hold option on any retrieval command. The REPEATING GROUP set in Hold status is still available for non-update retrieval. There are two types of Hold available: Global and Local. The former is a temporary Hold on the whole database, preventing an update retrieval by any other user. The Local Hold is a temporary Hold on a specific REPEATING GROUP. Neither Ancestors nor Descendants of the REPEATING GROUP are affected by the Hold.

The Local Hold is activated by an IMMEDIATE ACCESS user preventing other users from obtaining a Global or Local Hold on the specific database or REPEATING GROUP. In general, the Global Hold is activated by a QUEUE ACCESS user and prevents all other users from obtaining either a Global or Local Hold in the database. A program may never have more than one Global Hold at any point in time.

A Local Hold is released as soon as the REPEATING GROUP with the Hold is modified or a Hold is issued by the same program for another REPEATING GROUP, in the same database. The Global Hold can be retained for a whole-series of updates and is only ended by:

– a retrieval command without the Hold option, or
– a retrieval command with the Hold option for another database, or
– the TERMINATE command

The IMMEDIATE ACCESS user can only set a number of REPEATING GROUP occurrences from one database in Hold Status simultaneously by issuing a FRAME command which changes the Local Hold to a Global Hold.

If a non-key update operation is in progress in Immediate Mode, for a particular database when a Local Hold is requested for the same database, the request is honoured. However, if a key update is being performed, the Local Hold is postponed until the Global Hold is ended. A requested Global Hold is postponed until after any current update operation is completed or any current Local and Global Hold is ended. Fig. 5.7 shows the contention resolution table for Hold Logic. The DROP HOLD command releases all REPEATING GROUPS in HOLD status held by the issuing program.

S2000 offers a fairly flexible approach to back-up and recovery. As has already been explained in detail – see Section 5.6 – the user can group a series of updates to form a logical unit, a FRAME. The updates involved need not be limited to a single database, and a FRAME may consist of a single update. As soon as an update within a FRAME fails to execute correctly due to a hardware or software failure, all the updates within the FRAME will be backed out. There is no facility for the user to cause a transaction (FRAME) to be backed out if a logic error occurs, nor can the user include a message in the checkpoint. If a database does not have the ROLLBACK FILE enabled, an archival copy of the database together with the relevant Log files are needed to reconstruct the database. This can be a time-consuming activity.

The System 2000 commands used to dump and recreate a database are SAVE and RESTORE respectively. Providing the user knows the master password, these commands can be used in both Self-Contained Language and HLI. To recover a database from a catastrophic disc error, the following actions must be undertaken:

– delete/define the database files
– restore the database from the archival copy
– roll forward using the log tape to the last successful transaction.

These operations can be initiated via the Self-Contained Language or HLI. All other databases can be processed normally during this process.

		ACTIVE			
		R	LH	GH	U
REQUEST	R	Y	Y	Y	N
	LH	Y	Y*	N	N
	GH	Y	N	N	N
	U	N	Y	N	N

R- Retrieval, LH - Local Hold, GH - Global Hold, U - Update (except for concurrent MODIFY/REMOVE for non-key elements)
Y- Allow request to be processed
Y*- Allow request unless to same RG
N - Suspend request until current status is dropped

Fig. 5.7: Resolution Table for the HOLD Logic

5.8 Privacy and Security Controls

Security within System 2000 is based on a non-hierarchical system of passwords with the master password held by the DBA. Access authority may be allocated down to the individual field level. Any combination of fields may be allocated a secondary password, thereby granting retrieval update and/or qualification authority.

A further security feature offered by S2000 is the 'Security by Entry' facility. This provides security based on a data value, so that in order to access a particular logical entry, the user must supply a valid unique key for the entry. The secondary password security still applies when using 'Security by Entry'. To prevent unauthorized access to the passwords, they are encrypted and scattered within one of the six database tables. All access attempts with an invalid password are recorded on the system log. A second attempted access with an invalid password from an HLI program results in an ABEND with System Error Code 24.

5.9 Performance

The structure and interrelation of the six BDAM-organised files of a S2000 database are completely transparent to both user and the DBA. There are no specification parameters at the DBA's disposal to influence the physical organisation. Nevertheless, the DBA is responsible for allocating the size of each S2000 file, and this will have a direct bearing on performance.

There is only one limit on the number of REPEATING GROUP (RG) types and the number of fields in an RG, namely, that a database may not be composed of more than 1000 Components. Choosing more Components than necessary will have only a trivial impact on the size of the Database Definition Table, but a much larger negative impact on efficiency.

The size of each S2000 file has to be calculated by the DBA – either manually from a set of formulae, or semiautomatically using a program ESTIMAT. The DBA must allocate sufficient extra space to allow for anticipated data growth and the inevitable fragmentation. If, however, the allocated space should prove too small, it is a simple task to enlarge the database. The database can be copied using the SAVE command. The data space must be deleted and reallocated (enlarged), after which the database is copied back using the RESTORE command. The SAVE command must be issued periodically to provide a database archival copy for backup purposes. A brief space occupancy report is printed after either the SAVE or RESTORE commands have been executed. A further command is available to give more detailed occupancy information at any time.

The area in which the DBA can most directly influence performance is in the allocation of key fields. There is one 14 byte entry in the Directory for each page of the Unique Value Table (UVT). This means that unique keys (eg. personnel number) would require large amounts of space in the Directory and the UVT, but none in the Multiple Values Table (MVT). On the other hand, if the marital status field (containing 4 possible values: married, divorced, widower, single) were to be declared a key field, only one Directory page and one UVT page would be needed, but with each of the four pointers in the UVT pointing to the start of a long list in the MVT. Furthermore, it is unlikely that the database would be accessed solely on this key. It is much more likely that marital status would be used in conjunction with other key fields eg. locate all single programmers between the ages of 20 and 30 years with S2000 experience. This would result in all the 'single' pointers having to be merged with the other sets of pointers – although only a few people would be identified as satisfying all criteria. A much more sensible approach would be to define marital status as a non-key field using the WHERE option for this criterium. This approach would reduce both file size and seek time.

Since each RG type can have a different length, and all RG types are stored in a common data space, the Data Table (DT) must be composed of variable length records. At load time, all RGs belonging to one logical entry are grouped together physically. The space management algorithm endeavours to maintain this order, but fragmentation must be anticipated. It is recommended that the Structure and Data Tables of a database should be on separate units, as should the UV and MV Tables.

Owing to the interrelated nature of the S2000 files, reorganising one of the files in the database means that all files containing pointers into the reorganised file must also be modified.

The Database Definition Table should seldom require reorganisation, and occurs only when insufficient data space is available to accommodate new Component information.

The Unique Value Table will be modified whenever an RG occurrence is modified or inserted with a new key value. A high rate of new key values could exhaust the Padding (free) space, and when this happens, the UVT must be reorganised.

The Multiple Value Table contains variable length records composed of groups of pointers. The order of the groups of pointers is immaterial and this does not affect performance; but fragmentation will, and this is what determines the need for reorganisation.

As the Structure Table contains only fixed length records, it should never be necessary to reorganise it.

The Data Table, being composed of variable length records, and being the most volatile of all the S2000 files, is very prone to fragmentation. In order to minimise the need for reorganisation of this file and the consequent reorganisation of the preceding S2000 files, S2000 employs special techniques to reuse space in the Structure and Data Tables made available as the result of RG occurrence deletions. Following a deletion in the Data Table, the associated Structure Table is marked as deleted and incorporated in a chain of free entries for the particular RG type. The pointer within the entry to the Data Table space is maintained. An insertion of the same RG type then uses this Structure Table entry together with the associated Data Table space, thus efficiently re-using deleted space. Nevertheless, performance will in time degrade and a RELOAD will be necessary.

Using S2000 databases imposes no special skill, although the HLI requires somewhat greater skill than the Self-Contained Language. This is due to the greater flexibility of the former. The greatest difficulty is, most probably, understanding the power of the WHERE command.

The overlay structure and the size of the overlay areas chosen are extremely important with S2000 as are the I/O buffer and work area sizes. Unfortunately, no aids are available to help with the tuning of S2000.

S2000 is designed for fast data retrieval. Complex queries are resolved, as far as possible, in the Unique and Multiple Value Tables, thus reducing I/O traffic to a minimum. With the Database Definition Table and the Unique Value Table Directory held permanently in memory, query resolution will be even faster.

5.10 Conclusion

S2000 offers the user a flexible DBMS with superb query facilities for both the host language programmer and the end-user. The major features offered are:

- a report writer which will generate up to 100 separate reports in a single pass
- a Rollback feature
- a Multi-Thread feature capable of servicing up to nine threads simultaneously
- security provisions with which non-hierarchical password lockout can be applied separately for updating and retrieval of specific data fields
- a text search facility, allowing the user to search data values for a character string
- a Self-Contained Language which permits direct (or queued) update or retrieval, either on-line or in batch
- a Host Language Interface for COBOL, FORTRAN, PL/1 and Assembler, offering more powerful data manipulation facilities than the Self-Contained Language

- a LINK command in the Host Language Interface which allows the user to establish temporary network relationships between different databases so that the retrieval of one record automatically initiates the retrieval of the next
- a WHERE clause which can include non-key fields
- Control 2000, a data dictionary
- TP 2000, a TP monitor

S2000 is certainly not the 'fastest' of the DBMSs examined, but then it is not claimed to be. It is far more a general purpose DBMS which can be used in most commercial areas. It is particularly well suited to complex query type application, and is least suited to a production environment where speed of retrieval on single key fields is the main criterion – although even this area will be covered by a direct access retrieval method to be made available with Version 2.10.

The transaction-oriented processing first introduced in Version 2.9 must be considered somewhat provisional in nature. No checkpoint can be written from a program and the ROLLBACK FILE for a particular database can only be used by one program at any one time.

In the past, the vendors of S2000 have laid great emphasis on the end-user facilities of the system – NATURAL LANGUAGE, which at one time was without parallel. Great efforts have been made in the last few versions to improve the performance as well as to offer new facilities, and if the promised improvements are realised with Version 2.10, then S2000 will be able to count itself amongst the most flexible of the DBMSs available.

5.11 Advantages of SYSTEM 2000

- Excellent end-user query language facilities.
- Field level security.
- Good documentation.
- Data dictionary (CONTROL 2000).
- A TP Monitor – TP 2000 is available, but only in USA.
- A report writer.
- powerful selection criteria
- A multithreading feature is available.
- A simple system to use from the DBA's point-of-view
  - he cannot influence space management.
  - he can only generate hierarchical structures explicitly, thus file definition is a simple task. More complicated structures can be generated implicitly using keys as symbolic pointers.
  - the utilities eg. DB unload, are activated using a single command. No JCL is required.

- Interfaces (see Appendix III).
- The DBMS is somewhat more complicated from the programmer's point-of-view because of the different languages available. This is normally only a problem in the beginning whereafter they start to appreciate the flexibility offered by having both stand-alone and host programming languages. They are: –
  - NATURAL language – with two variations, both are stand-alone languages: –
    - QUEUE ACCESS – for batch applications.
    - IMMEDIATE ACCESS – for on-line use (can also be used in batch mode).
  - HOST LANGUAGE INTERFACE allows largely the same commands as NATURAL language to be used in any programming language supporting a CALL command. The HLI user is automatically in IMMEDIATE ACCESS mode but can change to QUEUE ACCESS mode by issuing the QUEUE command.
- Plans to fully intergrate the DBMS into the Data Dictionary such that all access is via the IDD.
  All DBA operations will also be implemented via the Integrated Data Dictionary (IDD).
- The SUBSCHEMA does not have to have the ELEMENTS in the same order as they are specified in the SCHEMA; nor do the ELEMENT format descriptions have to be the same, merely compatible.
- It is possible to access the hierarchy at any level and then navigate up, down or along the structure.
- No key field – even at the ENTRY LEVEL – need be unique.
- All fields including key fields may be modified.
- A REPEATING GROUP may exist (and hence all its dependents) even after all its fields have been deleted. An interesting concept.
- Backing store of 500KB is required (excluding the INDEX TABLES).
- Autorollback.
- Format checks both during loading and updating.
- Password protection for each database. A DB may have a series of passwords each with different access controls.
- A new release, 2.10, will be available from early in 1981
  The extensions will include:
  - a Direct Access Method
  - a method of storing the network generated by a LINK command
  - improvements to NATURAL LANGUAGE to enable it to process a number of databases simultaneously
  - the report writer will be made more flexible.

5.12 Disadvantages of SYSTEM 2000

- Performance very sensitive to the overlay structure. There are no aids which directly help with the tuning of the overlay structure.
- NATURAL language can only operate on a single database. In order to use this feature, complex hierarchical structures must be used – this of course reduces flexibility.
- The report writer can only process a single 'leg' of a hierarchical structure in one run.
- Network structures may only be generated by the LINK command, furthermore they only exist during the execution of the program that created them. To avoid networks, it would require extensive duplication of data in the tree structures.
- Performance degrades as data becomes fragmented; this leads to the need for regular reorganisation runs. One reason for this is that non-unique keys are stored in the Overflow Table.
- The insertion of a new REPEATING GROUP occurrence is totally dependent on the Current Position – this is weak.
- User-defined CHECKPOINTs cannot be written.
- S2000 is expensive in terms of price and system resources (although the new release 2.9 is reported to show a marked improvement in performance over earlier versions).
- S2000 is relatively slow in browsing along Sibling chains.
- There is no general data compression routine although INTEGER, DECIMAL and MONEY fields are always stored as packed decimal (the leading zeroes remain).
- Although it is possible to order the Sibling RGs on retrieval, it is not possible to order them in storage.
- NATURAL LANGUAGE users are responsible for their own integrity
- It is only possible to set one record per database in Hold status.
- Although S2000 can handle variable length records, the method used, an Overflow Table, leads to inefficient processing because of the extra I/O required.
- The transaction oriented processing, implemented in Version 2.9, is rather primitive. No checkpoints may be written from the user program. Only one program, at any one time, may use the ROLLBACK file for a particular database.
- Accessing of dependent REPEATING GROUPS using the hierarchical structure ist slow; particularly along SIBLING chains.

5.13 SYSTEM 2000 Glossary

ANCESTOR: Any DATA SET within a family of DATA SETS occurring at a level above the object DATA SET.

ARCHIVAL COPY: A backup copy of the database.

CHILD: A REPEATING GROUP occurrence one level lower in the hierarchy than the object REPEATING GROUP occurrence.

COMPONENT: 1. The term used to describe each of the four data definition types:

- ELEMENT
- REPEATING GROUP
- STRING
- user-defined function.

2. A database definition statement delimited by a statement number and a colon.

CONTROL 2000: MRI's data dictionary/directory.

DATA SET: A unit of data, composed of one or more ELEMENTS, normally a REPEATING GROUP.

DATA TREE: A DATA SET together with all its direct hierarchical DESCENDANTS.

DEFINITION TABLE: This S2000 internal file holds the COMPONENT numbers, names and descriptions.

DEPENDENT: A DATA SET that has at least one hierarchically higher LEVEL.

DESCENDANT: Any DATA SET within a family of DATA SETS occurring at a LEVEL below the object DATA SET.

ELEMENT: A named data field.

HIERARCHICAL TABLE: This internal file holds those pointers which expressed the PARENT, CHILD and SIBLING relationships for each REPEATING GROUP occurrence.

IMMEDIATE ACCESS: This option allows the user to perform data manipulation operations in batch, remote batch or interactive mode. Each instruction is, to a great extent, independent of the previously executed commands.

LEVEL: The relative position of a DATA SET within a hierarchy. The LEVELS are numbered from the top (zero) downwards. The LEVEL zero is the highest LEVEL of the hierarchy.

LOGICAL ENTRY: This is the set of DATA SETS dependent on a single DATA SET occurrence from the LEVEL zero.

MULTIPLE OCCURRENCE TABLE: This internal S2000 file contains pointers to all DATA SETS containing duplicate key values. In conjunction with the UNIQUE VALUE TABLE, it is possible to locate all occurrences of a particular key value.

NATURAL LANGUAGE: The very powerful query language.

PARENT: The DATA SET within a family of DATA SETS, occurring at the LEVEL above the object DATA SET.

POSITIONING: CURRENCY in S2000 terminology.

REPEATING GROUP: COMPONENTS used to indicate the hierarchical relationships between repeatable DATA SETS, ELEMENTS or other REPEATING GROUPS.

RETURN CODE: This field in the COMMBLOCK must be investigated after each database access. It will indicate the success or otherwise of the access.

SCHEMA: A database structural definition.

SIBLING: DATA SET occurrences with a common PARENT.

SUBSCHEMA: The user view.

TDMS: (Timeshared Data Management System). S2000's origins can be traced back to this product.

TP2000: S2000's TP monitor.

6. ADABAS (Adaptable Database System)

ADABAS emerged from a research project run by Software A.G. in the late 1960s. It was conceived as a host language DBMS, capable of handling large databases in batch mode.

The initial version of ADABAS was installed in March 1971. Version 2 followed in September 1972, and then in January 1974, Version 3 was introduced. The current version – 4 – was introduced in September 1979.

In 1972, Software AG of North America Inc was founded, an independent company which was also active in developing ADABAS, particularly in the on-line interface area. Their major developments were multi-user front end interfaces for various TP monitors. Software AG has also developed a procedural language macro interface, originally an idea of a user, and now fully supports it.

The ADABAS family of products now includes:

- ADABAS VERSION 4 with a multi-threading nucleus and ADAM, the new direct access method
- ADASCRIPT+, an on-line query language
- ADACOM, the successor to ADAWRITER, a batch report generator
- ADABOMP, a bill of materials processor
- ADABAS–M, a PDP–11 version of ADABAS
- ADABAS DATA DICTIONARY
- ADAMINT, a high level DML Macro Interface
- NATURAL, an on-line and batch communication system fully compatible with ADACOM and ADASCRIPT+
- COM–PLETE, a fully compatible TP monitor. Interfaces are available for the following TP monitors: TCAM, TSO, CICS, INTERCOMM, TASK/MASTER, ENVIRON/1, SHADOW II, for Siemens, ASMUS, and for about 20 homegrown TP monitors. An interface can also be made available for TP monitors developed by the customer himself. Interfaces also exist for the following report generators: EASYTRIEVE, MARK IV, SCORE, Quickjob, Data Analyser. It should not however be necessary to use an external report generator, since ADABAS has its own more than adequate on-line query and batch report generating facilities.

Software AG and Software AG of North America are now jointly responsible for the development of ADABAS and its associated products.

6.1 Classification

ADABAS is based on inverted file structures, which results in little or no formal structure being imposed on the data records. It is possible to define any number of record fields as DESCRIPTORS (keys). ADABAS does not recognise a primary key and a number of secondary keys, and it follows from this that the system does not try to maintain any particular key sequence when records are inserted. Nevertheless, if a particular key is used in sequential processing, it is possible to arrange that the physical and logical record orders are the same for this key.

One area where inverted list systems are weak is in fast response on-line applications where data is to be retrieved on a known key. This is because the index hierarchies that have to be followed before a record can be retrieved require between three and five accesses.

ADABAS now offers a direct access method integrated into the standard access method, thus allowing the required record to be retrieved with one access. This new direct access method (ADAM) only operates on unique keys, and if a second occurrence of an ADAM key value is offered for insertion, it is rejected. ADAM is completely transparent to the user. A further advantage of this unique key capability is that ADABAS now supports one-to-many relationships in addition to the many-to-many relationships which are implicit with any inverted list system.

One of the unique features offered by ADABAS is a phonetic retrieval capability. If a field is declared a phonetic DESCRIPTOR, then it is possible to retrieve phonetically similar DESCRIPTOR values, eg. 'FIND MEYER' would also retrieve 'MAYER' and 'MEIER'.

Version 4 of ADABAS offers a number of significant improvements over the previous version, the most important of which, without a doubt, being the fully multi-threading nucleus, although update commands are still only single-threaded. This restriction is necessary in order to guarantee data protection and the restart capability. The new transaction processing and its associated AUTOROLLBACK are amongst the best offered by any DBMS today. However, the identification and resolution of deadlock, although much improved, are still not as sophisticated as with some of the competing systems.

A deadlocked user is identified by the expiry of the 'Transaction Time Limit'. All resources held by the timed-out user will be released and the partially completed transaction will be rolled back. Thus, the other deadlocked transaction(s) can continue. It could be argued with a fair degree of justification that resource deadlock occurs so seldom that a simple solution must be found. If this were the aim, Software AG have been eminently successful.

ADABAS has been designed to accommodate databases of unthinkable proportions. Each database (file) can accommodate up to a maximum of over 16 million record, this limit being imposed by the 3 byte Address Converter entries. Moreover, 255 such files can be handled by ADABAS simultaneously, giving a maximum of 42 billion records. Each record can contain up to 500 data fields, of which up to 200 can be DESCRIPTORS.

ADABAS can be used with the following operation systems: IBM DOS, DOS/VS, DOS/VSE, OS/MFT, OS/MVT, OS/VS1, SVS, MVS, Siemens PBS, BS1000, BS2000 and BS3000. Recently, Software AG announced the ADABAS can also be used with OS/VM whereby only one copy is necessary. The maintenance of the version for the different operation systems has been simplified by removing the I/O instructions from ADABAS and the utilities; they are now contained solely in the ADAIOR module. Thus all Version 4 modules are operating system- and device-independent, except for ADAIOR, ADAMPM and ADARUN.

The ADABAS nucleus and all ADABAS utilities are invoked via the execution of the control module ADARUN, which performs the following functions:

- loading ADAIOR (the OS dependent I/O module)
- reading and processing ADARUN parameter cards
- dynamically loading required ADABAS modules
- passing control to the requested module.

The ADABAS utilities include:

1. ADAMER. The ADAM ESTIMATION utility produces statistics indicating the number of DATA STORAGE accesses required to FIND and READ a record. This information is used to determine: whether the ADAM option would be better than the ADABAS standard accessing method and the amount of data space required to produce optimal ADAM distribution.

2. AUDIT TRAIL. This utility selects information from the log file.

3. COMPRESSION. This utility compresses the raw input data. The data definitions which describe the input must also be supplied. The output of this program is used as input to the LOADER utility.

4. COUPLE. This utility constructs Inverted Lists for a common DESCRIPTOR in two files.

5. DB MODIFICATION. This utility performs the following functions:

- deleting a file
- ASSOCIATOR and DATA STORAGE expansion
- reordering the DATA STORAGE records
- file cluster definition and deletion, update prohibition and release of a locked cluster
- changing a database's name and the number assigned to a file

6. DECOMPRESS. This utility decompresses an ADABAS file.

7. DUMP/RESTORE. This utility dumps a database, a certain file or several selected files to a sequential data set for security purposes, and can copy it back.

8. FILE MODIFICATION. This utility performs the following functions:

- changing the standard length of a field
- adding 1 or more new fields to the FIELD DEFINITION TABLE
- creating a DESCRIPTOR
- releasing a DESCRIPTOR
- uncoupling two files.

9. FORMAT. This utility preformats those files (ASSOCIATOR, DATA STORAGE WORK, TEMP and SORT) which are accessed using the direct access method.

10. LOADER. This utility loads the output of the COMPRESSION utility into a database.

11. MAIN PRINT. This utility prints the contents of database physical blocks for special maintenance or verification purposes.

12. MASS UPDATE. This utility adds or deletes large volumes of records to or from the file with optimal speed. It is preferable to using single commands for this purpose.

13. REORDER ASSOCIATOR. This utility reorders the ASSOCIATOR, which may become fragmented owing to file deletion.

14. REPORT. This utility displays database status information including the physical space allocation for the ASSOCIATOR, DATA STORAGE and WORK; the field definitions for each file; the space allocation for each file and check-point information.

15. RESTART. This utility copies the log file to another file, which may be necessary when an ADABAS session terminates abnormally. It also performs the ROLLBACK and ROLLFORWARD functions.

16. UNLOAD. This utility unloads a file from the database in compressed form. The output from this utility may be used as input to the LOADER or DECOMPRESS utilities. The file may be unloaded in DESCRIPTOR, ISN or physical sequence.

6.2 Data Item Definition

An ADABAS database may consist of up to 255 files, each of which may hold up to nearly 17 million records. This limit is dictated by the 3 byte ISN of the

DEFINITION	EXPLANATION
01,GA	Group GA, consisting of fields AA and AB
02,AA,8,A,DE,NU	Elementary field AA; SL is 8, SF is alphanumeric, DESCRIPTOR, null value suppression.
02,AB,2,P,DE,NU	Elementary field AB; SL is 2, SF is packed, DESCRIPTOR, null value suppression.
01,AC,20,A,NU	Elementary field AC; SL is 20 SF is alphanumeric, null value suppression.
01,MF,3,A,MU,DE,NU	Multiple value field MF; SL is 3, SF is alphanumeric, DESCRIPTOR, null value suppression.
01,GB,PE	Periodic group GB
02,BA,1,B,DE,NU	Elementary field BA (within periodic group GB); SL is 1, SF is binary, DESCRIPTOR, null value suppression.
02,BB,5,P,NU	Elementary field BB (within periodic group GB), SL is 5, SF is packed null value suppression.
02,BC,10,A,NU	Elementary field BC (within periodic group GB); SL is 10, SF ist alphanumeric, null value suppression.
01,GC,PE	Periodic group GC
02,CA,7,A,DE,NU	Elementary field CA (within periodic group GC); SL is 7, SF is alphanumeric, DESCRIPTOR null value suppression.
02,CB,10,A,MU,NU	Multiple value field CB (within periodic group GC); SL is 10, SF is alphanumeric, null value suppression.

SL = Standard Length SF = Standard Format

Fig. 6.2a: File 'A' Record Description

Address Converter. A record type may consist of up to 500 fields of which a maximum of 200 may be DESCRIPTORS (keys) at any one time of which 12 fields may be defined as PHONETIC DESCRIPTORS.

Record definition in ADABAS is composed of Field Description Entries (see Fig. 6.2a and Fig. 6.2b). The following syntax is used to define each field:

LEVEL–NUMBER, FIELD–NAME(,STANDARD–LENGTH)(,STANDARD–FORMAT) (,ATTRIBUTES), EXTERNAL–FIELD–NAME

The restriction that a record description must consist of at least three fields, one of which must be a DESCRIPTOR no longer applies.

6.2.1 Level Number

The use of level numbers allows the DBA to specify hierarchical relationships between the fields. ADABAS uses the concept of the Group Field where a field is defined in terms of a number of subfields. A subfield has a higher level number than that of its associated Group Field. The level numbers range from 01 to 07.

6.2.2 Field Name

This is a two-character name, uniquely identifying the field. The first character must be alphabetic and the second alphanumeric. With ADASCRIPT+ and ADACOM, field names of up to 80 characters may be specified.

6.2.3 Standard Length and Format

The STANDARD–LENGTH and FORMAT of a field define the characteristics of the field when it is loaded and the default values when it is retrieved, (see FORMAT BUFFER). Data is normally stored in compressed form, all numeric fields are packed, leading zeros and trailing blanks are suppressed, (see the NU and FI attributes in this section). The FORMATS supported by ADABAS are shown in Fig. 6.2c.

6.2.4 Attributes

Each field in an ADABAS record must be assigned a particular field type, and optionally one or more field properties may also be assigned.

DEFINITION	EXPLANATION
01,RG	Group RG, consisting of all the fields in the record.
02,RA,8,A,DE,NU	Elementary field RA; SL is 8, SF is alphanumeric, DESCRIPTOR, null value suppression.
02,RB,10,A,DE	Elementary field RB; SL is 10, SF is alphanumeric, DESCRIPTOR, null value suppression.
02,GX	Group GX, consisting of the fields XA, XB, XC, XD and XE
03,XA,10,A	Elementary field XA; SL is 10, SF is alphanumeric.
03,XB,2,P,DE	Elementary field XB; SL is 2, SF is packed, DESCRIPTOR.
03,XC,6,U	Elementary field XC; SL is 6, SF is unpacked.
03,XD,8,P,DE,NU	Elementary field XD; SL is 8. SF is packed, DESCRIPTOR, null value suppression.
03,XE,5,A,DE,NU	Elementary field XE; SL is 5, SF is alpha-numeric, DESCRIPTOR, null value suppression.
SA=RA(1,4)	SUBDESCRIPTOR SA; derived from bytes 1–4 (incl.) of field RA, format is alphanumeric.
SB=RA(1,8), RB(1,4)	SUPERDESCRIPTOR SB; derived from bytes 1–8 (incl.) of field RA and bytes 1–4 (incl.) of field RB, format is alphanumeric.
SC=XB(1,2), XC(1,6)	SUPERDESCRIPTOR SC; derived from bytes 1–2 (incl.) of field XB and bytes 1–6 (incl.) of field XC, format is binary.

SL = Standard Length SF = Standard Format

Fig. 6.2b: File 'B' Record Description

CODE	MEANING	MAX. LENGTH in Bytes
A	alphanumeric left justified	253 (only 126 for a DESCRIPTOR)
B	binary right justified	126
F	fixed point	always 4 bytes in length
G	floating point	4 or 8
P	packed decimal	14
U	unpacked decimal	27

Fig. 6.2c: ADABAS Format Types

6.2.5 Field Types

Each field of an ADABAS record must have assigned to it one of the following types:

1. ELEMENTARY FIELDS allow only one value per record to be present.

2. MULTIPLE FIELDS (MU) allow a record to contain up to 191 values.

3. GROUP FIELDS allow compound fields to be defined, which are composed of one or more contiguous fields. Both ELEMENTARY and MULTIPLE FIELDS may be members of a GROUP FIELD. This mechanism allows seven levels of hierarchical structure to be defined with a record.

4. PERIODIC GROUPS (PE) are GROUP FIELDS which can occur up to 99 times within a record. A PERIODIC GROUP may not contain a further PERIODIC GROUP. Thus, a PERIODIC GROUP enables a two-dimensional table to be built, and a MULTIPLE FIELD within a PERIODIC GROUP enables a three-dimensional table to be built.

6.2.6 Field Properties

1. DESCRIPTOR (DE) defines the field as a key. If the DESCRIPTOR is unique, UQ must be specified in addition to DE.

2. NULL VALUE SUPPRESSION (NU) specifies that a numeric field containing zeroes or an alphanumeric field containing blanks should be handled as an empty field.

3. FIXED LENGTH (FI) specifies that the normal field compression should not operate on a field so described.

6.2.7 Descriptor Types

Beyond the normal DESCRIPTOR definition four further types of DESCRIPTOR are supported by ADABAS (see Fig. 6.2b).

1. SUBDESCRIPTOR describes a key field which consists of one part of a field, with the following syntax:

– field name (starting byte, ending byte)

2. SUPERDESCRIPTOR describes a key field composed of a number of fields or subfields, with the following syntax:

– field name (starting byte, ending byte) ..... field name (starting byte, ending byte)

3. PHONETIC DESCRIPTOR describes a key field which enables the user to retrieve data by "sound", ie. SMYTHE for SMITH.

4. ADAM DESCRIPTOR. This must be unique and be the first field in the record. The ISN value assigned may also be used as input to the randomizing routine. Neither MULTIPLE VALUE FIELDS nor fields within a PERIODIC GROUP may be used as ADAM DESCRIPTORS.

It is also possible to specify that a given number of bits are to be truncated from an ADAM DESCRIPTOR prior to it being submitted to the randomizer to optimize sequential reading of the file, or to remove insignificant information such as a check digit.

The use of the ADAM option is signalled to the ADABAS system in the LOADER module.

6.2.8 External Field Name

This is an 80 character field name used in ADASCRIPT+, ADACOM, NATURAL and ADAMINT.

6.3 Data Structures

Data in an ADABAS database is split into two distinct parts, primary and secondary data. The former is composed of pure (and usually compressed) user data, and the latter consists of all the internal data needed to manipulate the user data. Secondary data is held either in the ASSOCIATOR or in ADABAS WORK and contains:

- the global description of the database (STORAGE MANAGEMENT TABLES)
- the global description of the data (FIELD DEFINITION TABLES)
- the inverted lists (ASSOCIATION NETWORK)
- the Address Converter
- the randomizing algorithm
- the interfile relationships (COUPLING TABLES)
- the scratch files (in ADABAS WORK)
- security information (in ADABAS WORK).

1. The global description of the database is held in the STORAGE MANAGEMENT TABLES (SMT). They contain information whit which to locate the ASSOCIATOR and the other data files on physical storage, and also the free space tables. Management of the SMT is completely under the control of ADABAS. Should a file exhaust its originally allocated space, then ADABAS automatically assigns additional space from the general storage area.

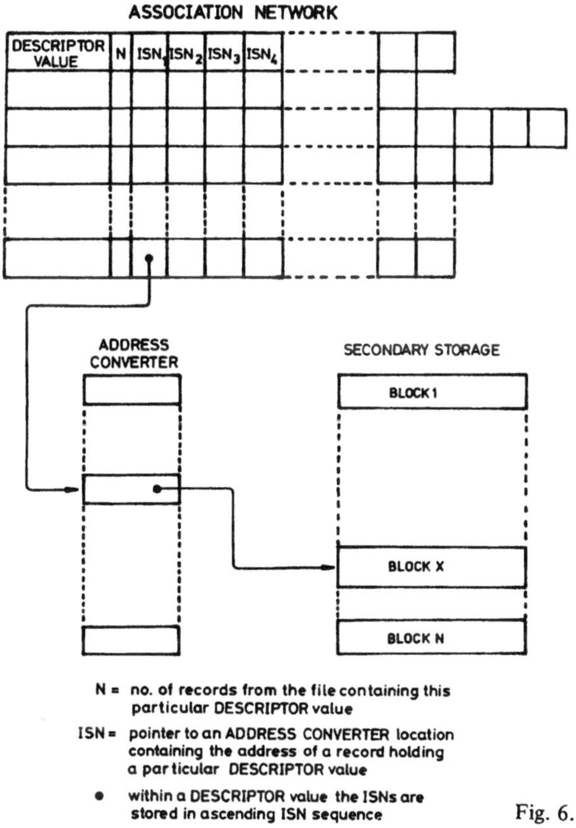

Fig. 6.3: Logical-to-Physical Mapping

2. The global description of the data is held in the FIELD DESCRIPTION TABLES (FDT). These descriptions are necessary for the compression/decompression routines. The 80 character EXTERNAL FIELD NAMES are also held in this data directory. The contents of the FDT can be retrieved via a special READ command, (see section 6.4). Extensions may be made to the FDT for a particular file even after the file has been loaded, without requiring any reorganisation at all, as long as the newly added field(s) are added to the end of the record.

3. The inverted lists, used by ADABAS to resolve queries and retrieve data, are held in a part of the ASSOCIATOR called the ASSOCIATION NETWORK. A separate ASSOCIATION NETWORK is generated for each DESCRIPTOR in each file within the database.

An ASSOCIATION NETWORK consists of a variable number of index hierarchy levels. The maximum allowed for is six: up to four Upper, the Main and the Normal index levels. The number of levels required depends upon such factors as the size of the DESCRIPTOR, the block size and the number of DESCRIPTOR values. The Upper and Main index levels contain the standard inverted list information, ie. each level carries a summary of the contents of the next lower level. This consists of the address of each block at the next lower level, together with the highest DESCRIPTOR value associated with the block.

The lowest index level, the Normal Index, contains all the DESCRIPTOR values together with pointers to all records containing each particular DESCRIPTOR value. These pointers are called INTERNAL SEQUENCE NUMBERS (ISN). Each record is assigned a unique ISN on being added to the database, and this ISN remains assigned to the record until it is removed from the database. The ISNs do not point directly to the object record, but point to an Address Converter entry, containing the actual object record address.

4. The Address Converter is a linear list of 3-byte address pointers to the user data records. An Address Converter entry can always be retrieved with, at most, one physical access, because ADABAS can calculate the block number containing the required entry. This separation of logical record identification from its physical location has one disadvantage – namely one extra retrieval operation, if the required block is not already in the I/O buffer. Set against this is the complete device independence, and, most important from the performance point of view, the reduced maintenance when a record changes its block owing to an update which causes the record to expand. Without an Address Converter, a number of entries in the Normal Index would have to be changed. These entries can only be located via the inverted list index hierarchy for each DESCRIPTOR, a process requiring 2 to 4 physical accesses per DESCRIPTOR (cf. 6.9 PERFORMANCE).

6.3.1 ADAM (ADABAS Direct Access Method)

This new access method, only available since Version 4 was released, was introduced to strengthen ADABAS in an area where it was lacking – namely in fast response TP applications. The new access method has been extremely cleverly 'grafted' onto the existing inverted list structure.

ADAM only operates on unique value DESCRIPTORS, and can retrieve a record with one access via a hashing algorithm instead of via the inverted list and Address Converter. This comparison is shown schematically in Fig. 6.3.1a and 6.3.1b.

A record is stored by using the hashing algorithm to generate a block address. If this block is full, then any other block (usually one already in the I/O buffer) is used. The normal inverted list entry etc. is built up for every DESCRIPTOR in the record, including one for the ADAM DESCRIPTOR. There is no chaining from the block where the ADAM DESCRIPTOR indicates a record should be stored to the block where it is actually stored.

When retrieving a record via an ADAM DESCRIPTOR, the same procedure is used. The hashing algorithm indicates where the object record is most probably stored. If the record is not in the indicated block, the Standard Access Method via the inverted lists must be used. ADAM offers a performance advantage only

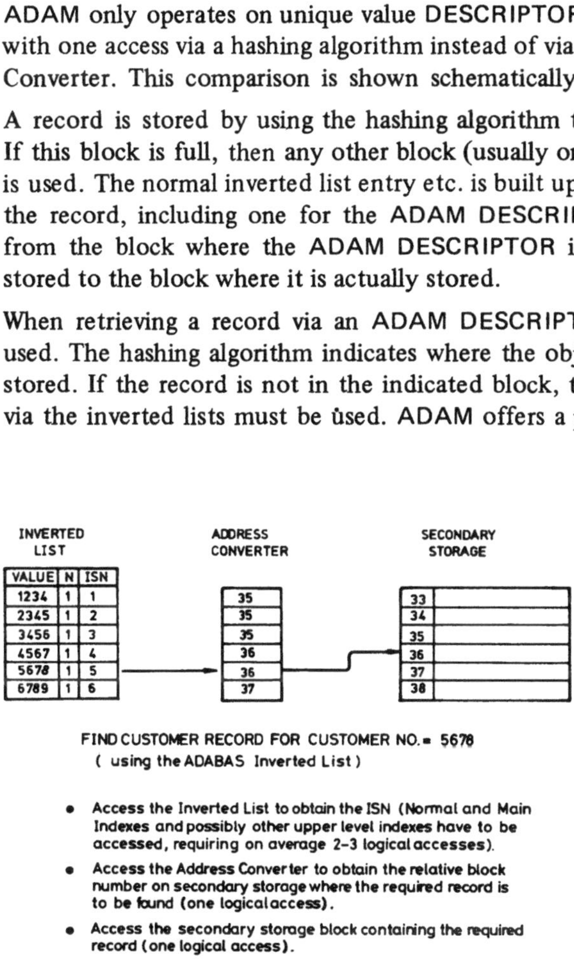

Fig. 6.3.1a: A Comparison of the Standard Access Method vs. ADAM (I)

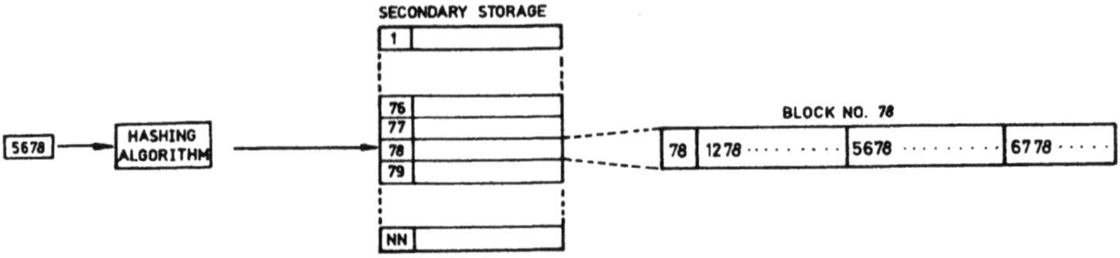

FIND CUSTOMER RECORD FOR CUSTOMER NO. 5678 (using ADAM)

- Calculate the relative block number on secondary storage (no logical access required)
- Access secondary storage block no. 78 (one logical access)
- Scan the block to determine whether the required customer record is present (no logical access required). Should the desired record is not in the block, then it must be located via the Inverted Lists using the ADABAS standard access method.
- The number of physical accesses necessary with ADAM will depend on:
  - the record density
  - the proficiency of the hashing (randomising) algorithm

  An average of 1-1.5 physical accesses can be expected.

  N.B. the record length and ISN fields have omitted from the diagram for simplicity.

Fig. 6.3.1b: A Comparison of the Standard Access Method vs. ADAM (II)

when the required record is found in its 'home' block in a great majority of cases. Factors which can negatively affect this are wildly expanding records following an update, and files more than ca. 80% full.

Therefore, although ADAM offers an undoubted improvement in one of the few areas where ADABAS was weak, it has added a degree of complexity and responsibility to the DBA function previously unknown to ADABAS users.

6.3.2 Logical Relationships

Logical data structures can be generated in ADABAS via the inter-file and inter-field relationships. It is possible to generate both network and hierarchical relationships between files, and these relationships may be implicit or explicit.

The implicit relationships are established by the user in his program, and it is these relationships which can achieve the best performance when using the normal ADABAS DML commands. For the ADAMINT interface, and for the self-contained and report writer facilities, it is often necessary to explicitly relate files. The great disadvantage with this is that new Inverted Lists, linking the related files, have to be built and maintained.

Explicit relationships are established by a process called FILE COUPLING. One DESCRIPTOR field in each file must be declared as the basis for the COUPLING. The advantage is that the contents of both files can be included in a single search request. The relationship is bidirectional, and it is not possible to limit COUPLING to unidirectional relationships.

These interfile relationships can be created and deleted at will, with no preparation having to be made when the files are loaded. Using the COUPLE utility, two files can be COUPLED simply by specifying the file names and the DESCRIPTORS – one from each file. The COUPLE utility creates two Inverted Lists (COUPLING TABLES), which are held within the ASSOCIATOR. The COUPLING Inverted Lists are almost identical to the normal Inverted Lists, except that instead of a series of DESCRIPTOR values in the Normal Index, the ISNs of file A are used, with all ISNs from file B containing the same DESCRIPTOR value (see Fig. 6.3.2). A second COUPLED TABLE is also created, with the roles of file A and file B exchanged. A single file can be COUPLED with up to 80 other files. Up to a maximum of five Coupled files can be referenced in a single query. Even using the standard DML, COUPLING can achieve a performance advantage over standard processing in an on-line environment. However, Inverted List maintenance resulting from insertion and deletion of records in the same environment could sometimes seriously affect performance.

Within a record, hierarchical relationships can be established between the fields by defining a GROUP FIELD (see Section 6.2). The hierarchy of up to 7 levels can be used with a GROUP FIELD. A repeating GROUP FIELD is known as a PERIODIC GROUP and can occur up to 99 times. A PERIODIC GROUP may contain MULTIPLE FIELDS but not PERIODIC GROUPS. This 'limits' ADABAS to being able to express two-dimensional arrays. However if every field in a PERIODIC GROUP is multiple (MU), ADABAS is able to express three-dimensional arrays.

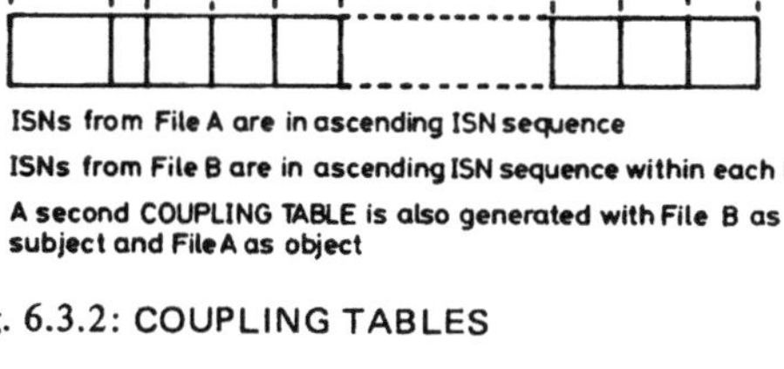

- ISNs from File A are in ascending ISN sequence
- ISNs from File B are in ascending ISN sequence within each Entry
- A second COUPLING TABLE is also generated with File B as subject and File A as object

Fig. 6.3.2: COUPLING TABLES

6.3.3 Space Management

All physical blocks are stored using BDAM. Both ASSOCIATOR and the data files are of fixed block length, but not necessarily of the same length. The block sizes are decided by the DBA. Both the user and the ASSOCIATOR records are compressed. Within a fixed length block, a number of variable length records can be stored. Each record is prefixed by a record length field and the record's ISN.

It is possible to suppress field compression and it is consequently possible to store a record in its uncompressed length. This should be done when the compressed length would be larger than the uncompressed length. ADABAS does not itself check for this. However, it must be added that this is a fairly exceptional circumstance.

Normally, the standard compression techniques of suppressing all empty fields, packing all numeric data and compressing out leading zeroes in numeric fields, as well as trailing blanks in alphanumeric fields results in a space saving of up to 80% in exceptional circumstances, with around 50% being quite normal.

The format of a data block and a compressed record are shown in Fig. 6.3.3. All compressed fields start with a length field, and empty fields with NULL VALUE SUPPRESSION are represented by a count field indicating how many of these fields are suppressed at that point in the RECORD.

When loading a file, the DBA can specify how much free space should be left for future expansion of the compressed records. If compression is not operating, no free space should be reserved. Normally, about 10% of the space should be held free. Space need not be reserved in each block for later addition to the file, because ADABAS does not recognise any block as being preferable to any other block, since the system views all DESCRIPTORS as being equal. This in turn means that even if an ADABAS file is loaded in a particular DESCRIPTOR

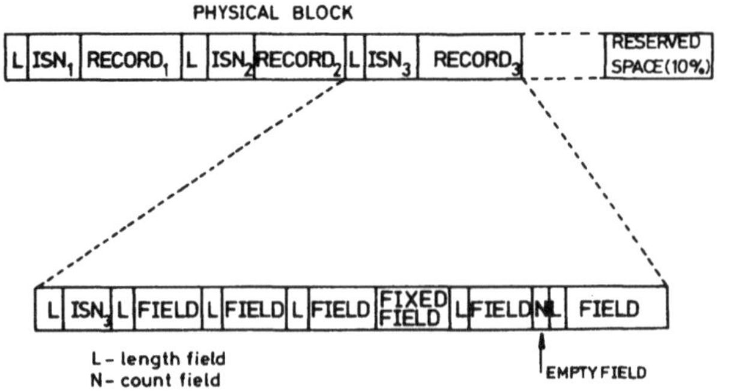

Fig. 6.3.3: Physical Block/Record Layout

sequence, this order will degrade with time, assuming insertion and deletion activity.

Nevertheless, the developers of ADABAS recognised that some applications do require skip-sequential processing and having the file ordered on this DESCRIPTOR would lead to much more efficient processing. A utility is available to resequence – rather than reorganise – a file.

A list of space available in each block is held in the ASSOCIATOR. This space-available count has to be updated continuously as records expand or shrink, and as they are added to and deleted from the files. When a record expands, all records following the expanded record are moved to make room. If there is not sufficient free space, the last record(s) in the block will be moved to a block where space is available. This is usually one of the other blocks in the I/O buffer. This permits ADABAS to maintain all free space at the end of each block.

6.3.4 Reorganisation

An ADABAS database does not become progressively more disorganised with time, simply because there is no order in the placement of the records. ADABAS does not recognise one main DESCRIPTOR and a series of subsidiary DESCRIPTORS. Even when a file contains only one DESCRIPTOR, no effort is made to keep the records in DATA STORAGE physically ordered on the DESCRIPTOR value. An ADABAS database, therefore, by definition never needs reorganising.

It has been recognised that some applications must process a complete file, retrieving the records in a logical sequence dictated by the values of one particular DESCRIPTOR. While this presents no problem for ADABAS, the performance can be enhanced by physically resequencing the contents of the file on the required DESCRIPTOR's values. Normally this is not necessary because such sequential processing takes place in batch and all records can be retrieved in their physical sequence and then, if necessary, sorted afterwards.

When an ADABAS file is loaded, the user may determine a particular sequence by a preload sort. This sequence will only be degraded by insertions to the file, and by updates which significantly increase the size of the compressed record, so that it no longer fits into the orginal block from which it was retrieved.

Where records are retrieved in a purely random sequence, performance degradation will never take place in the DATA STORAGE part of the database.

6.4 Data Manipulation

ADABAS was originally conceived as a host language system which could be interfaced to any procedural language that has a subroutine CALL command which passes an address list. Some users found these powerful low level commands too complicated to use, and in response to the request for a higher level interface, ADAMINT – the ADABAS Macro Interface – was introduced.

ADAMINT was based on a product of the same name developed initially by Shell Oil in Houston, Texas. It uses a CALL command with parameters to specify a record area, key values and response code. The advantages claimed for ADAMINT include:

- reduced programmer effort because of the simplified interface causing fewer errors and thus shorter development time.
- better control over the use of the database, because the DBA generates the ADAMINT access modules and so knows how the data is accessed by whom, and for what purpose. This is a great help in checking that standards are not infringed.
- simplified program maintenance, because the user program contains only the user logic, with an interface to the data source.
- good degree of separation between the user program and the database, and consequently excellent data independence. Data from various ADABAS files can be delivered to the user in the single record area in one ADAMINT access.

The ADAMINT module for each program can only be created by the DBA and the application programmer, the latter specifying which data is required and the former deciding how best to retrieve it. This leaves the application programmer free to concentrate on solving the application problems, since he does not have to be aware of the source or sources of the required data, record structures (PERIODIC GROUPS), or logical file relationships (COUPLED FILES).

The ADAMINT commands that the DBA has at his disposal are shown in Fig. 6.4a.

The ADABAS self-contained interface is provided by 3 languages: ADASCRIPT+, ADACOM and NATURAL.

1. ADASCRIPT+ is an interactive query language using commands based on English. It is intended for use by non-EDP personnel to interrogate ADABAS databases, and can be used both on-line or in batch as a report generator. An example of ADASCRIPT+ is shown in Fig. 6.4b.

2. ADACOM is a batch report generator which offers the user powerful report generation capabilities. In timing tests against COBOL, it was found that ADACOM executes just as quickly, but the programs require only a fraction of the time and effort to produce.

ADACOM executes in 70K of main memory, including a 10K user area and ca. 5K of file description. It does not use separate program overlays. It is written in Assembler and is available for IBM OS and DOS operating systems.

ADAMINT FUNCTION	EXPLANATION OF FUNCTION
ADDNEW	adds a new record occurrence to the file
CHEKPNT	writes a checkpoint to the log file
COMPSET	manipulates one or more ISN sets
DELETER	removes record occurrences from the file
FINDSET	finds a set of record occurrences based on a specific search argument
LOKATE	establishes position prior to processing
LOGTAPE	writes a record to the log file
LOKVAL	positions on first value, satisfying the user's selection criteria
MINTET	signals the end of a logical transaction
READSET	retrieves from a previously found set
READVAL	sequential retrieval of each value, along with number of records with that value, start at position specified in LOKVAL macro
REREAD	reads a previously read record again
RELEASER	frees a record occurrence held for update
RETISN	returns current ISN(s) to the user
SEQREAD	sequentially retrieves record occurrences starting from an established position.
SIGNOFF	ends a session
SIGNON	starts a session
SNAPINT	dumps the user view of the communications area
SORTSET	sorts the results of a FINDSET/COMPSET command
UPDATER	changes at least one field in a record occurrence.

Fig. 6.4a: The ADAMINT Commands

3. NATURAL is an on-line and batch communications language that is intended to offer the user all the functions for application program creation that are available in COBOL and PL/1. It is fully compatible with ADACOM, and offers the end-user a high level interface which contains all the ADABAS commands, without requiring the user to get involved with the technical aspects of the DBMS,

eg. Control Blocks, user-identification, Opening and Closing of files. The commands which are available include:

- read in physical sequence
- read in logical sequence by DESCRIPTOR value
- read by ISN
- read DESCRIPTOR values
- read individual records by ISN
- find, COUPLED, sorted
- update record
- store record
- delete record.

NATURAL allows the user to follow any logical path through the data that might include several different files, or use one file several times under different aspects. Establishing a logical path through several files does not require that the files be COUPLED.

NATURAL contains elements of BASIC, COBOL, FORTRAN and PL/1, together with some of its own, the aim being to give the end-user the greatest degree of flexiblility and power, while at the same time reducing the 'mechanics' of programming to a minimum. A request can thus be formulated rather than requested, and only 10–20% of the effort required with a conventional programming language is needed. A simple example of NATURAL is shown in Fig. 6.4c.

FIND ALL RECORDS IN FILE PERSONNEL WITH DEPT EQ SERVICE AND LANGUAGE EQ ENGLISH OR GERMAN AND NOT JOB EQ TRANSLATOR SORT BY NAME AND DISPLAY PERS–NO SURNAME CHRISTIAN–NAME START–YEAR BIRTHDAY

The results would be as follows:

3 RECORDS FOUND
REPORT READY FOR OUTPUT
24 DEC 79 10:20 PM PAGE 1

PERS–NO	SURNAME	CHRISTIAN NAME	START YEAR	BIRTHDAY
2537928	BROWN	PETER	1940	07.12.20
7830724	GREEN	JOHN	1963	15.09.45
8462206	BLACK	CHARLES	1959	25.01.38

Fig. 6.4b: An Example of an ADASCRIPT+ QUERY

Example showing how the following question would be formulated using NATURAL:

WHAT PERCENTAGE OF EMPLOYEES WERE ILL FOR MORE THAN 60 DAYS LAST YEAR?

```
0010  MOVE 0 TO TOTAL HISTOGRAM PERSONNEL
0020  FOR NAME ADD *NUMBER TO TOTAL LOOP
0030  FIND PERSONNEL WITH DAYS–ILL GREATER THAN 60 LOOP
0040  COMPUTE PERCENT (N2.7) = *NUMBER (0020)/ TOTAL * 100
0050  WRITE 'PERCENTAGE OF PEOPLE WHO WERE ILL FOR MORE
0060  THAN 60 DAYS IS: 'PERCENT.
PAGE 1                                  80–09–12   14:18:45
 PERCENTAGE OF PEOPLE WHO WERE ILL FOR MORE THAN 60 DAYS
 IS:
   65.806400
REPORT DONE
```

Fig. 6.4c: Example of NATURAL

6.4.1 The Standard ADABAS DML

Each ADABAS CALL must be accompanied by a parameter list. Each entry in the parameter list refers to a specific area (buffer) defined in the user program. These buffers allow for the transfer of information between ADABAS and the application program. These areas consist of a CONTROL BLOCK and five CONTROL BUFFERS. The format of the CONTROL BLOCK for a COBOL program and the CALL command are shown in Fig. 6.4.1a.

6.4.1.1 The CONTROL BLOCK

This is always present in every ADABAS CALL, and specifies which command is to be executed in the COMMAND CODE field. The COMMAND TIME field returns to the user the time that elapses between the application issuing the command and ADABAS returning control to the application. The RESPONSE CODE indicates the success or otherwise of the request.

6.4.1.2 The FORMAT and RECORD BUFFERS

The FORMAT BUFFER specifies the fields to be retrieved or modified during the execution of the ADABAS command. The RECORD BUFFER will contain the values of the fields to be stored in the database for ADD/UPDATE commands. The RECORD BUFFER will receive the contents of the specified fields during the execution of a READ command.

```
**----------------------------------------------------------------
****CONTROL BLOCK
 01  CONTROL-BLOCK.
     05  FILLER                     PIC XX     VALUE '  '.
     05  COMMAND-CODE               PIC XX     VALUE '  '.
     05  COMMAND-ID                 PIC X(4)   VALUE SPACES.
     05  FILE-NO                    PIC S9(4)  COMP   VALUE +0.
     05  RESPONSE-CODE              PIC S9(4)  COMP   VALUE +0.
     05  ISN                        PIC S9(8)  COMP   VALUE +0.
     05  ISN-LOWER-LIMIT            PIC S9(8)  COMP   VALUE +0.
     05  ISN-QUANTITY               PIC S9(8)  COMP   VALUE +0.
     05  FORMAT-BUFFER-LENGTH       PIC S9(4)  COMP   VALUE +100.
     05  RECORD-BUFFER-LENGTH       PIC S9(4)  COMP   VALUE +250.
     05  SEARCH-BUFFER-LENGTH       PIC S9(4)  COMP   VALUE +50.
     05  VALUE-BUFFER-LENGTH        PIC S9(4)  COMP   VALUE +100.
     05  ISN-BUFFER-LENGTH          PIC S9(4)  COMP   VALUE +20.
     05  COMMAND-OPTION-1           PIC X      VALUE '  '.
     05  COMMAND-OPTION-2           PIC X      VALUE '  '.
     05  ADDITIONS-1                PIC X(8)   VALUE SPACES.
     05  ADDITIONS-2                PIC X(4)   VALUE SPACES.
     05  ADDITIONS-3                PIC X(8)   VALUE SPACES.
     05  ADDITIONS-4                PIC X(8)   VALUE SPACES.
     05  FILLER                     PIC X(8)   VALUE SPACES.
     05  COMMAND-TIME               PIC S9(8)  COMP   VALUE +10.
     05  USER-AREA                  PIC X(4)   VALUE SPACES.
**----------------------------------------------------------------
****USER BUFFER AREAS
 01  FORMAT-BUFFER                  PIC X(100) VALUE SPACES.
 01  RECORD-BUFFER                  PIC X(250) VALUE SPACES.
 01  SEARCH-BUFFER                  PIC X(50)  VALUE SPACES.
 01  VALUE-BUFFER                   PIC X(100) VALUE SPACES.
 01  ISN-BUFFER                     PIC X(20)  VALUE SPACES.
**----------------------------------------------------------------
     CALL 'ADABAS' USING  CONTROL-BLOCK
                          FORMAT-BUFFER
                          RECORD-BUFFER
                          SEARCH-BUFFER
                          VALUE-BUFFER.
```

Fig. 6.4.1a: CONTROL BLOCK, BUFFERS and CALL Formats

The syntax of the FORMAT BUFFER is as follows:

[nX,] ['literal',] [field-name (i)] [,length] [{,format / ,edit-mask}]

The 'nX' parameter can be used to specify how many blank characters are to be inserted before a field, prior to it being moved to the RECORD BUFFER. With an ADD/UPDATE command, it indicates how many blanks in front of a field are to be ignored by ADABAS. For READ commands, the character string contained within the quotation marks is to be inserted into the RECORD BUFFER immediately before the next field value.

For UPDATE commands, the number of positions enclosed within the quotation marks will be ignored in the corresponding positions of the RECORD BUFFER. The 'field-name' parameter refers to the two-character field identifier. Should the 'field-name' refer to a PERIODIC GROUP or a field within a PERIODIC GROUP, a particular occurrence must be indicated with the 'i' parameter, eg. GB3 – the third occurrence of the PERIODIC GROUP GB (see Fig. 6.2a). A range of occurrences of a PERIODIC GROUP (or field within a PERIODIC GROUP) are selected by specifying the first and last occurrence (eg. GB2–4). MULTIPLE VALUE fields are referenced in a similar manner, eg. MF2, the second value. They may also be referenced by simply repeating the name, eg. AA, MF, AB, MF, AC, MF. This would result in the first three values of the MULTIPLE VALUE field being referenced.

If a MULTIPLE VALUE field is referenced within a PERIODIC GROUP, the PG occurrence number must be mentioned first, followed by the desired MULTIPLE VALUE field. The final, most complex variation is to reference a range of MULTIPLE VALUE field values within a range of PERIODIC GROUP occurrences, eg. CB1–2(1–4). Here, the first four values of the MULTIPLE VALUE field CB in the first occurrence of the PERIODIC GROUP GC is followed by the first four values of the MULTIPLE VALUE field CB in the second occurrence of GC. To reference a series of consecutive fields (as ordered in the FIELD DEFINITION TABLE), the first and last field names connected by a hyphen must be quoted eg. AA–AC. No MULTIPLE VALUE or PERIODIC GROUP field may be present within the series. The 'length' and 'format' parameters allow the user to specify a different length and/or format for each field from that held in the FIELD DEFINITION TABLE.

An edit mask may be specified for a numeric field. The edit mask rules are those used in COBOL, and users may specify their own masks. A number of FORMAT BUFFER/RECORD BUFFER examples are shown in Fig. 6.4.1b.

Naturally all deviations from standard length format and position affect performance, so that only those conversions which are absolutely necessary should be

Using elementary fields (standard length and format):

FORMAT BUFFER AA,5X,AB.

RECORD BUFFER

AA value 8 bytes alphanumeric	5 spaces	AB value 2 bytes packed

Using elementary fields (length and format override):

FORMAT BUFFER AA,5X,AB,3,U.

RECORD BUFFER

AA value 8 bytes alphanumeric	5 spaces	AB value 3 bytes unpacked

The first two values of the multiple value field MF are referenced:

FORMAT BUFFER MF01–02.

RECORD BUFFER

MF Value 1 3 bytes alphan.	MF Value 2 3 bytes alphan.

A reference to a periodic group:

FORMAT BUFFER GB1.

RECORD BUFFER

BA1 value 1 byte binary	BB1 value 5 bytes packed	BC1 value 10 bytes alphanumeric

Fig. 6.4.1b: FORMAT/RECORD BUFFER Examples

made. Equally, only those fields required should be specified, both for reasons of performance and data independence.

6.4.1.3 The SEARCH and VALUE BUFFERS

The SEARCH and VALUE BUFFERS are used together to define the search criterion to be used to select a set of records using a FIND command (S1, S2, S4). The search expressions are held in the SEARCH BUFFER, the corresponding values in the VALUE BUFFER.

These buffers are also used with the READ LOGICAL SEQUENTIAL (L3/L6) and the READ DESCRIPTOR VALUES (L9) commands, to indicate the starting value for a given sequential pass of a file.

The SEARCH BUFFER as used with the S1, S2 and S4 commands has the following format:

[/file/] {search-expression [,operator ,search expression . . . .]}

search-expression = name (i) [,length] [,format] [,value operator]

The '/file/' parameter is only necessary if the FIND command contains a file COUPLING criterion. If used, it must contain the ADABAS file number.

The 'name' must be a DESCRIPTOR, SUPERDESCRIPTOR, SUBDESCRIPTOR or a PHONETIC DESCRIPTOR. If the DESCRIPTOR is in a PERIODIC GROUP, a subscript may be used to limit the search to one occurrence, otherwise all occurrence will be searched.

The 'length' and 'format' are available when the values in the VALUE BUFFER do not correspond with those in the FIELD DEFINITION TABLE.

The 'value-operator' is the boolean operator that links the DESCRIPTOR in the SEARCH BUFFER to the value held in the VALUE BUFFER. The permissable operators are:

- greater than or equal to (GE)
- greater than (GT)
- less than or equal to (LE)
- less than (LT)
- 'equal to' is assumed when no operator is present.

The possible connecting operators are given in Fig. 6.4.1.9.

The VALUE BUFFER contains the values for each DESCRIPTOR specified in the SEARCH BUFFER. The values must be provided in the same sequence. Examples of the SEARCH/VALUE BUFFER are shown in Fig. 6.4.1c.

6.4.1.4 The ISN BUFFER

This buffer holds the ISNs which have satisfied a given search criterion after ADABAS has executed a FIND command.

A search which uses a single search expression.

SEARCH BUFFER	AA.
VALUE BUFFER	C'12345bbb' X'F1F2F3F4F5404040'

Result: This search returns the ISNs of all the records in file 1 which contain the value 12345 for field AA. The same search may be performed using AA,5. in the SEARCH BUFFER and the value 12345 (without trailing blanks) in the VALUE BUFFER.

A search which uses two search expressions connected by the AND operator.

SEARCH BUFFER	AA,D,AB.
VALUE BUFFER	X'F1F2F3F4F5F6F7F8002C'

Result: This search returns the ISNs of all the records in file 1 which contain the value 12345678 for the field AA and the value +2 for the field AB.

A search in which a multiple value field is used.

SEARCH BUFFER	MF.
VALUE BUFFER	C'ABC' X'C1C2C3'

Result: This search returns the ISNs of all the records in file 1 which contain the value ABC for any value of the multiple value field MF.

A search in which a DESCRIPTOR within a periodic group is used.

SEARCH BUFFER	BA3
VALUE BUFFER	X'04'

Result: This search returns all the records in file 1 which contain the value 4 in the third occurrence of the DESCRIPTOR BA (which is contained within a periodic group).

Fig. 6.4.1c: SEARCH/VALUE BUFFER Examples

The ISNs are normally provided in ascending sequence. When the FIND SORTED (S2 and S9) commands are used, the ISNs are provided according to a user-specified sort sequence ie. sorted on some other DESCRIPTOR in the record.

If the ISN BUFFER is not large enough to hold the entire resulting ISN list, ADABAS will store (if requested) the overflow ISNs on a scratch file, ADABAS WORK. These ISNs may be retrieved later. If the resulting ISNs are to be read using the GET NEXT option of the L1/L4 command, an ISN BUFFER is superfluous.

If a FIND command is issued with a non-blank, non-zero COMMAND–ID, and the SAVE–ISN–LIST option is specified, (a character 'H' in the COMMAND–OPTION–1 field), then the entire ISN list is stored on ADABAS WORK. If the SAVE–ISN–LIST option is not invoked and the resulting ISN list is too large for the ISN BUFFER, only the overflow ISNs will be stored on ADABAS WORK. If the COMMAND–ID is blank or zero, the ISNs are not stored on ADABAS WORK and simply lost after the execution of the FIND command.

The ISNs held on ADABAS WORK may be retrieved by issuing a FIND command with the same COMMAND–ID as originally used when the ISN list was created. ADABAS returns as many ISNs as will fit into the ISN BUFFER.

If the SAVE–ISN–LIST option was used in the original FIND command, the user can control which ISNs are to be retrieved by quoting the first ISN in the ISN–LOWER–LIMIT field. The next group of ISNs retrieved begins with the first ISN larger than the one specified. With the S2 command, the specified ISN must be present in the list and the ISN BUFFER is loaded, beginning with the next ISN list position. This is necessary because the ISNs are not in ascending sequence, as a result of a sort.

If the SAVE–ISN–LIST option was not specified in the original FIND COMMAND, the ISN groups will be deleted from ADABAS WORK after they have been moved to the ISN–BUFFER. The COMMAND–ID is released as soon as the ISN list is empty. The ISN–LOWER–LIMIT field may not be used with this variation.

The user may determine when all the ISNs have been processed – or whether or not too many ISNs have been retrieved – by using the ISN–QUANTITY field. As a result of the original FIND command, this field will contain the number of ISNs stored on ADABAS WORK. ADABAS returns, as a result of subsequent FIND commands used to retrieve ISNs from the ADABAS WORK, the number of ISNs which were moved to the ISN BUFFER. An example of ISN List Processing, using the SAVE–ISN–LIST option is shown in Fig. 6.4.1d.

When a command involving a FORMAT BUFFER is executed, ADABAS converts the contents of the FORMAT BUFFER to its own internal format. If a COMMAND–ID is present in the CONTROL BLOCK, then this Internal Format

Initial Sx call using SAVE ISN LIST option

COMMAND = Sx
COMMAND ID = SX01
COMMAND OPTION 1 = H
ISN LOWER LIMIT = 0
ISN BUFFER LENGTH = 20
CALL ADABAS . . .

Resulting ISN QUANTITY = 7

Resulting ISN list: (all ISNs are stored)

8	12	14	15	24	31	33

Resulting ISN BUFFER:

8	12	14	15	24

Subsequent Sx Call

COMMAND = Sx
COMMAND ID = SX01
ISN LOWER LIMIT = 24
ISN BUFFER LENGTH = 20
CALL ADABAS . . .

Resulting ISN QUANTITY = 2

Resulting ISN BUFFER:

31	33	14	15	24

Subsequent Sx Call

COMMAND = Sx
COMMAND ID = SX01
ISN LOWER LIMIT = 0
ISN BUFFER LENGTH = 20
CALL ADABAS . . .

Resulting ISN QUANTITY = 5

Resulting ISB BUFFER:

8	12	14	15	24

Fig. 6.4.1d: ISN List Processing Using the SAVE ISN LIST Option

Buffer will be stored in the Internal Format Buffer Pool (if it was not already present). If the pool is full, ADABAS will overwrite the least active entry. This procedure can achieve a significant decrease in processing time when a number of READ commands (L1–L6, L9) and/or UPDATE commands (A1/A4, N1/N2) are used with the same FORMAT BUFFER contents.

The READ SEQUENTIAL command requires a non-blank, non-zero COMMAND–ID to be specified so that positioning within the file can be maintained internally. The COMMAND–ID is automatically released when an EOF condition is detected during READ SEQUENTIAL processing. The user may release a COMMAND–ID and its associated entries or ISN lists with the RC or CL commands. The RC command contains options which call for the release of only those COMMAND–IDS contained in the Internal Format Buffer Pool, the TABLE of SEQUENTIAL COMMANDS or the Table of ISN Lists. The CL command causes all the COMMAND–IDs held for the user to be released.

Currency indicators are now available with ADABAS. It is not necessary to use them, as there are always alternative ways of processing with positioning under user control. They have been implemented to offer the user more 'comfort'. Positioning is available for:

- GET NEXT processing
- READ SEQUENTIAL processing
- processing of ISN Lists.

6.4.1.5 Control Commands

1. The OP Command (OPEN). This command informs ADABAS that a user session has begun. Those files which the user wishes to process, together with the processing authority, should be in the RECORD BUFFER when this command is issued.

This command is mandatory for Access Only users or for Exclusive File Control and File Cluster users who expect to update files. For all other users, an OP command is optional, as an implicit OP command is executed by ADABAS as soon as the first command is issued.

During the time a user is active, ADABAS maintains a USER QUEUE ELEMENT (UQE) for the user. It contains a list of the files the user is currently accessing, together with a processing authority, ie. access only, update, exclusive use, etc. If a user tries to access a file not in his UQE, the file will be allocated to him with access-only processing authority as long as no ADABAS utility is using the file. If a user tries to update a file to which he has no access permission, ADABAS must first check whether or not the request conflicts with the user type and also whether or not the file is under another user's Exclusive Control.

Permission may then be issued by including the file in the user's UQE with update processing authority.

2. The CL Command (CLOSE). This command informs ADABAS that a user session is over. It causes data to be written to the DATA PROTECTION LOG, the buffers to be flushed for this user, all records held by the user to be freed, and a SYN CHECKPOINT for the Cluster to be initiated for File Cluster users.

3. The C5 Command. This command writes data to the Data Protection Log. The data may be read and displayed by using the AUDIT TRAIL utility. User records are ignored by recovery processing. The user should provide a unique identifier in the first thirty characters of each record so that it can be properly identified and selected by the user.

4. The RC Command. This command releases one or more COMMAND–IDs currently assigned to the user. A COMMAND–ID should be released immediately under any of the following circumstances:

– the user has completed the processing of an ISN List stored on ADABAS WORK as the result of a FIND command with the SAVE–ISN–LIST option active.
– the user wishes to terminate a sequential pass of a file prior to reaching EOF.
– a sequence of commands has terminated, which used a common FORMAT BUFFER.

5. The RI Command. This command allows a user to release one or all records from hold status. If only one record is to be released, the user must specify both file number and ISN. If all records are to be released, the FILE–NUMBER field should be set to binary zero.

This command should never be used by an ET logic user if any updating has taken place during the current transaction, otherwise a ROLLBACK TRANSACTION could overwrite an update (from another transaction) to a released record.

6. The RE Command. This command may be used to retrieve user date which has been previously stored in an ADABAS system file by a CL, C3 or ET command.

6.4.1.6. Logical Transaction Processing Commands

1. The BT Command (BACKOUT TRANSACTION). This command removes all modification made by the current logical transaction and releases all resources held by the user. This may be necessary because of:

– a program error
– a conscious decision in the program logic
– deadly embrace

The user may exclude a particular file from BACKOUT processing; nevertheless, all records for this file in hold status for this user will be released.

2. The ET Command (END TRANSACTION). This command informs ADABAS that a logical transaction has ended. It causes ADABAS to write data protection information to the log. This information may be needed by ADABAS at the start of the next session if the current session has terminated abnormally before all ASSOCIATOR and DATA STORAGE modifications have been physically applied. Data may optionally be stored in the system file, and may be retrieved subsequently using an OP or RE command. It may also be used to help with program restart. All resources held by the user are released except for ISN Lists on ADABAS WORK.

ADABAS returns a unique sequence number which may be used to identify the last successfully processed transaction, should a restart be necessary.

6.4.1.7 Checkpoint Commands

1. The C1 Command. This command causes ADABAS to make a non-synchronized checkpoint. Normally, it is only issued by Exclusive Controls users (who are not using ET logic), and users operating in single-user mode.

A C1 command is automatically executed at the beginning of a program requesting Exclusive File Control or File Control updating.

The result of the C1 command is an entry in the Checkpoint Table. This entry contains the checkpoint identifier (supplied by the user in COMMAND–ID field) and the current log number and log block number. This checkpoint may be used to restore the database or certain files to the status in effect at the time the checkpoint was taken.

2. The C2 Command. This command requests that a synchronized checkpoint should be taken, and may only be used by File Cluster users. The command will be accepted only if the threshhold limit for synchronized checkpoints for the Cluster has been reached. This parameter is set by the DBA.

3. The C3 Command. This command indicates that a user is ready to participate in a synchronized checkpoint, and may be used only by File Cluster users. Before performing a synchronized checkpoint for a File Cluster, ADABAS asks all active Cluster users if they wish to participate in the synchronized checkpoint, by returning a Response Code = 5 to the next command issued. (The command itself is not executed and must be resubmitted).

Each Cluster user must submit a C3 (or CL) at the next logical break in processing, to be included in the checkpoint. The user who issues a C2 command to initiate the synchronized checkpoint will not receive a Response Code = 5, but should immediately issue a C3 command upon successful completion of the C2 command.

User data may be included with the checkpoint. The C3 command causes all records for the user with hold status to be released.

A C3 command can be used to initiate a synchronized checkpoint just like a C2 command, so that a C3 command can have the same effect as issuing a C2 then a C3 command. ADABAS will automatically issue a synchronized checkpoint after a certain number of updates have been executed; this is a Cluster parameter. The synchronised checkpoint will be taken after a specified time has elapsed – this is an installation parameter – and all programs not taking part in the synchronized checkpoint are logged on the operator's console.

6.4.1.8 Modification Commands

1. The A1/A4 Commands (Update). These commands modify one or more fields within a record. The object record is identified by both file number and ISN, the fields to be changed are specified in the FORMAT BUFFER, and the new values are in the RECORD BUFFER.

ADABAS will:

- update the data record
- update the Inverted Lists if a DESCRIPTOR was modified
- update the Coupling Tables if a DESCRIPTOR was involved in Coupling
- update SUB/SUPERDESCRIPTORS as necessary.

If the user is operating in multi-user mode, the UPDATE command (A4) will only be executed if the object record is in hold status. If the user is not using ET logic, the record will be released upon the update completing successfully.

A new length for a field may also be defined. If it is longer than before, all subsequent references must use the new length.

2. The E1/E4 Commands (Delete). These commands are used to delete a record, the E4 being used in multi-user mode. The record is physically removed from the DATA STORAGE area and all mention of it is removed from the ASSOCIATOR, including freeing the ISN. The space thus freed is immediately available for re-use.

If the user is operating in multi-user mode, and the record to be deleted is not in hold status, it will be placed in hold status for the user, unless it is in hold status for another user. In this case, the DELETE request is queued until the record becomes available. However, if the RETURN option is specified, control is returned to the user with a corresponding Response Code.

Unless the user is an ET logic user, the record will be released from hold status after successful completion of the command.

3. The N1/N2 Commands (Insert). These commands add a new record to an existing file. The FORMAT BUFFER specifies which fields are to be inserted,

and the RECORD BUFFER holds their values. All fields not specified will contain their default value.

If the N1 command is being used, ADABAS assigns the record an ISN, but if the N2 command is used, an ISN must be supplied. This is normally done when the USER ISN is in effect. Any necessary ASSOCIATOR updating is automatically executed. For ET logic users, operating in multi-user mode, the new records are placed in hold status.

6.4.1.9 Retrieval Commands

1. The S1/S2/S4 Commands (FIND). These commands are used to identify a set of records which satisfy given search criteria. The search criteria may consist of one or more DESCRIPTORS from a single file. A series of files may only be used if these files are COUPLED. The DESCRIPTORS must be connected with the logical operators shown in Fig. 6.4.1.9.

The result of any of these commands is a list of the addresses (ISN) of all records satisfying the criteria, and a field – the ISN–QUANTITY – containing a count of these records. The S1 and S4 commands result in an ISN list in ascending ISN sequence. The S2 command results in an ISN list sorted on the contents of up to three DESCRIPTOR fields, although not necessarily those DESCRIPTORS used for retrieval. Ascending or descending sequence may be specified in the COMMAND–ADDITION–2 field.

The various ways of processing the ISN List have already been dealt with earlier in the section under the heading 'The ISN Buffer'. If it is intended to process these records with the GET NEXT option of the L1/L4 commands, the ISN buffer is not required. ADABAS retrieves the records via the ISN List held on ADABAS WORK. If the record corresponding to the first entry in the ISN List is

OPERATOR	MEANING
D	AND
O	OR
S	TO
N	BUT NOT

Fig. 6.4.1.9: ADABAS QUERY Logical Operators

not to be retrieved by the FIND COMMAND, then the first non-blank character in the FORMAT BUFFER must be '.'.

The only difference between the S1 and the S4 commands is that the latter will place the first ISN of the ISN List in 'hold status'.

2. The S5 Command (FIND COUPLED). This command is used to retrieve all ISNs in one file which are COUPLED to a given record in another file. The record corresponding to the first ISN is not retrieved.

The FILE–NUMBER field must contain the number of the file to be searched and the ADDITIONS–1 field must contain the number of the file which contains the ISN held in the ISN field. This is the ISN of the record for which the COUPLED ISNs are to be returned. Here again, the ISN List can be returned to the user or managed by the system. This is described in this section under the heading 'The ISN Buffer'.

3. The S8 Command. This command performs logical processing on two ISN LISTs resulting from previous FIND commands, and which must be stored on ADABAS WORK. The lists must be in ascending ISN sequence, and their COMMAND–IDs must be placed in the ADDITIONS–1 field. ISN Lists resulting from S2 and S9 commands are not usually in ISN sequence. The ISN Lists should contain ISNs from the same file.

The following logical operations may be performed:

- AND. The resulting ISN List will contain only those ISNs present in both ISN Lists.
- OR. The resulting ISN List will contain all the ISNs from each ISN List.
- NOT. The resulting ISN List will contain those ISNs from the first list which do not appear in the second list.

The resulting ISN List is returned in ascending ISN sequence, and the number of entries appearing in it is returned in the ISN–QUANTITY field. The normal options are available for handling the resulting ISN List.

4. The S9 Command (SORT). This command causes a user-supplied ISN List to be sorted. The list to be sorted may be taken either from ADABAS WORK or from the ISN BUFFER. The list may be sorted on ISN in ascending sequence, or on one to three DESCRIPTORS. In the latter case, ascending or descending sequence may be specified in COMMAND–OPTION–2 field. The choice of ISN or DESCRIPTOR sort is specified in the ADDITIONS–1 field. All the normal options are available for processing the resulting ISN List.

5. The L1/L4 Commands (READ ISN). These commands retrieve a single record from DATA STORAGE. The file number and the ISN of the desired record must be specified in the FILE–NUMBER and ISN–NUMBER fields of the CONTROL BLOCK respectively.

The L1 and L4 commands have the same function, except that the latter also places the retrieved record in hold status. This action is only necessary in a multi-user environment, when the record is to be updated. If the record is already in hold status for another user, the user requesting the hold will be suspended until the record becomes free. However, if the L4 command was issued with the RETURN option, a RESPONSE–CODE of 145 is immediately returned to the user.

The GET NEXT option provides for the retrieving of records identified by the entries of an ISN List – which has been previously created by a FIND command. The user does not have to maintain position in the ISN List, and ADABAS automatically selects the next ISN and retrieves the corresponding record.

The READ ISN SEQUENCE option provides for the retrieving of a record identified by an ISN, but if the record is not present, ADABAS automatically retrieves the record with the next higher ISN.

6. The L2/L5 Commands (READ PHYSICAL SEQUENCE). These commands retrieve records from DATA STORAGE in the sequence that they are physically stored. The L5 command places the retrieved record in hold status.

Normally, the physical order of the records in a file bears little relationship to any logical order. There is a resequencing utility available which will order the logic sequence to the physical sequence for a particular DESCRIPTOR.

These commands allow the file to be processed at maximum speed because each physical access typically satisfies between 15 and 30 retrieval requests and no reference is made either to the ASSOCIATION NETWORK or to the ADDRESS CONVERTER.

If processing is to be started part-way through a file, this is achieved by placing the ISN of the record before the starting point in the ISN field.

7. The L3/L6 Commands (READ LOGICAL SEQUENCE). These commands retrieve records from a file in logically sequential order, based on the values of a specified DESCRIPTOR. The L6 command places the retrieved record in hold status. The user must specify the file to be read in the FILE–NUMBER field, and also the DESCRIPTOR to be used to control the retrieval sequence, (PHONETIC DESCRIPTORS, and those contained in or derived from PERIODIC GROUPS may not be used).

The VALUE START option allows processing to start retrieval with any DESCRIPTOR value. The option is specified by a 'V' in the COMMAND–OPTION–2 field. Normally, the first record (the lowest ISN) with the specified value is retrieved. This action can be modified by using the ISN field, then the first record containing the specified value with an ISN greater than that held in the ISN field is retrieved.

Resetting the last six bytes of the ADDITIONS–2 field to blank will cause the sequential processing to be broken off and restarted at the point indicated by the contents of the VALUE BUFFER.

8. The L9 Command (READ VALUES). This command enables the user to determine the range of values present for a DESCRIPTOR, and the number of records containing each value. Only the Inverted Lists are required to furnish this information.

The user must define the file and the DESCRIPTOR to be processed. The value of the DESCRIPTOR must also be specified. ADABAS returns the next value of the DESCRIPTOR in the RECORD BUFFER after each L9 command. The number of records containing the current value is returned in the ISN–QUANTITY field.

9. The LF Command (READ FIELD DESCRIPTION). This command retrieves field description entries from the FIELD DESCRIPTION TABLE. The user must specify the file number, and ADABAS returns the information in the RECORD BUFFER.

The following information is returned for each field:

– standard length and format
– definition options
– level number
– name

With this command it is possible to create FORMAT and SEARCH BUFFERS dynamically, by retrieving the standard length and format for a field during program execution.

6.4.2 ADAMINT

ADAMINT consists of Interface Definition Macros (IDMs) and the Data Manipulation Interface (DMI), or user interface. The DBA uses IDMs to generate the individual user interfaces dependent on the data elements and data manipulation functions required. The DMI, which is embedded in the user program, passes parameters to the interface module by means of a standard subroutine CALL.

The IDM USERVIEW defines the files required by the program and the relationships between the files. A USERVIEW may contain a single file or a linear hierarchy of up to 50 files. The USERVIEW together with the associated data selection, retrieval and manipulation functions, define the Access module. As only one USERVIEW can be defined in an Access module, it is often necessary to have a number of separate USERVIEWS – particularly if the overhead of Coupling files is to be avoided.

Each USERVIEW supports either a single or multi-file view; the multiple files can only be related in a 'linear hierarchical' fashion (see Fig. 6.4.2a.).

Although the structure in Fig. 6.4.2a (i) is valid in ADAMINT terms, it may produce somewhat unexpected results. If records exist in a finance file related to records in the personnel file, but no corresponding automobile file records exist, then the finance records will never be processed. Records from the automobile and finance files will be returned in ISN order. This may or may not be desirable.

In any hierarchy of two or more levels, unwanted records from the second (or lower) levels may be retrieved. For example, retrieving all persons in the personnel file with blue eyes who have red Minis (in the automobile file) may result in retrieving automobile records containing unwanted makes and colours. This is because the ADABAS FIND command identifies records only on the first level of the hierarchy, after which the FIND COUPLED commands will find records across all levels. Thus, people who own a red Mini may also own a blue Rolls-Royce. This latter record would have to be excluded from the processing by program logic.

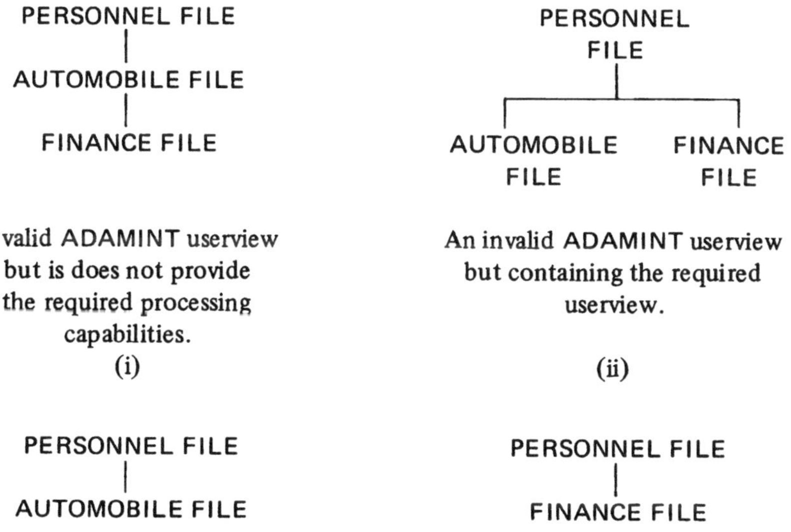

(i) A valid ADAMINT userview but is does not provide the required processing capabilities.

(ii) An invalid ADAMINT userview but containing the required userview.

(iii) A valid ADAMINT userview. It contains part of the required userview.

(iv) A valid ADAMINT userview. It contains part of the required userview.

Fig. 6.4.2a: Valid and Invalid ADAMINT Userviews

If more than one file is contained within a particular USERVIEW, then ADAMINT assumes the hierarchical data access method, and the files must be Coupled. Having two files Coupled, however, does not necessitate having both files in a USERVIEW. Even if the two Coupled files are used in the same application, they may be represented as two separate single file USERVIEWS.

6.4.2.1 Interface Definition Macro

The ADAMINT macros act in a similar manner to a high-level language compiler. The syntax of each macro parameter is analysed; code and an output listing are generated. Assembly language code is generated by the ADAMINT module generation process. It consists of a series of named common sections (CSECTS). The contents include:

- ADABAS control block data areas
- ADABAS buffers
- the ADABAS code necessary for each ADAMINT function.

The Access module definition control is accomplished with the AMPARMS, USERVIEW and GENERATE macros. The first describes the ADAMINT environment and is totally under the control of the DBA. The USERVIEW macro contains a list of the ADABAS file numbers, the sequence left to right indicating the hierarchical relationship.

The GENERATE macro is used simply to signal the end of macro processing.

The ADAMINT commands available to the DBA are listed in Fig. 6.4a, and an example of an Access module generation is shown in Fig. 6.4.2b. Also shown is the DMI (data manipulation interface) to this module to a COBOL program. Note that the labels in the Access module for each of the ADAMINT commands is the same as the name of the CALLED subroutine from the COBOL program.

6.4.2.2 Multiple ADAMINT Modules

ADAMINT offers a degree of simplification in the user interface when multiple USERVIEWS are required in a single program. This has the advantage that the programmer does not need to be aware of the ADABAS file structure.

These IDMs make what is called the ADAMINT 'Mult' module, which is capable of interfacing an application program to the SIGNON, SNAPINT and SIGNOFF commands. This results, for example, in multiple SIGNON commands being executed from a single CALL to the MULTOPEN subroutine. The 'Mult' module IDMs currently available are:

- MULTOPEN, multiple open (SIGNON)
- MULTSNAP, multiple snap (SNAPINT)
- MULTCLOS, multiple close (SIGNOFF)

```
//*    AN EXAMPLE OF AN ADAMINT MODULE CREATED FOR AN
//*    APPLICATION PROGRAM WHICH READS THE FIRST 100
//*    RECORDS OF A PERSONNEL FILE ONLY FIELDS AB TO DE
//*    (INCL') ARE TO BE RETRIEVED. COBOL FORTRAN AND
//*    PL/1 PROGRAMS MAY USE THIS ADAMINT MODULE
//*
//ASM           EXEC PGM=IEUASM,
//              PARM=(LIST,NOLOAD,DECK,XREF,TERM,NUM,STMT)
//SYSTERM       DD SYSOUT=A
//SYSPRINT      DD SYSOUT=A
//SYSLIB        DD DSN=SYS1.MACLIB, DISP=SHR
//              DD DSN=ADAMINT.V13.MAC, DISP=SHR
//SYSUT1        DD UNIT=(SYSDA,SEP=SYSLIB,SPACE=(CYL(5,5))
//SYSUT2        DD UNIT=(SYSDA,SEP=(SYSLIB,SYSUT1)),
//              SPACE=(CYL,(2,1))
//SYSUT3        DD UNIT=(SYSDA,SEP=(SYSLIB,SYSUT1)),
//              SPACE=(CYL,(2,1))
//SYSPUNCH      DD DSN=ADAMINT.V13.OBJ(TSTM01), DISP=SHR
//SYSIN         DD *
         AMPARMS CSNAME=TSTM01,PRINT=NOGEN
         USERVIEW 1
TSOP01   SIGNON
TSLK01   LOKATE SORTCN=NOTHING,READR=TSR01
TSRD01   SEQREAD (1, BA–DE, *98)
TSSN01   SNAPINT
TSCL01   SIGNOFF
         GENERATE
         END
//*  – AS THE FILE IS TO BE READ IN PHYSICAL SEQUENCE, THE
       LOKATE FUNCTION HAS SIMPLY TO FIND THE PHYSICALLY
       FIRST RECORD. THIS IS SPECIFIED BY SETTING THE 'KEY–
       VALUE' PARAMETER TO DUMMY.
     – THE ADAMINT FUNCTIONS WOULD BE CALLED
       IN THE FOLLOWING SEQUENCE. COBOL IS USED
       FOR ALL EXAMPLES

       CALL 'TSOP01' USING RUN–MODE RETURN–CODE.

       CALL 'TSLK01' USING KEY–VALUE RETURN–CODE.

       CALL 'TSRD01' USING RECORD–BUFFER RETURN–CODE.

       (should an error occur in the processing)
       CALL 'TSSN01'

       CALL 'TSCL01' USING RETURN–CODE.
```

Fig. 6.4.2b: ADAMINT Example

6.4.2.3 Data Manipulation Interface

This interface defines the syntax of the CALLS to the ADAMINT functions. The subroutine name in the CALL (the user-name) is predefined by the DBA at module creation time. It is the entry point, or label, coded in the corresponding ADAMINT function. Depending on the function being addressed, the number and meaning of the CALL parameters vary, but a Response-Code parameter must always be included. The other possible parameters are data-area, key-area and quantity-count.

6.4.2.4 Response Code Analysis

Response Code analysis is available in an ADAMINT subroutine. There are five different routines available:

1. RCANAL determines the 'cause' of the response's code; it is the standard subroutine.

2. ERSTAT returns four items of general information about the response code text, that is:

- total number of bytes for all response codes text
- maximum number of text lines used by any response code
- number of bytes in largest response code line
- number of bytes in smallest Response Code line.

3. MGSINF returns the text length of a specific response code text.

4. MSGUN retrieves the specific response code text.

5. ANALER retrieves class and cause statistics.

6.4.2.5 Retrieval of Fields From More Than One File

An ADABAS read command is limited to retrieving one record from one file. With a multifile hierarchical ADAMINT USERVIEW, data can be retrieved from all files using one ADAMINT CALL.

6.4.3 ADASCRIPT+

This is an interactive language which enables the user to interrogate and update the data, using English language commands. It can also be operated in batch mode. Standard ADABAS commands may also be used in an ADASCRIPT+ transaction. For complicated end user requirements, it is possible to give general predefined instruction sequences which can be executed within a transaction. Thus, programming personnel can make pretested routines available to the end user.

It is also possible to activate a stored query via a key text, eg.

WHERE DOES JOHN SMITH FROM DEPARTMENT 18 LIVE?
would activate a stored query in the form:
FIND PERSON WITH DEPARTMENT = 18 AND NAME = SMITH AND CHRISTIAN NAME = JOHN AND DISPLAY ADDRESS

An ADASCRIPT+ transaction can consist of up to 10 lines of up to 80 characters per line. Each ADASCRIPT+ user requires a separate copy of ADASCRIPT+ code.

The ADASCRIPT+ commands fall into three general groups:

1. The FIND command (see Fig. 6.4.3a)

2. The General Processing Commands (see Fig. 6.4.3b)

3. The Transaction Modification Commands. This group enables the user to modify and then execute a transaction.

- SHOW. This command causes a transaction to be displayed at the terminal
- CHANGE. This command enables the user to replace a line of a transaction. The user is required initially to type in sufficient of the line to enable ADASCRIPT+ to identify it, then the user must type in a replacement line.
- EXECUTE. This command starts the execution of a transaction.

```
FIND [ALL] [RECORDS] IN file name
      [AND COUPLED TO FILE file name ]
      [WITH search criteria AND . . . . .]
      [AND SORT THEM BY field name [field name field name]]
      [AND UPDATE WITH field name=value AND . . . . ]
      [AND DISPLAY IN FORMAT format specification]

   file name = internal file no. or external file name
   field name = internal or external field name
   format specification = field name [length] [format]
   search criteria = search criterion AND search criterion
   search criterion =

                          { EQ }           [ OR value   ]
      field name [NOT]  { { LT }   value   [ THRU value ] }
                          { GT }
```

Fig. 6.4.3a: The ADASCRIPT+ FIND Command Format

ACCEPT REJECT	record selection dependent on specified criteria
ACCUM	accumulation of a specified field's contents in all selected records
COMPUTE	arithmetic commands (+–x/)
CONTROL	automatic level–break processing
HISTOGRAM	listing of the distribution of the values of a DESCRIPTOR
IF	execution of commands dependent on specified criteria
PRINT	print predetermined fields from selected records
TITLE	headings for listing/reports
UPDATE	modify field contents in selected records

Fig. 6.4.3b: The ADASCRIPT+ General Commands

6.4.4 ADACOM

ADACOM is a batch mode report writer designed for the end-user with little or no EDP experience. Nevertheless, the language is sufficiently powerful to allow programming personnel the same flexibility as is available in high level languages, and with much less effort. In this respect, it has a number of features in common with BASIC. The user may reference several different ADABAS files in one request.

Prior to programming with ADACOM, the user must define a CNAMES module. This module contains synonym names, and attributes information for each ADABAS file and field to be referenced in the ADACOM request.

One of the most important aspects of the language is the processing loop. Contrary to most current programming languages, there is no 'branch' command, but instead a processing loop is introduced by one of the following commands: FIND, SORT, READ/BROWSE, CALL LOOP, CALL FILE. The commands which are to be processed repeatedly are all the commands which appear between the command introducing the loop and an AT END, AT BREAK, or END command. The number of repititions for a processing loop may be limited through the LT parameter of the SET GLOBALS command, or through the LIMIT command. Without the limit, the processing loop is dependent on the file being processed or on the program logic.

An example of a simple ADACOM request can clarify this processing loop concept and at the same time show how best an ADACOM request should be written. The concept of 'refer back' will also be introduced. Although statements can be assigned explicitly or implicitly with line number, the former method is recommended, since this avoids maintenance problems with refer-backs. It is also recommended to use one line per command, as in the example: List the first names and the car model and year of all people called STURDY.

```
0001FIND PERSONNEL WITH NAME = 'STURDY'
0005FIND CARS WITH OWNER–PERSONNEL–NUMBER =
0010PERSONNEL–NUMBER (0001)
0015DISPLAY FIRST–NAME (0001) MODEL COLOUR
0020END
```

This example functions as follows. All people in FILE 1 (PERSONNEL) named STURDY will be retrieved, and then records would be retrieved from FILE 2 (CARS), using the PERSONNEL–NUMBER from each of the retrieved records as a key. The resulting report would show the first-names (from FILE 1) and the model and colour from FILE 2. Since the fields PERSONNEL–NUMBER and FIRST–NAME appear in a previous file access initiated by the FIND in explicitly numbered statement 0001, the references number (0001) must be added to both these fields. MODEL and COLOUR are fields in the file being currently processed, and hence require no refer-back reference. If more than one FIND instructions were to be written on one line, then the refer-back reference would be ambiguous.

The ADACOM commands can be split into six functional groups:

- initialization commands
- record selection commands
- output commands
- processing control commands
- condition commands
- arithmetic/assign commands.

6.4.4.1 Initialization Commands

1. SET GLOBAL. This command allows the user to override default values assigned at system generation time. The values include:

- the number of characters per report line
- the number of lines per report page

– the number of active positions per input request line
– a loop processing limit (see LOOP command).

2. Password (PASSWORD). A password must be used to gain access to ADABAS files which have been password-protected using the SECURITY utility.

6.4.4.2 Record Selection Commands

1. The FIND Command. This command allows the user to select records from the ADABAS database. An ADACOM request may involve multiple FIND statements against the same or different files. The FIND command format is shown in Fig. 6.4.4a. The CYPHER clause is necessary when the file contents have been encrypted using the LOADER utility.

ADACOM recognises two types of search criteria, Basic and Extended. The former is limited to DESCRIPTOR fields ie. the query can be resolved using only the ASSOCIATION NETWORK, whereas the latter may search on any field type. The Extended Search Criterion, used in the WHERE clauses of the FIND and READ/BROWSE commands and in the IF and ACCEPT/REJECT commands, allows the three Boolean operators AND, OR and WHILE to connect the conditions.

ADACOM allows conditions in up to five Coupled files to be interrogated within one FIND command, although only data from the primary file is retrieved.

Two separate SORT facilities are available. The ADABAS sort is used via the SORT clause in the FIND command. This allows for sorting on up to three DESCRIPTORS in ascending sequence only. The second type of SORT is described in the SORT command.

2. The READ/BROWSE Commands. These commands enable the user to select a sequential range of records from a file. They may be retrieved in physical ISN or logical (ascending DESCRIPTOR value) sequence.

3. The ACCEPT/REJECT Commands. These commands are used to decide whether the processing should be continued or terminated. Because both statements use the Extended Search Criterion, it should be necessary for only one of these statements to appear in any processing loop. If a Limit has been specified, containing an ACCEPT/REJECT command, then all records processed are counted against this limit whether or not they are 'accepted' or 'rejected'.

4. The SORT Command. This command, the stand-alone SORT, invokes a post-election external sort. Any field or fields, DESCRIPTOR or otherwise, can be used to sort the records in ascending or descending sequence.

6.4.4.3 Output Commands

1. The FORMAT Command. This command causes all default values of output formats to be overridden in a single ADACOM request. It can also be used at the

```
FIND [ALL] [RECORDS] [IN] [FILE] filename [CIPHER= nnnnnnnn]
    { [WITH basic-search-criterial]
    { [AND COUPLED [TO] [FILE] filename      }
    {          WITH basic-search-criteria]   }
      [SORTED [BY] descriptor . . . . .]
      [WHERE extended-search-criteria]

basic-search-criteria
    basic-search-criterion [AND basic-search-criterion . . . .]
basic-search-criterion
    descriptor[(index)] operator expression
extended-search-criteria

    extended-    [ {  AND  }  extended- ]
    search-      [ {  OR   }  search-   ]
    criterion    [ { WHILE }  criterion ]

extended-search-criterion
    fieldname operator expression

              { EQ }
              { NE }
              { LT }
operator      { LE }
              { GT }
              { GE }

expression

    { constant  }  [ [OR=   { constant  } ]                                      ]
    {           }  [ [      { fieldname } ]                                      ]
    { fieldname }  [                                                             ]
                   [  THRU  { constant  }     BUT NOT { constant  }              ]
                   [        { fieldname }             { fieldname }              ]

fieldname
    - a database field name (cf CNAMES)
    - a user-defined temporary variable field
constant
    a numeric or literal constant
```

Fig. 6.4.4: The ADACOM FIND Command Format

single field level in conjunction with the DISPLAY, WRITE TITLE, and WRITE commands. The format entries that can be defined are:

- Line Size
- Page Size
- Maximum Number of Pages
- Spacing Factor
- Underlining Character
- Multiple Count
- Periodic Count
- Filler Count
- Header Centring Character (DISPLAY only)
- Leading Character (DISPLAY only)
- Insertion (floating) Character (DISPLAY only)
- Trailing Character (DISPLAY only)
- Alphanumeric Length
- Numeric Length.

2. The DISPLAY Command. This command specifies the output format to be produced for each processed record. Titles, heading and edit masks can also be included in this powerful command.

3. The WRITE Command. This command writes the output in free format allowing for line overflow by wrapping a report over multiple lines if the report width (line size) is exceeded.

4. The WRITE TITLE Command. This command overrides the default page title line which contains the page number (left-justified) and current data and time (right-justified).

5. The WRITE TRAILER Command. This command causes a line to be printed at the bottom of each page after the last line of the page has been printed.

6. The NEWPAGE Command. This command causes a page advance and the Page Count to be incremented.

7. The EJECT Command. This command can be used to suppress all page advancing, and can be used during testing to save paper.

8. The SKIP Command. This command causes blank lines to be produced when used in conjunction with the WRITE, WRITE TITLE and DISPLAY commands.

6.4.4.4 Control Commands

1. The LIMIT Command. This command limits the number of records processed in a loop, ie. when the limit is reached, an exit from the loop is effected. Any record entering the processing loop is counted against the limit even if it is rejected by the ACCEPT/REJECT command. However, only records which pass the WHERE clause will be counted against the limit.

This command is used in conjunction with FIND and READ/BROWSE commands to limit the number of records read.

2. The REDEFINE Command. This command restructures a numeric or alphanumeric field, which may be a database or user-defined variable field. The field may be separated into a number of fields or rearranged into a new field. This command can also be used to construct new fields for use in Basic and Extended Search Criteria.

3. The CALL Command. This command allows a program to pass control to another program or subroutine written in any language. A called program may contain ADABAS commands, as long as the files and fields referenced are in the CNAMES module.

4. The CALL LOOP Command. This command is used to repeatedly pass control to a user-written subroutine. The loop can only be exited via an ESCAPE command. A loop may contain any number of ESCAPE commands.

5. The CALL FILE Command. This command creates a processing loop and passes two parameter addresses to a user-written subroutine which reads a record and passes the whole record to the ADACOM request program.

6. The ESCAPE Command. This command terminates the execution of a loop which has been initiated by the CALL LOOP or CALL FILE commands.

7. The END Command. This command signals the end of an ADACOM request. A period may be used instead of an END command.

6.4.4.5 Condition Commands

1. The IF Command. This command conditionally controls the execution of a following group of commands, or directs processing to one of two groups of commands based on the Extended Search Criteria specified. Each group of commands is introduced by the DO key word and is terminated by the DOEND key word. No nesting of IF clauses is possible. The DO/DOEND construction is not needed if only one command instead of a group is to be executed.

2. The AT BREAK Command. This command causes a group of statements enclosed within a DO/DOEND construction to be executed when a level-break condition is reached.

3. The following four commands are similar and self-explanatory. A dependent group of commands delimited by the DO/DOEND key words is executed when the condition applies.

- AT START OF DATA
- AT END OF DATA
- AT TOP OF PAGE
- AT END OF PAGE

6.4.4.6 The Arithmetic/Assign Commands

1. The ASSIGN/MOVE Commands. These commands allocate values to existing or newly defined fields.

2. The Arithmetic Commands. The following commands are available for mathematical manipulation:

- ADD
- COMPUTE
- DIVIDE
- MULTIPLY
- SUBTRACT.

6.4.5 NATURAL

NATURAL offers many powerful features which should make it a very attractive tool for both programmers and end-users alike. Its full compatibility with ADACOM means that it is relatively easy to graduate from ADACOM to NATURAL.

The NATURAL features include:

- screen formatting which automatically does the necessary mapping to read screen fields into program variables
- storing and editing of NATURAL source programs from TP and batch
- full multi-file capability to support all ADABAS commands
- full support of ADABAS and intermediate fields as variables including data conversion from numeric to alphanumeric
- capability to defer on-line query to batch
- creation of multiple reports in one run
- enquiry, page and time limit options
- built-in performance measurement tools, giving differences in time from any point in the program execution
- powerful system standard functions for dates, times, maximum, minimum, average, count etc.
- access to system variables such as ISN, MF/PE counters
- using variables to index MF/PE fields
- full decimal arithmetic, including exponentation and square root
- creation of output files which can be reprocessed with other programs
- full floating point support for arithmetic and formatting facilities
- two dimensional array processing for non-ADABAS fields
- enhanced macro capability (similar to ADASCRIPT+)
- possibility to prompt the user of a pre-stored program to include additional source lines, (eg. search criteria or fields to be displayed) at execution time

– the full BASIC language as a subset of NATURAL
– support for the ET logic of ADABAS, including an automatic restart procedure.

6.5 Data Independence

The degree of data independence offered by ADABAS depends upon the language chosen to access the data. The standard access method (described in section 6.4.1 etc) offers the lesser degree of data independence. Even so, no competing system offers a higher degree of data independence, and most are markedly inferior.

The programmer is required to know only which files contain the fields of interest; their format, length and position are all of little or no interest to him, since program-oriented definitions can be made in the FORMAT BUFFER. The programmer is almost completely insulated from the way the data is physically stored and structured. The two limitations are: fields from only one file may be retrieved with one access; only DESCRIPTOR fields may be used as search criteria.

The ADABAS nucleus is first informed of the fields required by the application program in the CALL command, the binding of data therefore taking place at run time. Both fields and files may be added to the database, field characteristics may be changed, field positions may be changed (with the record type), new DESCRIPTORS defined, new COUPLING relationships added, all without impacting on existing programs.

The removal of DESCRIPTOR status from a field, or the removal of a COUPLING relationship, would only affect those programs using these particular characteristics of the fields involved. A program is always affected by the removal of a field from the record, but as this inevitably means a change in the logic, compilation is necessary anyway.

With ADAMINT, a much higher degree of data independence is achieved because the application program can retrieve fields from records in different files, with one CALL. Even if a restructuring of the files were to take place, only the ADAMINT interface module would have to be changed. This degree of data independence is bought at a high performance cost. The maintenance of the Inverted Lists is increased dramatically by the COUPLE FILES option.

6.6 Concurrent Usage

Version 4 of ADABAS is completely multithreading and is able to overlap any number of database commands. The 'number-of-threads' parameter determines how many threads are to be available for the session. Update commands cannot be overlapped with other update commands because of data protection and restart considerations. Multithread processing is completely transparent to the application program. The only visible results are improved response times.

The ADABAS nucleus can handle batch and on-line applications simultaneously. The nucleus, together with the buffer pool, is located in a separate region from the application programs. All application programs issue subroutine CALL commands to a linkage routine called ADABAS. The linkage routines communicate with the nucleus via a type 2 or 3 SVC.

The are a number of ADABAS session parameters which help co-ordinate the usage of resources in a multi-user environment.

1. User Non-Activity Time Limit. If an application program fails to issue an ADABAS command within this time limit, ADABAS will automatically issue a CL command for that user. If the user is using ET logic, the transaction will be backed out, prior to the CL command being issued.

2. Transaction Time Limit. If an ET logic application program exceeds the time limit, ADABAS will automatically back out the current transaction. This feature resolves the deadly embrace problem, and results in the automatic removal of partially completed transactions which have terminated abnormally.

3. File Cluster Synchronized Checkpointing. If File Cluster updating is to be performed during the session, the threshold limits to be used by ADABAS (to determine how often synchronized checkpoints are to be taken for each File Cluster) must be specified by the DBA. The threshold times specified are:

- minimum and maximum elapsed time since last synchronized checkpoint for the Cluster
- minimum and maximum number of updates processed for the Cluster since the last synchronized checkpoint.

4. Number of Threads. This parameter will determine the maximum number of ADABAS commands which may be overlapped. One thread is reserved for updating commands. Each thread defined requires ca. 4K.

6.7 Data Integrity Protection and Recovery

Data to be stored in the DATA STORAGE, whether as a result of a modify or insert command, will be checked to see that it is of the correct format etc. This is done by comparing the format with that held in the FIELD DESCRIPTION TABLE and, where necessary, with the contents of the FORMAT BUFFER.

As no structural data is made available to the application program, corruption from this quarter is impossible. Users wishing to modify the database are separated into two basic protection categories: transaction oriented (ET logic) users, and the rest. The basic data protection rule is that two or more users performing competitive updating (simultaneous updating of the same fields) must belong to the same data protection category. ET logic users need not necessarily be on-line applications.

ET logic users perform database updating based on the logical transaction concept. A logical transaction may consist of one or more ADABAS commands to one or more files, but the transaction represents the smallest logical unit to work.

A logical transaction begins with the first HOLD or ADD command, and ends with an ET (MINET) or CL (SIGNOFF) command. ET logic users must place each record to be modified in hold status. All database changes are held on the ADABAS WORK file, and all records which are either modified or inserted by the ET user in the current transaction are kept in hold status until the ET command is issued. At this time, the database changes are made permanent and all this user's records are released from hold status. Successful completion of an ET command guarantees that all database changes made during the transaction have been physically applied to the database. ADABAS returns to the user the transaction sequence number. The ET logic user should never use the RI (RELEASE) command as this can compromise the database integrity.

The ET (MINTET) command may store user data on an ADABAS log file. This information can be retrieved with an OP (SIGNON) or RE (READET) command. The primary purpose of generating ET data is to enable the user to subsequently identify the last successfully completed transaction. Other uses of ET data are to pass data from one on-line user to another, and also to establish a programmed checkpoint-restart capability for batch mode users.

Files being competitively updated by a group of users may be clustered for data protection and synchronization purposes. Files within a given Cluster may only be updated by users belonging to the cluster. File Clusters may not be updated by ET logic users. Each user updating the File Cluster must participate in synchronous checkpointing.

In the event of an abnormal termination during File Cluster updating, the BACKOUT CLUSTER function of the RESTART utility can be used to remove all updates performed subsequent to the last synchronized checkpoint. All cluster update programs may then be restarted at the last synchronized checkpoint. ADABAS automatically takes a synchronized checkpoint when a CL (SIGNOFF) command is issued by a cluster user. This prevents successfully completed cluster users from having to be restarted.

File Cluster users must place a record in hold status before updating it. The record is released from hold status after the user has updated or deleted it. Records are also released when the user issues a CL (SIGNOFF) command (a synchronized checkpoint is taken) or a Cluster user terminates abnormally.

A user may obtain exclusive control over a file for the purpose of preventing the other users from performing competitive updating to the file. This does not prevent other users from reading the file. Exclusive control users may, but do not have to, use ET logic. Non-ET logic exclusive control users performing updates may issue C1 (CHECKPOINT) commands which result in non-synchronized checkpoints.

In the event of an abnormal termination of an ADABAS session in which only ET logic users were updating the database, the new session may simply be restarted. AUTOBACKOUT will automatically backout all partially completed transactions. Each ET logic user may either reprocess the backed out transaction, or start a completely new one. AUTOBACKOUT uses data protection information maintained on ADABAS WORK and does not require the Data Protection Log or the RESTART utility nor does it require a TP Error Recovery data set. If all the updates made during a particular session are to be removed, then the BACKOUT function of the RESTART utility together with the Data Protection Log can achieve this end. ADABAS automatically takes a session initialization checkpoint which can be used for the BACKOUT checkpoint specification.

If, as a result of a catastrophic system failure, the physical integrity of the database has been compromised, the database can be reconstructed from a complete database copy created by the DUMP/RESTORE utility and the Data Protection Log, using the REGENERATE function of the RESTART utility. It is not possible to apply updates selectively with this utility. Furthermore, it is impossible to remove/regenerate updates for a particular ET user if competitive updating with other ET users was in effect during the session.

In the event of an abnormal termination of a Cluster user ADABAS session during file cluster updating, ADABAS will terminate all updating of the File Cluster automatically, each Cluster user will reveive a Response Code to this effect, and then each Cluster user will be closed by ADABAS. The operator is also notified that the File Cluster updating terminated abnormally.

Following a user- or ADABAS-session abnormal termination in which file cluster updating was in effect, the normal procedure is to execute the BACKOUT CLUSTER function of the RESTART utility. This function removes all updates made subsequent to the last synchronized checkpoint for the File Cluster. All Cluster update programs may be started at the first command which was processed subsequent to the last synchronized checkpoint.

Should it be necessary to remove updates applied prior to the last synchronized checkpoint, the BACKOUT function of the RESTART utility may be used. The synchronized checkpoint must be specified as must the files in the Cluster. The log file will be required for this and the previous case.

If exclusive updating was in effect at the time of a user or ADABAS session termination, then the BACKOUT function of the RESTART utility must be executed for each exclusive update user. If CHECKPOINT commands were used, the BACKOUT can be to the last successful checkpoint issued; otherwise, the BACKOUT must be to the beginning of the user program. ADABAS automatically issues a non-synchronized checkpoint at the beginning of each update program, operating in exclusive mode.

ADABAS records BEFORE and AFTER images of all records changed during the course of a session on the DATA PROTECTION FILE which can be either a disc or tape file. The changes are recorded in internal compressed form at the record, not block level. The DUMP/RESTORE utility can copy either individual files or the whole database for backup purposes.

Deadly embrace is automatically resolved by ADABAS by the simple expedient of a transaction duration time limit. The time starts when the first record is placed in hold status and ends when an ET, BT or CL command is issued. As soon as the time limit is exceeded, ADABAS automatically generates a BACKOUT TRANSACTION (BT) command. This results in all the updates made during the current transaction being removed, and all of the user's records in hold status being released. The user is informed that the transaction has been backed out; it may now be repeated, or a completely new one may be started. This transaction duration time limit applies only to programs employing Transaction Logic. The time limit may be set by the DBA at the start of each ADABAS session.

All users are subject to a non-activity time limit. Different time limits may be defined for each user type:

For a Transaction (ET) Logic user, a BACKOUT TRANSACTION command is issued, if necessary, which releases all resources held by the user. The next command issued by the user will not be executed and a Response Code of '9' will be returned to indicate what has happened.

For File Cluster users, ADABAS suspends all updating of the Cluster, returns a non-zero Response Code to each active Cluster user, initiates AUTO–CLUSTER–BACKOUT for the Cluster, and this results in the Cluster being returned to the conditions when the last synchronized checkpoint was taken. The operator is informed of the jobs which were abnormally terminated, and they may be restarted at that point in processing which pertained at the time the synchronized checkpoint was taken.

Exclusive File Control users simply lose exclusive control.

6.8 Access Control

Although it is possible to protect user data from unauthorized access and update at the field, file, database and/or dataset levels, it is not mandatory to do so on non-sensitive data.

6.8.1 File Level Protection

Each file can be assigned a password, and each command accessing a security protected file must specify a valid password. This is in addition to specifying a password when the OP command is issued. Not all classes of user are required to issue the OP command, but it is good programming practice to do so.

6.8.2 Field Level Protection

A pair of Permission Levels are assigned to each password for each associated file, one for retrieval and one for update. Permission Levels can be assigned in a range 0–14. Each field in a file has a pair of Security Levels assigned to it, one for retrieval and one for update. Security levels can be assigned in a range 0–15. A command is not executed if the Permission Level is lower than the Security Level.

Field level security can also be provided by the FORMAT BUFFER. This method is normally not so easy to control, although with ADAMINT this reservation does not apply.

A further security measure available is based on one or more field values. Security by Value usage results in the determination by ADABAS of the validity of a user FIND, READ or UPDATE command based on the value content of one or more fields in the record(s) involved. The specific values associated with each password must be specified together with the combination of criteria which must apply before allowing the various commands to be executed.

6.8.3 Data Set Level Protection

Protecting a database via passwords is of course only a protection when the databases are accessed via ADABAS. Dumping the data sets used to store the database is completely unprotected. DATA STORAGE is in compressed form and cannot therefore be read easily. Nevertheless, it presents no great obstacle to a determined attempt to read it. In order to prevent this, ADABAS enables the DBA to cypher-protect files.

Users retrieving encyphered records without quoting the 8 digit cypher key are simply presented with the encyphered record itself. When adding records to a encyphered file, the cypher code must be specified. An audit trail can be optionally produced for each ADABAS session which contains such information as which programs issued which commands and which commands resulted in which Response Codes.

Transaction-oriented processing also uses a form of access control. A user's updated records are held on ADABAS WORK until the transaction is completed. All a user's updated records are kept in hold status until the transaction has completed. When that transaction completes, the changes to the database are copied from the ADABAS WORK to the DATA PROTECTION LOG and the hold status is released for all the user's updated records.

6.9 Performance

ADABAS, being based on inverted lists, naturally excels at resolving complex queries, without reference to primary data. The number of physical accesses required to retrieve a record (using one DESCRIPTOR) is dependent on the size of the DESCRIPTOR and the number of DESCRIPTOR values. These two parameters determine the number of index levels. An average value is between 3 and 4 accesses; this is largely dependent on the size of the buffers. Resolution of complex queries will require correspondingly more physical accesses. If the required block is already in the buffer, an access is saved. In this way, ADABAS's performance is sensitive to buffer size.

If the DESCRIPTORS are unique then the new direct access method ADAM should be considered, as this can in general retrieve a record with one access. However, this depends on the density of records in the file, because ADAM cannot retrieve a record which is not stored in the calculated block, which can occur when this block is full. When the ADAM access does not find the required record, the standard Inverted List must be used. This, of course, requires one extra access, over and above standard methods. This means that ADAM (and its occasional reference via the Inverted Lists) is superior to the standard method (using solely the Inverted Lists) unless 80% of the records are not to be found in their home blocks (assuming 4 physical accesses for the standard access method).

Data compression is used both for the Data Protection Log and the DATA STORAGE. On average, the original data can be compressed to between 20% and 60% of its original size. This means that an I/O transfer moves on average roughly twice the data of a system not using compression. Moreover, for the same buffer size, it is at least twice as likely that the required data is in the buffer as with a DBMS which does not use compression.

Naturally, there is a small overhead, because when a record is inserted it must be compressed, and when it is retrieved it must be expanded. The latter can be kept to a minimum because ADABAS expands only those fields which are requested in the FORMAT BUFFER. In the interests of efficient processing, therefore, only those fields which are required should be retrieved.

It is possible, because ADABAS does not check, for a compressed file to be larger than the uncompressed size. If this happens, the DBA should specify that the fields should not be compressed. This is, however, an exceptional case, and normally the Inverted Lists and the DATA STORAGE together occupy less space than the original file.

COUPLING TABLES can be created to link a common DESCRIPTOR in two files. COUPLING TABLES consist of two extra Inverted Lists. They offer the user the chance of resolving a query spanning the two COUPLED files in one standard DML FIND command. The query could still be resolved with the standard DML, without COUPLING TABLES, but would need program logic and a series of standard DML commands.

The great disadvantage with COUPLING TABLES is that they have to be maintained whenever the common DESCRIPTOR is modified in a record occurrence in either file. It is therefore recommended that COUPLING should not be used, or used very sparingly, when DESCRIPTOR values are constantly being modified.

The ADABAS standard DML is somewhat complicated to learn initially, principally because of the terseness of the commands and the variety of options available with some of the commands. As with most DMLs, the programmer is able to learn a subset of the DML initially, and then the more complicated options as the necessity arises. The greatest problem when examining any DML is to judge the amount of support offered to the programmer: a very simple DML can require far more supporting code than a more complex one. The ADABAS standard DML offers the programmer a high order of flexible support, particularly in manipulating ISN lists from FIND commands under system control. This feature is especially useful for on-line applications where paging backwards and forwards is required.

The READ and UPDATE commands require a FORMAT BUFFER specifying the fields to be operated on. The contents of the FORMAT BUFFER must be converted into an internal FORMAT BUFFER. A non-zero non-blank COMMAND–ID may be used to avoid repetitive interpretation and conversion during a series of commands all using the same FORMAT BUFFER. Any READ or UPDATE command containing a valid COMMAND–ID causes ADABAS to scan the Internal Format Buffer Pool for this value. If it is found, no FORMAT BUFFER interpretation and conversion is necessary, thus achieving a significant decrease in processing time.

From a performance point of view, the Address Converter can be a great disadvantage. It is used to save having to update all the Inverted Lists in a multi-DESCRIPTOR environment when, due to record expansion, a record changes block. Nevertheless, all records which have not been updated and even those which have (but where sufficient space was available in the block) require an extra and unnecessary retrieval access for the Address Converter block. In a file where one or more of the following apply, the Address Converter is simply a disadvantage:

- a single non-unique DESCRIPTOR is used
- the file contains no compressed fields
- no updates will change the length of the records.

Even while it is recognised that these constitute only a small percentage of the total number of applications, in any case, the vast majority of applications only require an Address Converter for migrated records as explained above.

An alternative would be to use a pointer in the block from which the record was moved to where it was stored, which would mean that only those records which had actually changed block would need the extra access. In the worst case, where every record had changed block, the implicit Address Converter would contain as many entries as the normal ADABAS Address Converter. Even if a record had to change block a second time (or more), the pointer in the original block would point directly to the block currently holding the object record. This would not cause any extra accessing, because the record can only be accessed via the pointer in its original block, so this block is always in the I/O buffer when needed. The ideal solution would be to allow the DBA to decide whether an explicit of implicit Address Converter should be used with each file.

A similar situation arises with DESCRIPTORS. If an application requires a primary key or even if only a single key is necessary, then it would be advantageous if the DBA was able to define whether space management was to attempt to keep the data records in a specified order or not.

I realise that the nature of the criticisms departs radically from the original concepts of ADABAS. Nevertheless, the incorporation of such departures from the original partially inverted file concept would be no more radical than the recent inclusion of the direct access method ADAM.

6.10 Conclusion

ADABAS and its associated products offer the user the most comprehensive set of tools for data management available anywhere. Coupled to this, ADABAS with its new direct access method ADAM, can be used effectively in any environment, making the system a leading contender, if not the leading contender, in any DBMS selection.

ADABAS is conceptually the simplest DBMS examined, but nonetheless – or perhaps because of this – it offers the user processing power and flexibility second to none. The inherent simplicity of the system means that both the DBA and programming functions can concentrate on solving user problems, not on maintenance and manipulation of the database. This leads to a lower level of manning, particularly in the DBA function, in comparison with some competing products, but without any corresponding increase in the responsibility or workload of the programming function.

The end-user languages ADASCRIPT+ and ADACOM make ADABAS databases available to non-programming staff to produce adhoc queries and reports. This helps alleviate the time delay and bottleneck of having all processing against the database implemented by professional programming staff.

ADAMINT, the high level DML interface, offers programmers the opportunity of accessing an ADABAS database without having to be involved with the different buffers.

ADABAS offers each class of potential user a powerful tool with which to access and manipulate the database. Experience has shown that most users find the ADABAS DMLs and end-user languages relatively simple to learn and use. This is perhaps best borne out by the manufactures's offer of a three day demonstration of ADABAS, during which a program and its associated files will be converted to ADABAS. This shows another adavantage of the system, namely that it is extremely simple to convert running applications.

Two unusual features of ADABAS which are not found in most of the competing products are the phonetic DESCRIPTOR used to retrieve like-'sounding' values, and the file cyphering facility to protect the information from unauthorized access. These features indicate the thoroughness with which ADABAS was designed, that is as a system which can express general network structures of the type m:n and also hierarchical structures of the type 1:n. Complete separation of user and internal relationship data leading to excellent data integrity and simple recovery; a data organisation which does not in general require reorganisation; data compression leading to very flexible record design and a minimum of secondary and buffer storage usage: all these characteristics show that ADABAS is not a DBMS of great strengths and weaknesses, but a DBMS incorporating almost all the worthwhile features required, with most of them having been optimally implemented.

6.11 Advantages of ADABAS

- No primary key has to be defined, thus reorganisation is not required unless very efficient sequential processing on a particular key is required.
- All key field types may be updated.
- No key has to have unique values, but a key can be defined as having unique values, thus both 1:M and M:N relationships can be generated.
- Direct access for fast response real-time applications.
- Synchronized DB/DC checkpoints.
- Multithreading nucleus.
- Integrated DB/DC using the TP Monitor (COM–PLETE).
- Data Dictionary available.
- On-line query/update language (ADASCRIPT+); it can also be used in batch mode.
- Batch report writer (ADACOM).
- Self-contained language (NATURAL) which enables the user to develop both batch and online programs interactively. It requires less that half the coding effort for the same results compared to COBOL.
- Both LOGICAL and PHYSICAL sequential retrieval possible.
- The application programs can write messages to a system file and retrieve them.
- Security violation audit facilities.
- Training costs lower than with most other leading DBMSs; the training course costs are included in the purchase price.
- The most powerful, flexible and concise (perhaps too concise) DML commands of any of the DBMSs examined.
- Simplicity and ease of database design.
- Interfaces – see Appendix III.
- Password security at the field level, with different security levels for access and modification.
- Direct Access using ADAM (ADABAS Direct Access Method).
- A phonetic key can be generated, allowing retrieval of like-'sounding' values eg. Smythe and Smith. Two separate routines are available, one for English and one for German.
- Good data independence; the fields in the user-view may have different lengths and formats. The order may differ from that in the original record, and text (and blanks) may be inserted between the fields as they are retrieved.
- Data Compression reduces the user data file on average to less that half its original length. The compression routine packs all numeric fields and removes leading zeroes and trailing blanks on a field basis. Compression on a field basis has the advantage over string compression because only those fields requested

via the FORMAT BUFFER have to be decompressed, saving enormously on CPU time.
- Full transaction oriented processing with the control over what constitutes a transaction in the hands of the user.
- It also runs on DEC PDP–11 computers.
- Backward and forward paging for TP applications is possible without having to retrieve and manage the pointers within the program using the ISN LIST option.
- ADAMINT offers exceptionally good data independence – the user is no longer even aware of the file from which the data comes but this is achieved at a high performance cost because of the FILE–COUPLING feature.
- Automatic warm restart.
- Superb complex query resolution facilities.
- The FIND command results in a list of the addresses of all records satisfying the search criteria and a count of how many records were 'found'. It is possible to sort the resulting ISN LIST on up to three key fields – not necessarily those used in the search criteria. The FIND command can also optionally retrieve the record whose address is at the top of the ISN LIST.
- A new Inverted List can be created without even taking the file off-line.
- Good documentation, but the printing could be improved.
- A comprehensive set of utilities is offered as part of the basic package.
- The READ DESCRIPTOR VALUE command permits histograms to be easily constructed.
- Clear separation of user data from internal data helps with data security.
- The data encryption option offers extremely good external data security.
- Security by value capability checks on the validity of a retrieval or modification command based on the contents of one or more fields. (An application for this would be to protect salaries above a certain amount from general access).
- A Bill of Materials Processor package.
- Checkpoints can be written from the program.
- Backing store of ca. 2MB (excluding ASSOCIATOR)
- Easy to install and maintain.
- Data inserted into the database is subjected to a format check via the FORMAT BUFFER or by default via the FIELD DESCRIPTION TABLE.
- Loading the database can be done with a utility.
- Only that record in a block that has been modified is written to the log file (in compressed form).
- Many utilties can be run while the database is on-line.
- Dual logging is available on either disc or tape.
- Utilities for mass updating and deleting.

6.12 Disadvantages of ADABAS

- It is not possible to define a primary key such that the record placement strategy would try to maintain the order of the file based on the contents of this field.
- The use of the Coupling feature has a negative effect on performance.
- High initial cost – training is included in the price. Multicopy discount is available.
- Address Converter (see Appendix II – General Glossary).
- Deadly embrace resolution is time controlled.
- The use of ADAM in a situation where many requests result in a 'not found' status should be avoided because of the excess I/O caused by the use of both the ADAM and standard Access Methods. If ADAM files become too full (over 80%) then the performance will degrade because the number of records not located in their home block increases dramatically and they can only be retrieved via the standard access method (after ADAM has failed to locate the record) – again excessive I/O.
- The ADAMINT user-view is only capable of displaying a 'linear hierarchy'. This often results in multiple user-views being necessary.
- Multi-file User-views with ADAMINT have a negative affect on performance because the files must use the ADABAS Coupling feature.
- The update command is only single-threaded.

6.13 ADABAS Glossary

ADABOMP: A separate Software AG product based on ADABAS for 'Bill of Materials' processing.

ADACOM: A batch report generator.

ADAM: The new ADABAS DIRECT ACCESS METHOD, which operates only on unique DESCRIPTORS.

ADASCRIPT+: An on-line query language that can also be used in batch mode.

ADAWRITER: A batch report generator replaced by ADACOM.

ADDRESS CONVERTER: A linear file containing the relative addresses of the blocks in DATA STORAGE. This file is indexed by the ISN, thus translating it into a physical block address.

ASSOCIATOR: This database component contains the physical space allocation (STORAGE MANAGEMENT TABLES), the ADDRESS CONVERTER, the Inverted Lists for each file (ASSOCIATION NETWORK) and the field definitions for each type (FIELD DEFINITION TABLE).

BASIC SEARCH CRITERIA: An ADACOM term, indicating those search functions which are available via the ADABAS nucleus, ie. limited to DESCRIPTOR fields.

COUPLED FILE: see FILE COUPLING.

DATA CYPHERING: This relates to the storing of information in cyphered form, thus making the data unreadable even when printed directly from external storage. Only with the correct cypher code can the record be retrieved with meaningful information.

DATABASE: An ADABAS database consists of up to 255 logical files which are physically encompassed by the components ASSOCIATOR, DATA STORAGE and WORK.

DATA PROTECTION FILE: A log file held on either discor tape.

DATA STORAGE: This database component contains the compressed user records. Each record is prefixed with its ISN.

DESCRIPTOR: A key field. For each key type, an Inverted List is created, and maintained by ADABAS. DESCRIPTOR fields may be defined as holding unique or duplicate values. (ADAM DESCRIPTORS must be unique). DESCRIPTOR fields may be derived from an ELEMENTARY FIELD, MULTIPLE VALUE FIELD occurrence, a PERIODIC GROUP, a portion of an ELEMENTARY FIELD (SUBDESCRIPTOR), or a combination of several fields or portions of fields (SUPERDESCRIPTORS).

ELEMENTARY FIELD: The basic unit of information within an ADABAS database, having only one value per record occurrence.

EXTENDED SEARCH CRITERIA:	An ADACOM term, indicating that non-DESCRIPTOR fields may be included in the search. This means that the records must be retrieved before the search criteria can be satisfied.
FIELD DEFINITION TABLE:	see ASSOCIATOR
FILE:	An ADABAS file consists of a collection of logically related records all having the same structure. The records are stored in compressed form in DATA STORAGE.
FILE–COUPLING:	This is a means of physically representing the relationship between two files by establishing Coupled Lists based on a common DESCRIPTOR. The Coupled Lists are maintained by ADABAS.
GROUP FIELD:	This consists of one or more consecutive ELEMENTARY or MULTIPLE VALUE FIELDS. GROUP FIELDS offer a convenient and efficient method of referencing a series of fields. A GROUP may be contained within another GROUP. A hierarchy of up to seven levels may be generated.
ISN:	Each logical record is assigned an Internal Sequence Number (ISN) which serves as a logical identifier for the record. ISNs must be unique within a file and may be assigned either by ADABAS or the user.
LOGICAL RECORD:	This is a collection of logically related fields stored together.
MULTIPLE VALUE FIELD:	This is an ELEMENTARY FIELD which may contain up to 191 occurrences.
NATURAL:	This is an on-line and batch communication language fully compatible with ADABAS.
NULL VALUE SUPPRESSION:	If a DESCRIPTOR field is specified with this option, no entries will be made in the Inverted Lists for null value entries. All numeric fields

containing zeroes and alphanumeric fields containing blanks, which are assigned. NULL VALUE SUPPRESSION are treated as empty fields.

PERIODIC GROUP: This is a GROUP FIELD which may occur up to 99 times within a record occurrence. A PERIODIC GROUP may not contain another PERIODIC GROUP.

PHONETIC DESCRIPTOR: This is used to select a field on phonetic value, rather than on the exact contents of the field. The phonetic value consists of a 3-byte binary number derived from the first 20 bytes of each field value. Numeric values and special characters are ignored.

WORK: The WORK file (see ASSOCIATOR) is used by the nucleus to store data protection information and ISN Lists resulting from FIND commands.

7. IDMS (Integrated Database Management System)

IDMS was originally developed in 1971 by B.F. Goodrich Chemical Company to support their distribution billing and accounting applications. The commercial possibilities were soon realised by the company, but they felt they were in no position to offer the necessary support. It was therfore decided to sell the product. In September 1973, the Cullinane Corporation puchased the marketing and development rights to IDMS. Early in 1975, SCICON were given the UK marketing rights for the IBM 360/370 range, ICL bought the rights to IDMS for their computers and developed a separate version of IDMS for the 2900, which they market world-wide, as have UNIVAC for their 1100 and 90 series. ADV-Orga of West Germany hold the marketing rights for most of the German-speaking countries of Western Europe.

ADV-Orga have developed an IDMS version to run on the Siemens 4004 series, and its successor the UNIDATA/Siemens 7000 series.

IBM is the only major main-frame manufacturer not to offer a CODASYL-based DBMS. This gap has been filled by two developments: SIBAS and IDMS. The latter is by far the more successful.

The main advantage of the CODASYL DBMS is that the user interface remains the same irrespective of the hardware supporting the system. This protects the investment made in currently running applications and EDP training. This advantage is somewhat negated by the dramatic changes proposed in the 1978 CODASYL DBTG report.

While there is no necessity for IDMS to implement the 1978 recommendations, failure to do so would seriously detract from IDMS's portability, with a consequent negative impact on sales. On the other hand, current users will have a large amount of rewriting to do to upgrade their IDMS applications should the new recommendations be implemented.

This report examines the IBM 360/370 version. The comments may or may not apply to other versions. The newly announced PDP–11 version will almost certainly not contain all the functions of the main-frame version.

IDMS has been interfaced to the following TP monitors:

- SHADOW II
- CICS
- TASK/MASTER
- INTERCOM
- WESTI
- ENVIRON/1.

A few years ago, the Cullinane Corporation entered into an agreement with Altergo to market SHADOW II in North America. This would have obviated the necessity for Cullinane to develop their own TP monitor. However, about a year later, the agreement was nullified. Altergo set up their own marketing organisation in North America and Cullinane developed their own TP monitor IDMS–DC, which is fully integrated with IDMS–DB.

A Cullinane product, CULPRIT, a generalised report generator, has been interfaced to IDMS. The other two supporting software products required by any successful DBMS – a query language and a data dictionary – have both recently been introduced by Cullinane. They are both rather primitive when compared to the leading products in their respective fields. Nevertheless, it can be expected that they will be further developed over the next few years until they reach the high standard set by IDMS itself.

B.F. Goodrich has stated publicly that their agreement with Cullinane specifies that IDMS will only be developed in line with CODASYL ideals. This does not, however, mean that Cullinane must implement the whole of the 1978 CODASYL DBTG recommendations, merely that any extensions which are made will be in keeping with CODASYL recommendations. All these extensions have in any case to be agreed between Cullinane and representatives of the current users.

7.1 Classification

IDMS is a host language system using a preprocessor to produce a COBOL, FORTRAN, Assembler or PL/1 source program.

All other computer languages that contain a 'CALL' statement can also access an IDMS database.

IDMS is a pointer-based system, capable of implementing both hierarchies and networks. The pointer information is held within the record itself, but it is never made available to the user. The pointer contains a physical block address.

The network structures of IDMS are based on CODASYL SET relationships. A set consists of an OWNER record type and one or more MEMBER record types. The rules for relating OWNERS to MEMBERS are as follows:

- a set may have only one OWNER type record,
- a record type cannot be both OWNER and MEMBER in the same set,
- a set may contain multiple record types as MEMBERS,
- records may be OWNERS and MEMBERS in an unlimited number of different sets.

There are two main languages within IDMS: the DDL (Data Definition Language) and the DML (Data Manipulation Language). The DDL consists of three compilers: the schema compiler; the subschema compiler (see 7.5. Data Independence); and the DMCL (Device/Media Control Language) which is used to map the schema – the logical structure – onto physical storage.

7.2 Data Definitions (including Set and Pointer Definitions)

Data ITEM definitions are based on ANS COBOL. (For a detailed treatment of this subject, refer to the ITEM description in the IDMS 'Database Design and Definition Guide'.)

The LEVEL NUMBER must be the first entry in the ITEM description, immediately followed by the 'item-name'. The remaining entries can follow in any order.

- LEVEL NUMBER is an unsigned integer in the range 02–49 or 88, allowing logical relationships to be defined between ITEMs. 01 level is generated by the system with the record name.
- ITEM–NAME is up to 32 characters long, and should be unique
- REDEFINES clause enables a previously defined ITEM's representation in storage to be changed
- PICTURE clause describes the characteristics of the ITEM
- USAGE clause describes the way an ITEM is held in storage. The options are: DISPLAY, BINARY, LONG or SHORT PRECISION FLOATING POINT, PACKED DECIMAL.
- VALUE clause assigns an initial value to the ITEM
- SYNCHRONIZED clause is treated as comment by the SCHEMA DDL processor
- OCCURS clause is used to define repeating groups or ITEMS, between 2 and 9999 being permissible
- INDEXED clause is related to the OCCURS clause
- COMMENT clause is used to enter the text for inclusion in the data dictionary.

There is no limit to the number of ITEMS that can be defined within a logical record.

The logical record is itself described by five parameters in the RECORD DESCRIPTION:

- RECORD NAME is used to identify the record type uniquely within the SCHEMA. It can consist of up to 16 alphanumeric characters (a maximum of 8 characters are allowed for Assembler synonyms.)
- RECORD ID is a number between 100 and 9999 which may be used by the DBA to identify a record type within the SCHEMA. The RECORD IDs 1–99 are reserved for internal use within IDMS.

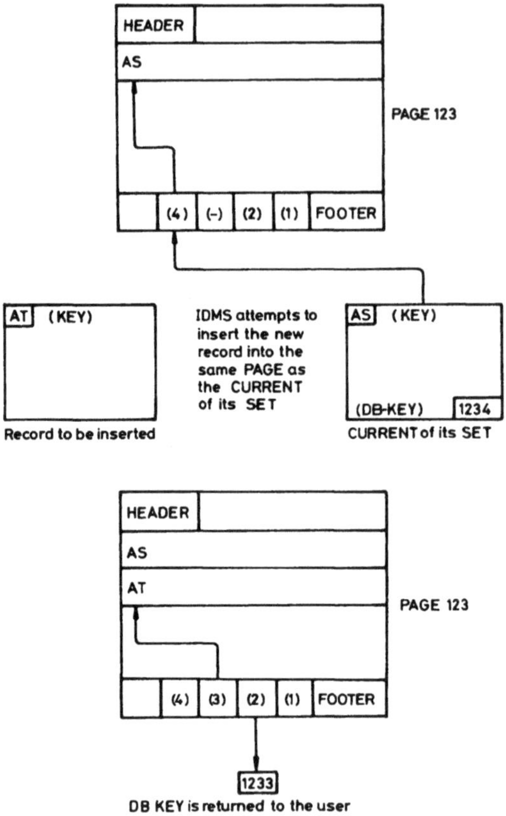

Fig. 7.2a: Storage Using LOCATION MODE 'VIA CURRENT of SET'

- WITHIN. This option allows the DBA to specify an AREA of the SCHEMA within which the record occurrence should be stored. A range of PAGES may also be specified.
- LOCATION MODE is the mechanism which allows the DBA to control the way the record occurrences are stored within the database. The efficiency of the database design will depend on the competence of the DBA in using this parameter. Three options are available:

  (1) CALC (RANDOM) is a placement method whereby a specified ITEM within the record occurrence is subjected to a hashing algorithm which produces a PAGE address. DUPLICATE ITEM values can be either allowed or disallowed (see Fig. 7.2b).

  (2) DIRECT. IDMS allocates a unique DATABASE KEY to every record stored within the database. With the DIRECT mode, it is possible for the user

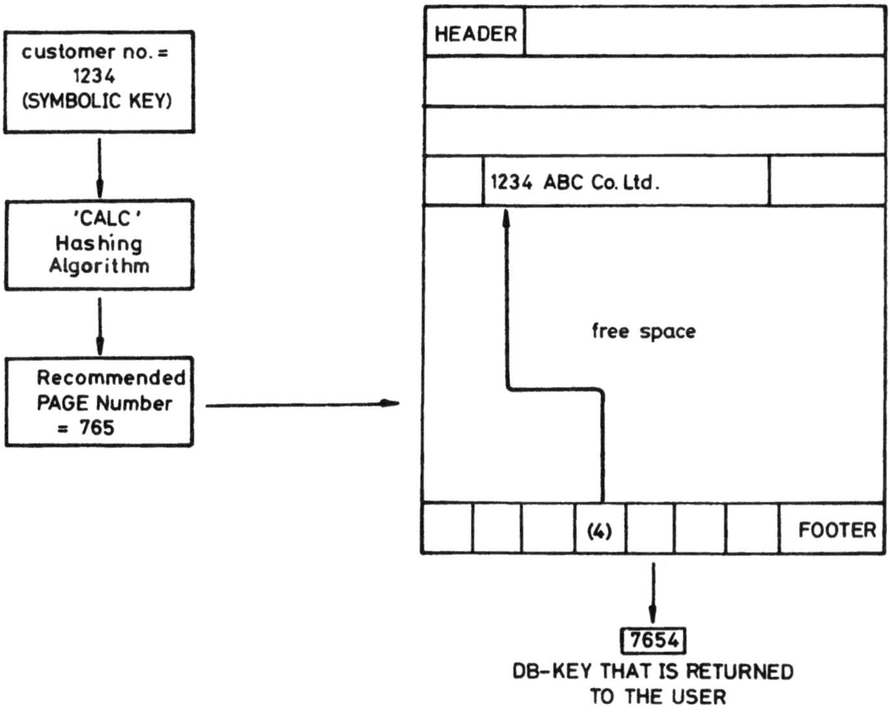

Fig. 7.2b: Storage Using CALC LOCATION MODE

to recommend a PAGE number to be allocated to the record on its being stored into the database. If this key has already been allocated, then IDMS will allocate the next available PAGE number to the record occurrence (see Fig. 7.2c).

(3) VIA. This placement mode allows record occurrences to be placed physically close to each other, eg. all MEMBER occurrences of a SET occurrence to be placed in the same PAGE (or an adjacent PAGE), so minimising the disc accesses for processing these records (see Fig. 7.2a).

(4) INDEXED SPF assigns a PAGE number to a record occurrence.

7.3 Data Storage Structures

7.3.1 Physical Representation

An IDMS database is held on direct storage and is accessed using BDAM (under DOS–DAM). Relative block BDAM addressing is used with IDMS, providing the

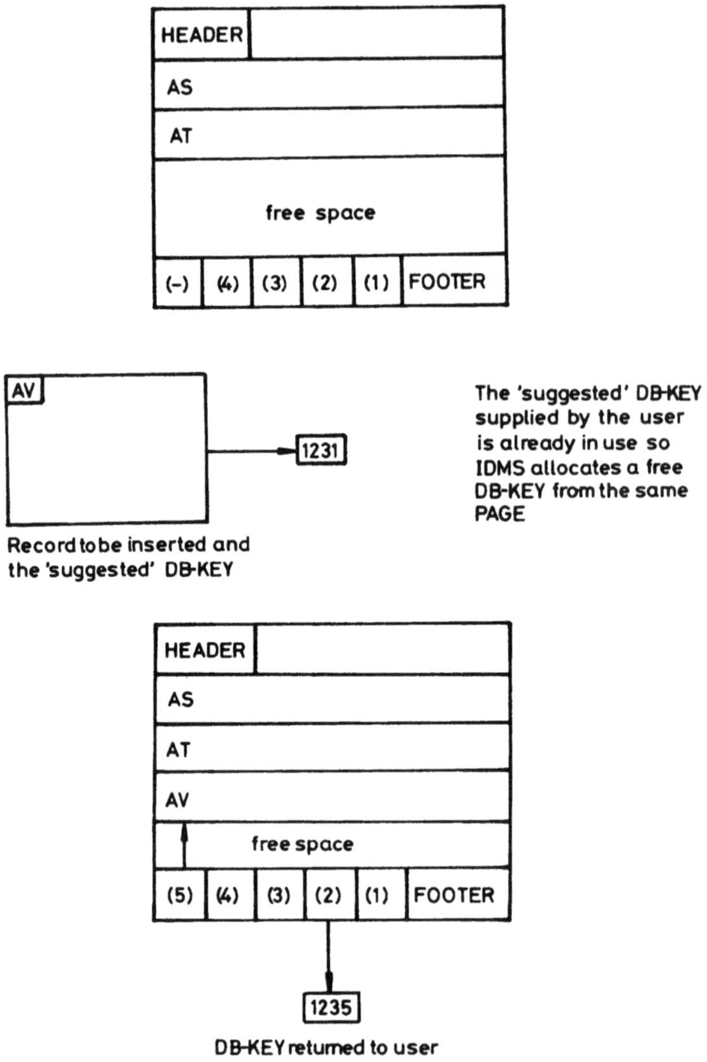

Fig. 7.2c: Storage Using DIRECT MODE

mapping from the schema AREAS to the physical storage.

VSAM is now also available as access method.

Each record occurrence stored in IDMS consists of two parts: a prefix for the structure data which contains a number of four-byte pointer fields; and the user data. If variable length records are being used, then the prefix will contain a further field of 8 bytes. Variable length records result either from data compression (via a user exit) or by using the OCCURS . . . DEPENDING ON construction. The length of the prefix can vary greatly depending on the number of relationships the particular record type participates in.

The records are stored in an IDMS PAGE, which is the basic unit of physical storage. The size of the PAGE is fixed by the DBA at system generation time for each AREA, and is typically between 2K and 6K bytes. An IDMS pointer (DATABASE KEY) is 4 bytes in length. This is broken into two parts: 23 bits to represent the LOGICAL PAGE NUMBER (which is unique across the whole SCHEMA), and 8 bits for the LINE (record) INDEX within the PAGE. An IDMS database can contain up to $2^{23}-1$ PAGES and each PAGE can hold up to 255 records.

Fixed length records must be stored wholly within one PAGE. Variable length records can be broken up into one root segment and a number of fragments which are all chained together.

Each PAGE consists of five parts (see Fig. 7.3.1):

- a 16-byte PAGE HEADER
- a number of data records
- free space
- control information to locate and manage each record
- a 16-byte PAGE FOOTER.

The PAGE HEADER holds the following information:

- the unique PAGE number (LPN)
- pointers for CALC record placement
- a free space indicatior
- switches to aid buffer management.

The 8-bit LINE INDEX in the DATABASE KEY does not point directly to the record but to the RECORD LOCATION POINTER at the foot of the PAGE. This is because the location of a record within a PAGE can vary, (see Fig. 7.3.2 Space Management).

7.3.2 Space Management

The RECORD LOCATION POINTERS (see Fig. 7.3.1) contain a record length field, which means the IDMS operates only on variable length records. Records are inserted into a PAGE directly after the header. No space is needed after a record to allow for future expansion. Should a record be deleted, then IDMS automatically reorganises the PAGE in order to maintain the largest possible area of contiguous free space. The record location pointer for the deleted record will be set to zero and is immediately available for reuse (see Fig. 7.3.2).

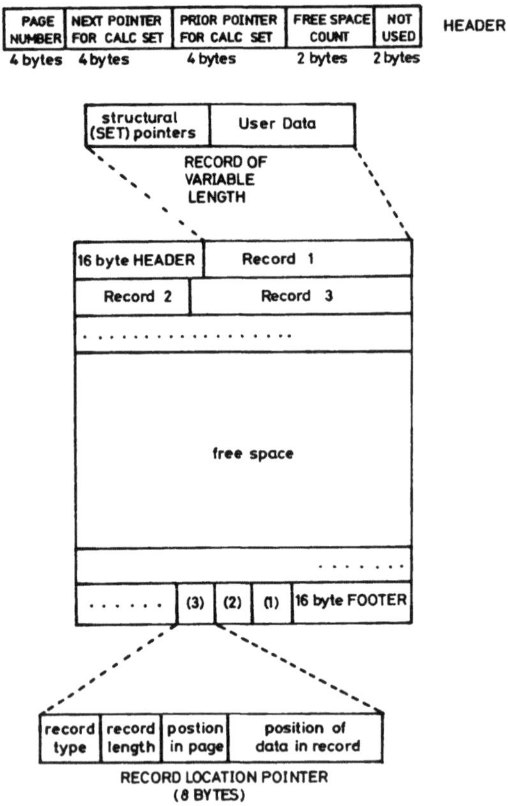

Fig. 7.3.1: Physical Storage PAGE Layout

If a variable length record expands and there is insufficient space within the PAGE for the new enlarged record, the record will be split into two parts, the root containing the principle key, and a pointer to the rest which will be accommodated in a neighbouring PAGE. This process can be repeated, resulting in a number of fragments linked together with pointers. Should pointer maintenance be necessary due to the deletion of a fragment, the system will try to reorganise the record to avoid or at least reduce the fragmentation.

The first 1000 PAGES of an IDMS database are reserved for use by the Data Dictionary. The first PAGE of each AREA is used for SPACE MANAGEMENT. They are only updated when the occupancy of a particular PAGE exceeds 70%.

There are no overflow PAGES within an IDMS database, although it is possible to specify that only a part of each PAGE will be occupied during an initial load;

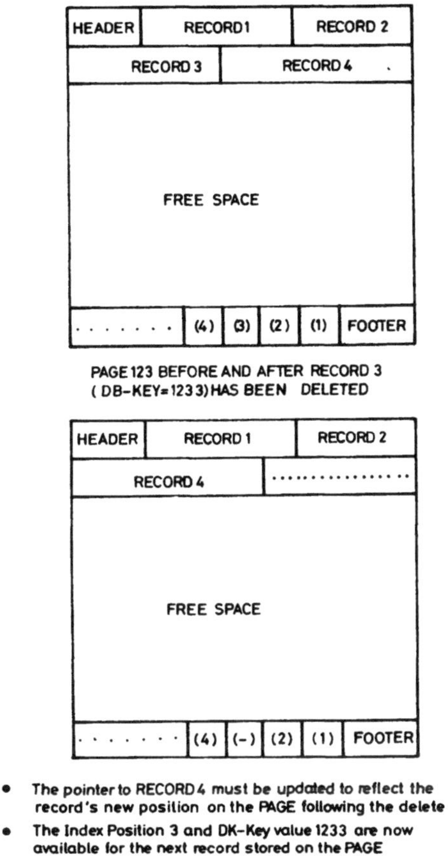

Fig. 7.3.2: Space Re-use After Deletion

this free space can be used later to accommodate expanded records and new records.

Essentially, space management is only necessary with the CALC records. The VIA or DIRECT LOCATION MODES only indicate where the record should be placed. If there is no space available, a neighbouring PAGE is equally acceptable. The actual DATABASE KEY is returned and can be used to retrieve these records. With CALC placement, however, the randomizing algorithm generates a particular PAGE as address. If this particular PAGE is full, an overflow condition occurs, and an overflow pointer must be maintained in this PAGE to the PAGE where the record is actually stored. This will adversely affect performance. The DBA must therefore either change the algorithm or change the PAGE size, should a large number of records be stored in a PAGE other than that indicated by the CALC algorithm.

The general objective with I/O buffers is to reduce to a minimum movement between main storage and secondary storage. PAGES are returned to secondary storage only when absolutely necessary. This can be caused by a COMMIT command, which requires that all PAGES containing record occurrences which have been changed by the RUN UNIT which has issued the command should be secured. A second possibility is that the buffer becomes full. Each PAGE would then be examined and that PAGE with the lowest priority, containing a modification, would be returned to secondary storage. BEFORE and AFTER IMAGE PAGES for the JOURNAL FILE are managed in a similar manner.

7.3.3 Logical Storage Structures

There are two ways of linking data within an IDMS database, either by inter-field or inter-record relationships.

- Inter-field Relationships. An ITEM within an IDMS logical record is equivalent to a field within COBOL. A hierarchical relationship between ITEMS is established by means of level numbers in the record description (in the SCHEMA DDL). A maximum of 48 levels is permitted.
- Inter-record Relationships. The CODASYL name for an inter-record relationship is a SET, which is defined using the SCHEMA DDL and implemented by physical pointers embedded within each record prefix.

  A SET can be used to define both network and hierarchical structures within the following constraints:

  (1) a SET has only one OWNER type record,
  (2) a record type cannot be both OWNER and MEMBER of the same SET,
  (3) a SET may consist of different types of MEMBER records,
  (4) records may be OWNERS and MEMBERS in an unlimited number of different SETS.

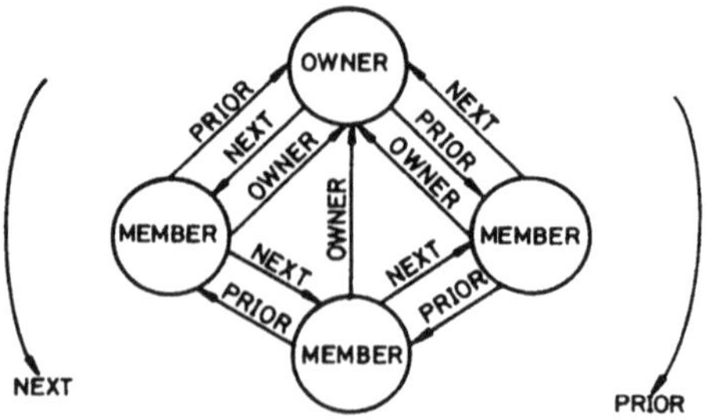

Fig. 7.3a: Types of pointer

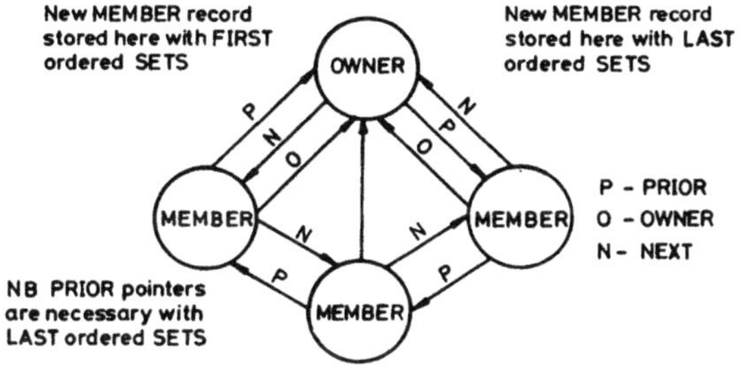

Fig. 7.3b: Insertion Rules 1

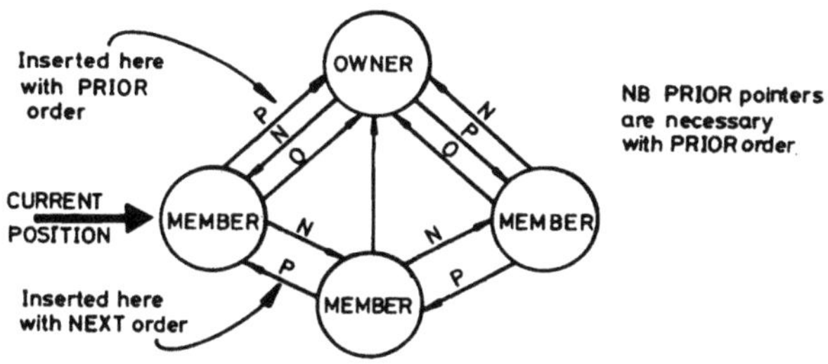

Fig. 7.3c: Insertion rules 2 (PRIOR/NEXT)

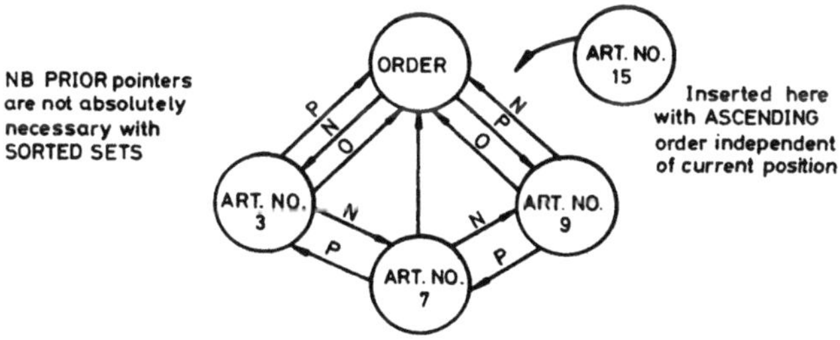

Fig. 7.3d: Insertion Rules 3 (ASCENDING/DESCENDING Order)

There are three different types of pointer (DATABASE KEY) used to relate OWNER and MEMBER within a SET (see Fig. 7.3a). NEXT pointers are automatically inserted by IDMS, PRIOR and OWNER pointers are optional. It is always possible to reach the 'prior' record to the current position simply by following the NEXT pointer chain. OWNER pointers can be used to increase access efficiency when the OWNER record occurrence is required of a MEM-

BER record occurrence which has been accessed via another SET relationship or a secondary index. The PRIOR pointer can save having to traverse the whole SET. It is particularly useful in volatile SETS where, for the same reason, it increases delete efficiency. (The NEXT pointer of the previous record has to be changed to point to the following record when the current record is to be deleted). Thus order in which records are inserted into SETS can be controlled (see Fig. 7.3b, c and d), and the following options are available:

(1) FIRST, the next record to be inserted will appear directly after the OWNER (giving LIFO sequence).
(2) LAST, the next record to be inserted will be placed at the end of the MEMBER chain (giving FIFO sequence).
(3) NEXT, the new record will be inserted immediately after the CURRENT record in the SET.
(4) PRIOR, the new MEMBER will be inserted immediately before the CURRENT record in the SET.
(5) Sorting on a field within the record, achieving an ascending or descending logical sequence within the SET occurrence.

The NEXT and PRIOR options leave the record sequence under programmer control.
There are two further qualifications required to fully define SET MEMBERSHIP, either AUTOMATIC or MANUAL and either MANDATORY or OPTIONAL. These parameters are concerned with establishment and termination of SET MEMBERSHIP:

(1) AUTOMATIC or MANUAL MEMBERSHIP. The former means what it implies ie. that as a result of a STORE command, this record becomes a MEMBER of all SETS in which it is defined. MANUAL MEMBERSHIP can only be established for a record occurrence after it has been stored in the database.
(2) MANDATORY or OPTIONAL MEMBERSHIP. With the former, an occurrence cannot be removed from a SET without being deleted from the database. With the latter an occurrence's participation in a SET can be deleted, without disturbing its MEMBERSHIP in any other SET. The commands associated with these different MEMBERSHIP types are explained in the 'Modification Commands' section of 7.4 'Data Manipulation'.

7.3.4 Secondary Processing Sequence

The SEQUENTIAL PROCESSING FACILITY (SPF) provides a secondary processing capability, so that any record may be declared a database entry record. This facility is implemented in IDMS as a normal SET, however, the user does not have to maintain it. The secondary index may be based on any field(s) within the desired record type. The designer must choose whether duplicated occurrences of a particular value are to be allowed. There is no restriction on the number or type of other relationships which the object record type may participate in. The SPF locates the desired entry record with a few accesses via a binary search of the sparse-to-dense hierarchically arranged index.

7.3.5 Generic Key Accessing

Partial key retrieval is available for both primary and secondary index values. However with a CALC key it has no meaning.

7.4 Data Manipulation

The original intention of the CODASYL database activities was to extend the COBOL language by providing database facilities. The commands necessary to access the database are provided within a DATA MANIPULATION LANGUAGE (DML). The commands are embedded in a COBOL program, in a way similar to the normal COBOL commands. However, as these commands are not yet (if ever) recognised as part of the COBOL language, they are translated into 'CALL' statements by a preprocessor. Preprocessors are also available for PL/1, FORTRAN and Assembler.

The logical structure that is available to the program is defined in the SCHEMA SECTION of the DATA DIVISION.

The IDMS interface module is link-edited to the user's relocatable object program prior to execution. Fig. 7.4 reflects the actions that occur during the execution of a typical DML statement:

1. The COBOL program issues a CALL instruction to the interface routine. Parameters of the CALL instruction identify what action, to which database, is required.

2. The interface routine passes the request to the IDMS nucleus which will carry out the required processing.

3. In order to be able to process the request, the nucleus will require the information held in the object SCHEMA. The object SCHEMA contains a representation of the data structure, CURRENCY status, record placement control, record and SET characteristics, database usage statistics and database usage limitations.

4. After the request has been processed, the contents of the object SCHEMA must be updated to reflect the new conditions. Should the processing request have involved the location of a record, then the DATABASE KEY and other record related information is moved from the IDMS system buffers to IDMS COMMUNICATIONS BLOCK in the user program.

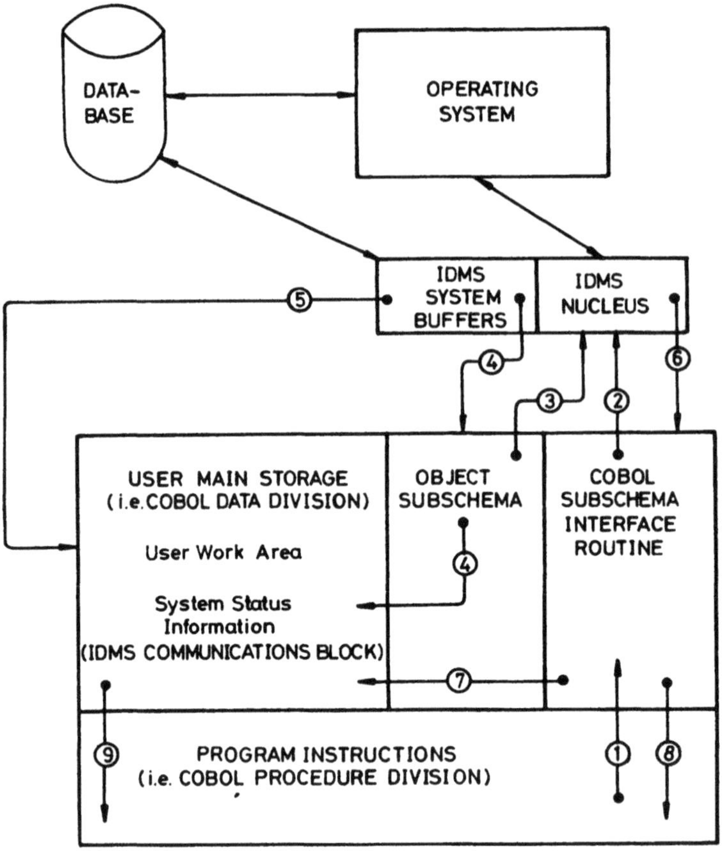

Fig. 7.4: Execution of a DML Command

5. If the processing request involved data retrieval (a GET command), the data will be moved from the IDMS system buffers to the program RECORD DELIVERY AREA. (Data movement in the reverse direction will occur in response to a STORE or MODIFY command.)

6. Control is returned to the interface routine with an indication as to the success or failure of the request.

7. The interface routine moves status information to the user's IDMS COMMUNICATIONS BLOCK!

8. Control is returned to the user program.

9. The user program can now continue processing. The results of the request are held in summarised form in the IDMS COMMUNICATIONS BLOCK.

The I/O area for the database resides in the program work area. Each record type specified in the SUBSCHEMA is included in the source program as a record level entry followed by the record contents description. On retrieval, a record occurrence is always placed in its like-named area in the program work area. The reverse is true when a record occurrence is to be stored in the database.

Three operations are required each time a database command is issued:

- initialisation of data items as required by the DML command to be issued
- DML command to initiate the required action
- error checking to determine the outcome of the DML command just executed.

7.4.1 CURRENCY

The concept of CURRENCY is used in a number of systems to identify the most recently accessed record, so as to be able to access NEXT, PRIOR, FIRST, LAST, OWNER etc records. IDMS takes this idea much further and has four types of CURRENCY:

- CURRENT OF RUN–UNIT (program). This is the last record successfully manipulated by a STORE or a FIND/OBTAIN DML command. The DATA-BASE KEY of this record is placed in a control location within the WORKING STORAGE SECTION.
- CURRENT OF AREA. This is the most recent record from the AREA that was CURRENT OF RUN–UNIT.
- CURRENT OF SET. For each SET, it is that record which was most recently the CURRENT OF RUN–UNIT.
- CURRENT OF RECORD TYPE. This is that record which last was CURRENT OF RUN–UNIT within each record type.

7.4.2 DML Commands

The DML commands are split into three categories: control, retrieval and modification.

- **Control Commands.** There are a number of commands available within IDMS's DML which do not cause any user data to be moved, but rather signal processing intention or retrieve metadata, ie. information about user data. The sequence of these commands is as follows:

BIND RUN–UNIT	issued once per RUN–UNIT
BIND RECORD NAME etc.	issued at least once
READY	issued at least once
IF	does not have to be used

manipulation (retrieval/modification) commands

KEEP	does not have to be used
COMMIT	does not have to be used
FINISH	issued once per RUN–UNIT
ROLLBACK	used to restore the database to its original state after an irrecoverable program error or at the end of a test run

(1) The BIND Command. This is used to sign-on the RUN–UNIT, and as such must precede all other DML commands. It informs IDMS of the location of the IDMS COMMUNICATIONS BLOCK and identifies the SUBSCHEMA which should be loaded for the subject RUN–UNIT. It is formulated as follows –

BIND RUN–UNIT [FOR subschema-name] [TO subschema-control identifier]

The command is further used to establish the addressability of any required record from within the 'signed-on' schema. It is formulated –

BIND { record-name [TO identifier] | identifier WITH record-name-identifier }

The final use of this command it to establish communication between the RUN–UNIT and a DBA-written database procedure. It is however unusual that more information is required by such routines. Normally these procedures are executed without the intervention of the RUN–UNIT. This final command is formulated –

BIND PROCEDURE FOR proc-name-ident TO proc-common-area

(2) The COMMIT Command. This creates a CHECKPOINT, releases all records held as the result of a KEEP command and flushes the buffers. The only difference between a COMMIT command and a FINISH–BIND–READY command sequence is that in the former, all CURRENCY pointers remain undisturbed. The COMMIT command is formulated –

COMMIT

(3) The FINISH Command. This causes the following actions to occur:
- control over all AREAS is withdrawn from the RUN–UNIT
- any other RUN–UNIT is permitted to assume control over the released AREAS
- a CHECKPOINT is written
- statistical information relating to those database operations performed during RUN–UNIT execution is released to the JOURNAL file.

The FINISH Command is formulated:

FINISH

(4) The IF Command. This falls between control commands and data manipulation commands. It operates on user data but does not manipulate it. It is used to:

– detect the presence of member record occurrence
– evaluate the membership status of a record occurrence in a specified SET occurrence.

It is formulated:

IF set-name IS [NOT] EMPTY imperative-statement

IF [NOT] set-name MEMBER imperative-statement

(5) The KEEP Command. This command can be used in stand-alone mode or as part of a FIND or OBTAIN command. It sets the select (KEEP) or update (KEEP EXCLUSIVE) lock for a record, SET or AREA. It is formulated:

KEEP [EXCLUSIVE] CURRENT [record-name | WITHIN set-name | WITHIN area-name]

(6) The READY Command. This command serves two purposes:

– to specify those AREAS to be accessed and the intent, ie. read/update
– to specify the initial CHECKPOINT condition for the RUN–UNIT for possible rollback/recovery operations following a system-failure.

It is formulated:

READY [area-name] [USAGE–MODE IS [PROTECTED | EXLUSIVE] {RETRIEVAL | UPDATE}]

– **Retrieval Commands.** These are: FIND/OBTAIN, GET, ACCEPT and the modification commands.

(1) The FIND/OBTAIN commands. The FIND command locates and the OBTAIN command both locates and retrieves a record according to the selection criteria specified. (Strictly speaking, the FIND command locates the record of interest and retrieves it into the IDMS buffer, and the GET command moves it into the program work area.) The OBTAIN command functions as if a FIND command followed by a GET command had been executed. The successful completion of a FIND/OBTAIN command results in the located record becoming CURRENT of AREA, all SETS in which the record participates and record name. Its DATABASE KEY is returned in a user-specified location. There are six main variation of this command:

(a) via DB–KEY. The record is located via a field in storage containing its key.

FIND [record-name] DB–KEY IS db-key-identifier

(b) CURRENT record. That record will be retrieved which is CURRENT of SET, record or AREA name.

```
             ┌record-name      ┐
FIND CURRENT │WITHIN set-name  │
             └WITHIN area-name ┘
```

NB. Issuing 'FIND CURRENT' without further qualification ie. for the CURRENT of RUN–UNIT, does not accomplish anything, as IDMS has not implemented the RETAINING CURRENCY option.

(c) from within a SET AREA or Index. Records from within SETS or AREAS are located with this command.

```
      ⎧NEXT      ⎫
      ⎪PRIOR     ⎪
      ⎪FIRST     ⎪                           ⎧set-name ⎫
FIND  ⎨LAST      ⎬  [record-name] WITHIN     ⎩area-name⎭
      ⎪integer   ⎪
      ⎩identifier⎭
```

The NEXT and PRIOR options are based on the CURRENCY of the specified AREA or SET; the FIRST and LAST options relate to logical order for SETS and to DB KEY order for AREAS; the 'integer' and 'identifier' options allow the retrieval of the nth record occurrence of a SET.

(d) OWNER record within a SET. This command retrieves the OWNER record of the CURRENT SET.

FIND OWNER WITHIN set-name

(e) CALC records. With this command, records whose LOCATION MODE is CALC can be retrieved.

```
      ⎧CALC (ANY)⎫
FIND  ⎩DUPLICATE ⎭  record-name
```

N.B. The 'CALC' option functions in conjunction with a specific 'CALC' key quoted in WORKING STORAGE. The 'DUPLIKATE' option accesses the next record with the same 'CALC' key as the CURRENT of record type.

(f) from an ordered SET. This command retrieves a MEMBER record from a sorted SET using a specific key.

FIND record-name WITHIN set-name [CURRENT] USING identifier

(2) The GET Command. This command simply transfers the CURRENT record of the RUN–UNIT or record name from the I/O buffer to the program work area.

GET [record-name]

(3) The ACCEPT Command. This allows the user to move CURRENCY indicators (DATABASE KEYS) and storage-address information to specified location in his program. It is formulated

$$\text{ACCEPT db-key-identifier FROM} \begin{bmatrix}\text{record-name}\\ \text{set-name}\\ \text{area-name}\end{bmatrix} \text{CURRENCY}$$

If neither record nor SET nor AREA name is specified, the DATABASE–KEY for the CURRENT record of RUN–UNIT is returned. It is also possible to retrieve the DATABASE–KEYS of the NEXT, PRIOR and OWNER records as follows

$$\text{ACCEPT db-key-identifier FROM set-name} \begin{Bmatrix}\text{NEXT}\\ \text{PRIOR}\\ \text{OWNER}\end{Bmatrix} \text{CURRENCY}$$

The other three variations of the ACCEPT command are beyond the scope of this report.

– **Modification Commands**. These are ERASE, CONNECT, MODIFY, DISCONNECT, STORE.

(1) The CONNECT command. With this command, a record occurrence (which must be CURRENT record of its record type) is made a MEMBER of a SET occurrence. The record type must be defined as OPTIONAL AUTOMATIC, OPTIONAL MANUAL or MANDATORY MANUAL. It is formulated:

CONNECT record-name TO set-name

(2) The DISCONNECT command. This removes a record occurrence from its participation in a SET occurrence. The record must be defined as an OPTIONAL MEMBER of the SET concerned. The record's occurrences in all other SET occurrences are totally unaffected. This command does not remove the record occurrence from the database. It is formulated:

DISCONNECT record-name FROM set-name

(3) The ERASE command. This enables the user:

(a) to disconnect the object record occurrence from all set occurrences in which it participates as a member

(b) to erase all those record occurrences which are MANDATORY MEMBERS of a particular SET owned by the object record.

(c) optionally to ERASE all record occurrences which are MANDATORY MEMBERS of SET occurrences where the object record is OWNER

(d) optionally to DISCONNECT or ERASE all record occurrences which are OPTIONAL MEMBERS of SET occurrences where the object record is OWNER.

The command is formulated:

$$\text{ERASE record-name} \left[\begin{Bmatrix} \text{PERMANENT} \\ \text{SELECTIVE} \\ \text{ALL} \end{Bmatrix} \text{MEMBERS} \right]$$

(4) The MODIFY command returns a previously accessed record occurrence to the database. Any or all of the data items within the object record may have been replaced with new values. It is formulated:

MODIFY record-name

(5) The STORE command inserts a record occurrence into all the SET occurrences in which it has been defined as an AUTOMATIC MEMBER. It is formulated:

STORE record-name

7.5 Data Independence

The DBA, having defined the global view of the database (SCHEMA) can define a subset (SUBSCHEMA) of this overall view for each user, thus limiting the user to only that information which is absolutely necessary. This insulates the user from changes to the database structure which do not affect his application.

7.5.1 The Local View

IDMS was originally designed (in keeping with CODASYL recommendation) to interface with COBOL via a preprocessor which would translate the DML command, embedded in the COBOL program into COBOL CALL commands. Preprocessors are now also available for Assembler PL/1 and FORTRAN.

Compiling the program only binds the specified DML commands. The SUBSCHEMA and the DMCL mapping statements are compiled separately and produce the SUBSCHEMA OBJECT MODULE and the DMCL OBJECT MODULE. These modules are bound to the program at run time. Data is bound to the program partly at compile time and partly at run time, the former generating relative addresses and the latter absolute addresses.

It is not possible to vary ITEM formats and/or lengths between SCHEMA and SUBSCHEMA. However, the user's view (SUBSCHEMA) of the database can be restricted to:

- particular SET types ie. logical relationships
- particular record types
- particular fields within record types

There is, however, one restriction when defining the SUBSCHEMA, namely that this local view must contain all record and item descriptions which could be affected by insertion and deletion activity.

7.6 Concurrent Usage

The latest version of IDMS – Release 5 – offers a dramatic improvement in throughput as a result of a multithreaded CENTRAL VERSION (CV). The SIGN–ON command issued by RUN–UNIT is received by the DATABASE–RESOURCE–CONTROLLER module (IDMSDBRC) which allocates an EXTERNAL–RUN–UNIT–SERVICE module (IDMSERUS). This latter serves as a link between the RUN–UNIT and the IDMS nucleus. The SUBSCHEMA TABLE is now part of the CV, whereas in previous releases it was attached to the RUN–

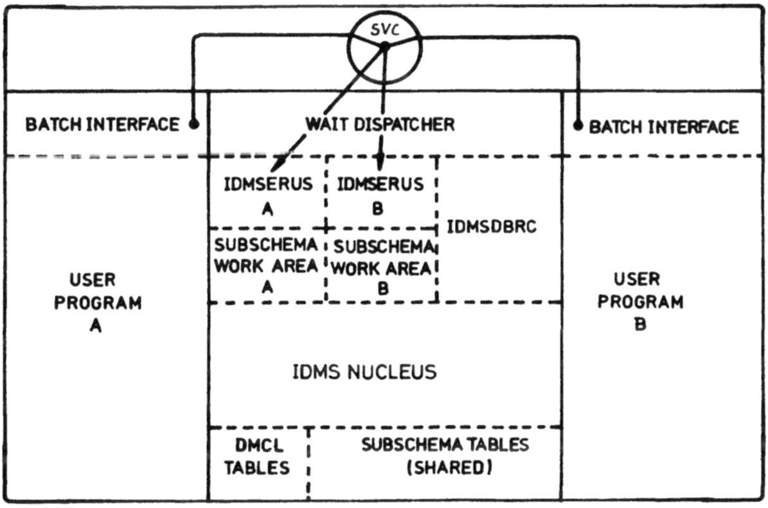

Fig. 7.6.1: BATCH MODE

UNIT. The advantage of the new configuration is that one SUBSCHEMA TABLE can be shared between RUN–UNITS. The SUBSCHEMA TABLES are held on secondary storage and read into main memory as required. It is possible, however, to make them resident to improve effeciency.

The SUBSCHEMA TABLES, which only contain database descriptions, are re-entrant, thus allowing a single copy to be used concurrently by multiple RUN–UNITS. Other data specific to each RUN–UNIT eg. CURRENCY pointers, is stored in its own 4K, dynamically-allocated, work-area held within the CV.

The IDMS–DC nucleus is resident in the CENTRAL VERSION functioning as a 'wait dispatcher', monitoring the activities of the master DATA–BASE–RESOURCE–CONTROLLER module and all EXTERNAL–RUN–UNIT–SERVICE modules. This step integrates the IDMS database and teleprocessing systems. The IDMSDBRC also communicates with the operator, and monitors the IDMSERUS module for abnormal RUN–UNIT termination.

The CENTRAL VERSION together with the integrated IDMS–DC nucleus is used in both batch and on-line modes of operation.

7.6.1 Batch Processing

Figure 7.6.1 shows programs A and B running in batch mode. If they have a common SUBSCHEMA, then only one copy of the SUBSCHEMA TABLES would be required. A SUBSCHEMA WORK AREA is present in the CV for each program. It is about 4KB large and holds CURRENCY information and communication block data. An EXTERNAL–RUN–UNIT–SERVICE module is available for each active application and provides communication between the application program and the required CV functions.

7.6.2 On-line Processing

IDMS supports two different modes of on-line operation. ATTACH mode (see Fig. 7.6.2a) allows the user programs to run in the same partition as the CENTRAL VERSION. There are two variations with ATTACH mode: ATTACH MONITOR and ATTACH CONTROL modes. The Control Routine acts as the main task in the latter case, the Communications Monitor in the former. Using the Control Routine has the advantage that the abnormal termination of the Communications Monitor does cause the DBMS to terminate.

It is also possible to run the DBMS in a separate partition from the Communications Monitor and its associated user programs (A and B) and this is called EXECUTE Mode (see Fig. 7.6.2b). The situation is similar when operating under MVS (see Fig. 7.6.2c and 7.6.2d) with the addition that a Packet-Data-Move-

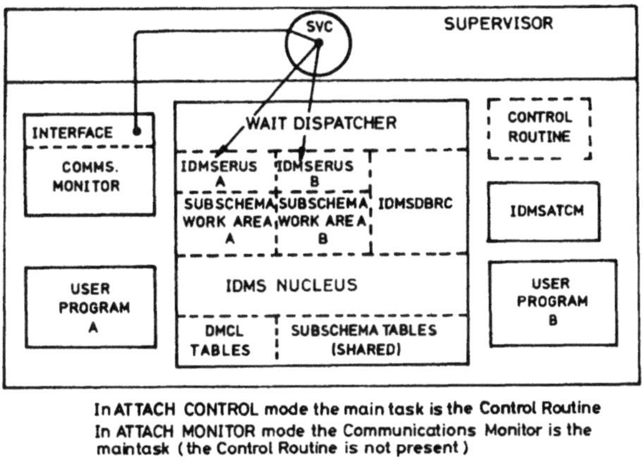

Fig. 7.6.2a: CENTRAL VERSION and Communications Monitor in ATTACH MODE

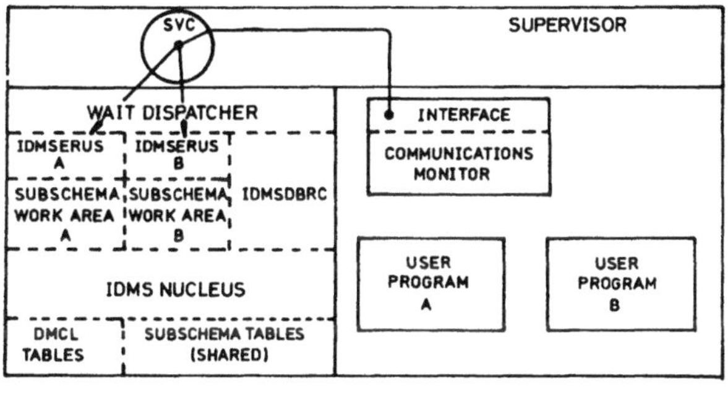

Fig. 7.6.2b. CENTRAL VERSION and Communication Monitor in EXECUTE MODE

ment-Buffer in the Common Storage Area must be made available to each program not executing in the same address space as the CENTRAL VERSION. In ATTACH mode, a buffer is made available to the batch user program 'C'. In EXECUTE mode, buffers must be made available for each user program.

The CENTRAL VERSION may run with a user protect key for all user programs using Packet-Data-Movement-Buffers, which protects against storage destruction outside that region controlled by the CV.

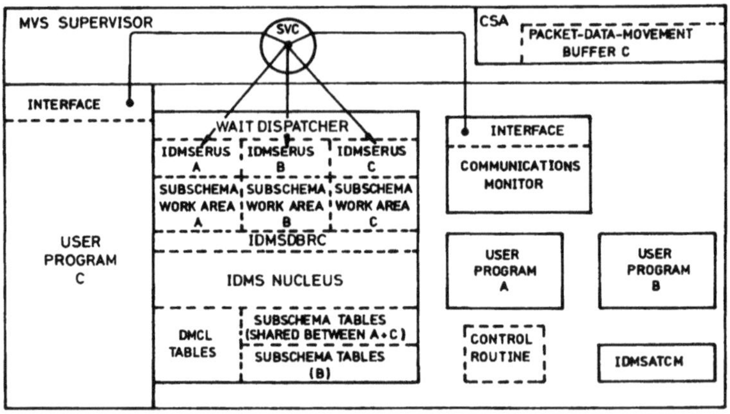

- ATTACH CONTROL mode – Control Routine is the main task
- ATTACH MONITOR mode – Communications Monitor is the main task
- The SVC is not necessary for programs running in the same Region as the CENTRAL VERSION, when using a SYSCTL file at run-time

Fig. 7.6.2c: MVS CENTRAL VERSION and Communication Monitor in ATTACH MODE

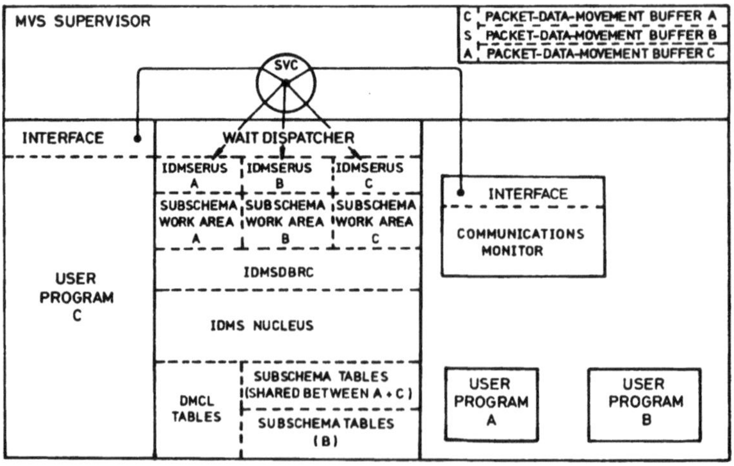

Fig. 7.6.2d: MVS CENTRAL VERSION and Communication Monitor in EXECUTE MODE

7.7 Integrity Controls and Recovery

Although IDMS does not perform format checks on user data, it is possible for the DBA (or user) to write such routines which could then be incorporated into IDMS via the PROCEDURES option. Structure data, which is physically stored in the record prefix, is protected simply by never making it available to the RUN UNIT. Concurrent updating can be prevented by specifying the appropriate AREA USAGE MODE.

The problem of not supplying obsolete data while one program is updating can be avoided by specifying EXCLUSIVE UPDATE USAGE MODE for the AREA and the updating program. This is particularly necessary if a RUN–UNIT reads a number of records for a processing unit while, during this time, some of them could be updated from another RUN–UNIT.

Deadly embrace (deadlock) is resolved by aborting and ROLLING BACK the offending program. The aborted RUN–UNIT is informed via a status code that the ROLL BACK has occurred. The program may decide to start the same transaction again, or a new transaction. In either case, the first command must be BIND RUN–UNIT.

IDMS may also abort and ROLL BACK a RUN–UNIT after a specified period of time, it it is waiting to update a record occurrence with a SELECT LOCK held by another program. Run-time LOCKS have the advantage over PROTECTED and EXCLUSIVE READY options as they tie up only those records required and not whole AREAS. This is true for short duration transactions, but less applicable for batch processing, where serious performance degradation could occur.

The whole JOURNALING and recovery conception has been changed in Release 5.0. JOURNAL entries are maintained at the record level – previously this was done at the PAGE level. Entries are made for CONNECT, DISCONNECT, MODIFY, ERASE and STORE commands.

The JOURNAL BUFFER is written to the JOURNAL file when:

- the buffer is full
- a PAGE containing an updated record occurrence, whose BEFORE IMAGE is in the JOURNAL BUFFER, is returned to the database
- a RUN UNIT aborts
- a RUN UNIT issues a COMMIT, ROLLBACK or FINISH command.

The JOURNAL file may be either on tape or disc. When a disc file is full, a new utility (IDMSAJNL) copies the contents to a tape file and also rebuilds the disc JOURNAL file putting all BEFORE IMAGES of active RECOVERY UNITS in new blocks at the beginning of the new JOURNAL file.

With the CENTRAL VERSION and disc JOURNAL file, automatic recovery can be accomplished in one of two ways:

- WARM RESTART. When the CENTRAL VERSION is restarted after a failure, it will recognise the previous failure and then ROLLBACK all incomplete RUN UNITS.
- ROLLBACK. This is the simpler case, where the CV continues processing other RUN UNITS while returning a RECOVERY UNIT to the last CHECKPOINT (ROLLBACK). This can be as a result of a ROLLBACK command, or when a RECOVERY UNIT fails.

7.8 Privacy (Access) Controls

IDMS provides various privacy and security control facilities at the program, AREA, SET and record levels.

7.8.1 Program Level

Each RUN–UNIT must invoke a SUBSCHEMA (via the SCHEMA SECTION in the program). The DBA should be the only person who has the authority and knowledge to generate SUBSCHEMAS. A program is only allowed to access those SCHEMA elements (AREAS, SETS, records ITEMS) copied into the SUBSCHEMA.

7.8.2 AREA Level

A separate PRIVACY LOCK may be allocated to each AREA specified in the SUBSCHEMA, for the USAGE MODES:

- RETRIEVAL
- PROTECTED RETRIEVAL
- EXCLUSIVE RETRIEVAL
- UPDATE
- EXCLUSIVE UPDATE
- PROTECTED UPDATE.

EXCLUSIVE USAGE MODE denies access to the specified AREA to all other RUN UNITS until that RUN–UNIT issues a FINISH command. PROTECTED USAGE MODE allows all other RUN–UNITS to access the specified AREA, but only for retrieval.

7.8.3 SET Level

It is possible to forbid the use of certain DML commands within SET types. This is done in the SUBSCHEMA with a PRIVACY LOCK. The DML commands are:

- CONNECT
- DISCONNECT
- FIND.

7.8.4 Record Level

The manipulation of each record type can be restricted to certain DML commands.

7.9 Performance

The performance of IDMS Release 5.0 should certainly prove to be better than previous releases simply by virtue of the multi-threading capability of the IDMS nucleus. However, the total performance of any DBMS is dependent on many aspects of the system and on external factors such as how easily it can be learned and used by EDP personnel.

7.9.1 Growth

An IDMS database can accommodate over 4 billion records, a database being limited to 8 million PAGES and each PAGE capable of holding a maximum of 255 record. This should pose no threat to almost any EDP environment. But as with all hierarchical/network- based systems, the initial design of the data structure is very important. However, utilities are available to help incorporate new logical relationships and new record types into existing databases. Data independence insulates existing application programs from later developments that do not affect their processing.

7.9.2 Programmer Skill

The concepts within the CODASYL DBMS are unambiguous and the terminology is clear if somewhat complicated. Nevertheless, even a moderately competent programmer would be quite capable of grasping the concepts of logical SETS and the method of navigating through the database structure with the help of the various CURRENCY pointers.

The flexibility of IDMS does however leave it open to abuse: a programmer can write substantially inefficient programs. The power and elegance of IDMS more than compensates for the complexity, but nevertheless, this gives the DBA an extra level of responsibility, that is, to guard against inefficient coding. Although it is not essential for the programmer to be aware of the physical placement of the records, this knowledge would definitely permit him to use IDMS more efficiently.

7.9.3 Reorganisation

IDMS continuously reorganises the database, which means that it degrades only very little with time. Space management ensures that the largest possible contiguous area of free space is available on each PAGE. This continuous reorganisation means that immediately after a record has been deleted, the free space is incorporated into the contiguous free space area for the PAGE, even when this means shifting records within the PAGE. This is possible because the location of any record occurrence within a PAGE is noted at the end of that PAGE. External to the PAGE, the pointers only indicate which PAGE contains the desired record occurrence. This solution has resulted in volatile databases not being reorganised for months or possible years, even when they contain variable length records.

Variable length records present no performance problem as long as there is sufficient space within the PAGE to accommodate any expansion. When no more space is available, IDMS splits the record into a root (which remains in the original PAGE) and a fragment (stored in some other PAGE in the vicinity). This process can be repeated infinitely, in theory at least, with pointers linking the root to the fragments. IDMS tries to reduce the number of fragments to a minimum at every opportunity, even when the record is just retrieved and not updated.

Although data compression facilities are not automatically included in IDMS, they can be included on a record type basis via a user exit. The record type to be compressed must be declared as of variable length. The compression routine is supplied by the vendor. As it is of a general nature, it does not operate on the separate fields of a record, but views the record as a continuous data string. All repeating characters and character pairs are suppressed.

7.9.4 Monitoring, Tuning and Utilities

Statistical information about database operations related to each RUN–UNIT is written both to the log (JOURNAL) file and to the CONTROL AREA when a FINISH (real or implied) command is executed. This information includes:

- PAGES read and updated
- which CALC records overflow the home PAGE
- VIA records placed with their OWNER and those placed in overflow
- those records which became CURRENT of RUN–UNIT
- the number of CALLS made to IDMS
- the number of LOCKS held.

The SECURITY DUMP, containing space-usage statistics, is used by the DBA to monitor the database. Neither this nor any other utility is available to assist the DBA to tune the system, which must be done on a hit-or-miss basis. One of the most critical points with most systems is the I/O buffer size, and IDMS is no exception. However, beyond a certain size, the search time will decrease the efficiency. Each DML retrieval command examines the contents of the buffer pool before issuing the necessary I/O command. This search time can become significant.

No matter how good a DBMS might be, it cannot be used to full advantage without an adequate set of supporting utilities. In this respect, IDMS is well provided for:

1. The IDMSAJNL facility will unload a disc log file to an archive magnetic tape.
2. IDMSCALC is accessed via a subroutine and returns to the user program a suggested PAGE number to store the record whose CALC key was supplied in the original CALL together with a target PAGE range.
3. IDMSCLUC is the data directory update utility.
4. IDMSDBLU assists the user to load a database. The user program which addresses this utility via a CALL statement must provide:

- one record occurrence descriptor
- one OWNER descriptor for each SET in which the object record participates as an AUTOMATIC MEMBER. OWNER descriptors may also be provided for MANUAL SETS at the user's or DBA's discretion.

All DMBSs using embedded pointers have more difficulty loading data, and IDMS is no exception. One particular weakness is apparent with this utility: violations of the DUPLICATES NOT ALLOWED clause cannot be detected in the first step but will be detected in the second.

5. IDMSDUMP performs any or all of the following functions:

- creating a space utilisation report, which contains information about space distribution per record type, space distribution per PAGE, file utilisation, and PAGE size or sizes.
- dumping to magnetic tape or disc file the database or data directory, either in their entirety or by AREA or file.
- punching the DATABASE KEYS of logically deleted records, for use by the IDMSLDEL utility.

6. IDMSINIT is responsible for the following activities:

- initialising the data directory
- initialising or re-initialising all or portions of a database.
- initialising the SYSCTL file, used by the Central Version under OS to pass parameters
- initialising the disc log file or files.

7. IDMSJFIX processes the tape log file which was in use at the time of a system crash. It can perform the following activites:

- writing ABRT checkpoints for all RUN–UNITS active at the time of the crash
- printing checkpoints and program statistics for RUN–UNITS on the log file.

8. IDMSLDEL physically erases from the database logically deleted records as listed in the punched output from the IDMSDUMP utility.

9. IDMSPFIX can perform all or any of the following activites:

- printing a specific PAGE or PAGES in display and/or hexadecimal characters
- printing the contents of a PAGE containing a specific CALC key in both display and hexadecimal characters
- removing an in-use lock from an AREA
- verifying the contents of a PAGE.

10. IDMSRBCK performs any or all of the following activities using a tape log file:

- restoring a database by processing the log file in a reverse direction and applying the BEFORE IMAGES and using the AFTER IMAGES to verify the contents of the database
- printing the BEFORE and AFTER IMAGES
- printing the checkpoints.

11. IDMSRFWD can perform one or more of the following functions:

- working in a forward direction, copying the AFTER IMAGES from the log file onto the database
- printing the BEFORE and AFTER IMAGES from the log file
- printing the checkpoints from the log file.

12. IDMSRPTS prints out the contents of the data directory.

13. IDMSRSTR can be used to restore a database (or data directory) in its entirety or by file or AREA. The database copy created by the utility IDMSDUMP is used as input.

14. IDMSRSTU offers the user the possibility of making a limited number of structural modification. These are:

- adding new data items to a record type
- changing the position of existing data items

- deleting existing data items
- expanding the record type prefix to include new SET relationships, new PRIOR pointers or new OWNER pointers.
- deleting NEXT, PRIOR and OWNER pointers
- changing fixed length records to variable length records and vice-versa.
- executing a new DP–PROCEDURE on existing record occurrences

None of these changes requires the database to be reloaded. This utility cannot be used on databases containing logically deleted records. When PRIOR or OWNER pointers are to be added, the utility IDMSPCON must be used additionally.

15. IDMSUNLD unloads, and, in conjunction with IDMSDBLU, reloads the database. It cannot be used on databases containing logically deleted records.

16. IDMSXPAG expands the database PAGE size.

The foregoing shows that IDMS is supported by all the necessary utilities.

7.10 Conclusion

One of the more difficult problems when examining a CODASYL-based DBMS is separating the CODASYL IDMS implementation from the CODASYL specification. This report is limited to examining IDMS, which is, coincidentally an implementation of a subset of the CODASYL recommendations. No comments are levelled directly at the CODASYL recommendations themselves, but some observations about IDMS do inevitably relate directly or indirectly to the origins of this system.

Systems based on embedded pointers are relatively easy to compare, using such criteria as:

- the system's ability to generate hierarchical/network structures
- how easily the structures can be defined
- how easy it is to change the structures
- the clarity and flexibility of the command layout
- which commands are available and their flexibility
- the flexibility of placing a record within a SET and within the data space.

IDMS is at least as good as its competitors in these areas, and normally superior. The IDMS implementation of secondary indexing is in some aspects, however, inferior to that offered by IMS.

The normally precise and clear terminology of IDMS has one particularly glaring irregularity, the LOCATION MODE clause. Historically, this clause stems from two separate concepts of IDS/1; namely the Storage Mode and Retrieval Mode.

Unfortunately it has been debased to mean simply Storage Mode and is therefore a misnomer.

One particular failing in the original CODASYL specification and hence in IDMS was the explicit exclusion of the capability of allowing an OWNER record occurrence to participate as a MEMBER record occurrence in its own SET occurrence. An example of where this type of relationship is necessary is in an electoral register, where the elected representative is OWNER of all the voters (MEMBERS) in an electoral area, but where the elected representative may also vote. He can therefore be both OWNER and MEMBER. This type of relationship is not currently offered by the main competing embedded pointer based systems. It is however offered by SIBAS, another CODASYL-based system available for IBM hardware. This relationship is often called Involuted or Incestuous.

An advantage of IDMS which should be mentioned is its literature, which is among the very best offered for any software product. This can, to some extent, be attributed to the clarity of the CODASYL specifications upon which it is based. However, Cullinane has expended considerable effort in producing manuals which reduce to a minimum the extremely high learning requirement needed before any embedded pointer system can be used competently. Once the complexity of IDMS is mastered, the user is rewarded with a degree of flexibility not available from any of the other DBMSs examined, which uses embedded pointers. This in no way means that the CODASYL concept is flawless; simply that IDMS offers the user a greater degree of flexibility for a lower hardware cost than any similar DBMS.

IDMS must now be considered a mature DBMS although some of the supporting products should be regarded as somewhat provisional. The Query Language, and the Sequential Processing Facility will certainly be improved extensively in the near future.

A full range of utilities is offered to cope with all ancillary functions from warm restart to reorganisation. Warm restart is completely automatic. Any DBMS evaluation which does not include IDMS cannot be considered complete.

7.11 Advantages of IDMS

- Clear and precise terminology.
- Both hierarchical and network structures can be expressed.
- Best documentation of all the systems examined.
- Good transaction-oriented processing capabilities.
- Commands easy to learn and use.
- Command formats are excellent because of preprocessor.

- Extremely good record placement and manipulation commands.
- Direct access for fast response real-time applications.
- Portability.
- On-going DB reorganisation (even on retrieval for variable length records) largely obviating the need for off-line reorganisation runs.
- Report writer (CULPRIT).
- Data dictionary.
- Interfaces – see Appendix III.
- Different SET types under one OWNER type may have different LOCATION MODES; so allowing very flexible tuning, with the LOCATION MODE chosen to suit the SET characteristics not the average DB characteristics.
- Logging file may be disc (recommended). It is preformatted so as to avoid recovery problems.
- IDMS requires relatively few system resources.
- Many utilities can be run on-line.
- It also runs on DEC PDP–11 hardware.
- Automatic warm restart.
- Multithreading nucleus.
- Fully integrated TP monitor.
- Backing storage of 2MB (excluding SPF).
- The 'CALC' record placement can accept unique or duplicate keys as the design requires.
- Data compression is available via a User-Exit – the routine is supplied by Cullinane. It treats the record as a string.
- Logging at record level.
- Field level sensitivity for the user-view, but although the order of the fields may differ, the characteristics must be the same as in the SCHEMA.

7.12 Disadvantages of IDMS

- The secondary indexing is somewhat clumsily implemented. It does not use inverted file techniques but internally generated SETS.
- Query language is somewhat primitive; no on-line 'ad-hoc' complex query facility.
- TP Monitor somewhat primitive.
- The uncertain pace of development to reach the level of the 1978 CODASYL recommendations.
- The learning and design difficulties associated with all complex embedded pointer systems.
- Dual logging only available via a user exit.
- No security violation audit.

- Intersection data is hard to handle in M:M relationships.
- Data is bound partly at compile time.
- The load program must be written by the user.
- No user-messages may be written to the log file.
- No format checks are made when records are loaded.
- Involuted relationships cannot be expressed directly.
- Data Independence is somewhat limited because the SUBSCHEMA cannot vary the SCHEMA'S ITEM characteristics.
- The data compression routine, if used, has to expand the whole record irrespective of the number of ITEMS requested by the SUBSCHEMA.

7.13 IDMS Glossary

AREA: A group of **PAGES** within an **IDMS** database.

AUTOMATIC: This is a rule of SET MEMBERSHIP (cf. MANUAL) which specifies that a record, on being entered into the database, will be placed in an occurrence of each SET type in which it is an AUTOMATIC MEMBER.

CALC: A method of storing records by using a randomizing routine on a particular field to produce a PAGE address. All records which map to a particular PAGE are chained together in ascending key sequence.

CURRENCY: Information held internally indicating the most recently located record of each RUN–UNIT, AREA, record-type and SET.

DATABASE KEY: Each record in an IDMS database is allocated a unique relative address, the DATABASE KEY. It is assigned for the life of the record and consists of a PAGE number and LINE number in the PAGE FOOTER where the address of the record is held. This method is used so that the actual location of the record may change, and has the great advantage that it avoids constant reorganisation runs.

(DATA) ITEM: This is the CODASYL name for a COBOL field. Both elementary and group ITEMS may be defined.

DDL: (DATA DEFINITION LANGUAGE). Used to define the data storage structure for the SCHEMAS and SUBSCHEMAS.

DIRECT: This LOCATION MODE gives the user the greatest degree of control over the placement of the records. The user specifies the DATABASE KEY, ie. the PAGE and LINE numbers where the record is to be stored. If this key is already in use, then IDMS will allocate the next available DATABASE KEY in the specified AREA.

DMCL: (DATA MEDIA CONTROL LANGUAGE). This language maps the database onto physical storage, defines the names and sizes of the I/O buffer pools, and names those files whose changes are to be logged.

DML: (DATA MANIPULATION LANGUAGE). This language, similar in format to COBOL statements, is used to insert, delete and modify the data in the databases.

LINE NUMBER: This is an index to a series of 8-byte addresses held at the end of each PAGE referring to all records stored on the PAGE. Each PAGE can hold a maximum 255 LINE NUMBERS ie. RECORDS.

LOCATION MODE: This term means 'storage mode'. There are three methods of storing – and hence retrieving – a record: CALC, DIRECT or VIA. This storage mode must be specified for every record type.

MANDATORY: This is a SET MEMBERSHIP rule (cf. OPTIONAL), which specifies that once a record occurrence has become a MEMBER of a SET, it must remain a MEMBER of that SET for as long as it remains in the database.

MANUAL: This is a SET MEMBERSHIP rule, (cf. AUTOMATIC), which specifies that a record occurrence only becomes a MEMBER of those SET occurrences in which it is explicitly placed.

MEMBER: A record occurrence together with more record occurrences of the same or of different types dependent on a particular OWNER record occurrence.

OPTIONAL: This is a SET MEMBERSHIP rule (cf. MANDATORY) which specifies that a record occurrence may be removed from a particular SET occurrence without affecting its MEMBERSHIP in any other SET occurrence.

OWNER: This is the record type which occurs only once in each SET occurrence and on which all SET occurrence MEMBERS are dependent.

PAGE: This is the CODASYL name for a physical block.

RECORD: Each record occurrence consists of a prefix containing SET information and user information, which are stored contiguously. The user never sees the prefix.

RUN–UNIT: This is an executing instance of a user program.

SCHEMA: This is the description of the structure of a database which includes all assoiated AREAS, records and SETS. The definition is effected using the DDL.

SET: A SET is the defined relationship between two or more record types. A SET occurrence consists of one, and only one, occurrence of the OWNER record type and one or more occurrence of the MEMBER record types.

SUBSCHEMA: This is a subset of the total user view as defined in the SCHEMA. It is used by a RUN–UNIT to supply the necessary view of the database. The DDL contains facilities for defining the SUB-SCHEMA.

VIA: This LOCATION MODE causes record occurrences to be placed as close as possible physically to their OWNER occurrence.

Appendix I: DBMS Questionnaire

1. Profile of Vendor and History of Product

- Where developed?
- When developed?
- Developed for what purpose?
- Developed by whom?
- Are the developer and vendor the same?
  When not:
  - What is the relationship between them?
  - How long have they worked together?
  - Is the contract between them of a limited nature?
- What will happen if the vendor/developer stops supporting the DBMS (or any associated product)?
- Developments planned?
- List of major developments introduced in the last one/two years.
- Active user group?
  - Number of members?
- Level of support available?
  - Nearest office?
  - Number of support personnel?
    Also as ratio to no. of systems installed.
  - When on call?
- Cost of the products?
  - DBMS
  - Data Dictionary
  - TP Monitor
  - Query Language
  - Report Generator
- Cost and length of training?
  - DBA
  - System Programmer
  - Programmer
  - Systems Analyst
  - Operator
- Installation costs?
- Time required for installation?

2. Classification and Environment

- In what language is the package written?
- DBMS/DMS
- Batch
- On-line
  - DB/DC synchronized checkpoints?
  - Logging done by DB or DC (or both)?
  - Is the TP monitor the Main Task?
- Main storage requirements

	CODING		BUFFERS	WORK AREA
	batch	on-line		
TYPICAL				
MINIMUM				

- Data Dictionary/Directory Facilities?
  - Integrated.
- Any device dependent restrictions?
- Is the DBMS overlaid?
- Which Operating Systems are supported?
  - Are there any changes necessary when changing from one to another?
- Which OS access method is used by the DBMS?
  - Is there any choice (eg. VSAM or BDAM)?

3. Programming

- Host Language?
  - Which are supported?
    (PL/1, FORTRAN, COBOL, BASIC, ALGOL, ASM, APL)
- Preprocessor?
- DDL?
- DMCL?
- Report Generator?
  - On-line input?
  - How many reports in a single pass?
  - Restrictions on the structure that can be processed?

- Query Language?
  - Interactive or simply on-line input?
  - Can data be updated?
- User Exits?
  - Data compression?
  - Index suppression?
  - Encyphering?

4. Data Item Definitions

- Fields
- Segments
- Repeating Items
  - maximum number?
- Repeating Groups
  - maximum number?
- Records
- Can the contents of a key field be modified
  - primary,
  - secondary?
- Are the contents of a field checked by the DBMS?
  - Loading
  - Updating
- Can a field be modified when the record is retrieved via the secondary index?
- Is there an appreciable performance penalty when all the fields are defined and not just key fields?
- Is there any limit on the number of ITEMs?
- What data ITEM characteristics can be defined?

5. Data Storage Structures

- Pointer Information
  - Embedded?
  - Tables?
- Structures
  - Flat files?
  - Hierarchies?
  - Networks?
  - Can the occurrences in a 'twin' chain be ordered?

- ascending and descending order,
- in front of and behind the current position,
- at the beginning and end of a chain?

- Space Management
  - Free space management
    - chain,
    - bit map.
  - Space reuse after record is deleted
    - primary,
    - secondary.

- Pointers
  - symbolic
  - direct
  - directly to record's position in the block (leads to framentation)
  - only to the block (block prefix holds exact position)
  - address converter (see General Glossary)
    - separate (requires an extra access)
    - integrated (only generated when needed)

- Variable Length Records
  - How are variable length records accommodated?
  - Fragmentation
    - How are fragments handled when space becomes available in the block holding the root (or a higher level) fragment?
      - not at all
      - only on update
      - with each access

- Secondary Indexing?
  - How implemented?
    - Is a count kept of the number of occurrences of each non-unique value?
  - Can it consist of more than one field?
  - Is the index compressed?
  - Is there any performance loss when the secondary index is not unique?
  - Where does the secondary index point to?
    - The primary index (for inverted file based systems).
      This saves on maintenance in a variable length record environment but requires an extra access.
    - Directly to the object record (with a further pointer should the record change location).
    - To an address converter entry.
    - Must the record which contains the value be the object of the secondary index or can it be any ancestor of the source record?

  - Can unwanted secondary index values be suppressed?

- Direct Access Methods
  - Must the primary key be unique?
  - Can more than one record be accommodated in the 'home block'?
  - Are synonyms in 'foreign blocks' removed to make way for records whose 'home block' it is?
  - Are synonyms chained in native key sequence?
  - How are synonym chains handled after the deletion of an entry?
  - Can the user supply his own hashing routine?
  - Can more than one hashing routine be used simultaneously (for different databases)?

- Is it possible to construct key fields from more than one field?
  - Must the fields be adjacent?
  - Can parts of fields be used?

- Compression
  - Single characters only?
  - Double characters?
  - Leading zeroes and trailing blanks?
  - Primary file compression?
  - Secondary file compression?

6. Data Independence

How does the DBMS cope with the following situations:

- Insertion of a new field type
  - at the end of the record/segment,
  - anywhere in the record/segment?

- Insertion of a new record/segment type
  - at the end of the structure,
  - anywhere in the structure?

- Change the characteristics of an existing field
  - lengthening of a field eg. introduction of a check digit,
  - changing packed data to binary?

- Introducing a new secondary index
  - Must the primary DB be reloaded or just read?

7. Data Manipulation

- Information retrieval commands
  - GET/READ
  - LOCATE/FIND

- Is it possible to change a primary key field value?
- Is it possible to process a chain or structure in both forward and backward directions ie.
  - READ NEXT and READ PREVIOUS?
  - READ PARENT and READ CHILD?
- Is it possible to retrieve all records satisfying a particular criterion (or at least their addresses) with one command?
  - Can these records be retrieved ordered on a field (key or non-key)?
- CURRENCY (Positioning)
  - How is it established?
  - How is it removed?
  - How many positions can be held simultaneously?
- Can a Boolean expression be formulated?
  - Are there any restrictions on the operators?
  - Is there any restriction on the complexity of the expression?
- Generic Key Searching available?
- Is it possible to search on non-key fields?
- Is it possible to retrieve data from different record types with one DML request?

8. Concurrent Usage and Integrity

- Multithreading
  - For retrieval?
  - For update?
- HOLD
  - How is the locking achieved?
    - Core table (with overflow written to disc)?
    - Ring table – with possibility of overwriting?
    - Only one record per type per database?
  - How is deadlock resolved?
    - Logic?
    - Timer?

9. Recovery

- Rollback
  - synchronized checkpointing
- Rollforward?
- Warm restart?

- How much operator/programmer intervention is necessary?
- How many log files can be used simultaneously?
- What information is written to the Log file?

10. Privacy Controls

- Subschema
  - Record level sensitivity
  - Field level sensitivity
  - Can the characteristics be different from the schema?
  - Can the field sequence be different from the schema?
- Password
- Encyphering
  - Field level
  - Record level
- Audit trail
  - Security violation audit

11. Performance Statistics and Tuning

- Is there a report on the following characteristics:
  - block splits,
  - percentage full,
  - length of chains,
  - record distribution statistics,
  - response times,
  - simulation for performance forecasting?

12. Reorganisation

- Running reorganisation
  - Only when updating the record
  - On every access to the record
- No effort made to reorganise
  - All insertions after initial load are placed in overflow
  - Any free space is used
- No need to reorganise (access method requires no order)
  - Possible to reorganise parts of a database separately eg. a secondary index or primary without having to reorganise the secondary

Appendix II: General Glossary of Database Terminology

For ease of use the terms and expressions directly related to a particular DBMS have been included in each report. It is quite possible for an expression to appear in different glossaries with different meanings.

The general glossary is provided to help with current technical database literature. It should not be viewed as a standardized database glossary: this does not exist. The nearest approach to an industry standard for database terminology is the work of the CODASYL Database Task Groups.

Those words within an explanation appearing in BLOCK CAPITALS are also the subject of an explanation in the glossary.

ACCESS: The act of seeking, reading or writing on a secondary storage unit.

ACCESS METHOD: A technique available, but external, to the application for moving data between the CPU and secondary storage. eg. VSAM, ISAM or BDAM.

ACCESS PATH: That route taken in traversing a logical structure to locate a given unit of data.

ACCESS TIME: The time interval between the RUN-UNIT requesting a unit of information be transferred to or from its communication area and the operation being completed.

ACTIVITY RATIO: The percentage of records in a file or DATABASE that have been retrieved in a given time period (cf. HIT RATE).

ADDRESS: The identification of a particular location on primary or secondary storage.

ADDRESS CONVERTER: From a performance point of view, the use of an Address Converter is poor as it leads to an extra access to locate the required record's address. It is used to avoid the necessity of having to update all the index pointers when a record is moved from one block to another, due, for example, to its compressed length increasing after an update. A better solution would be to have a pointer in the original block to the new location. Thus the extra access would only be necessary after a record had moved block. If the record moved a second time the pointer in the original block would be updated to reflect the new position. This would present no difficulty as this block would be in the buffer. Nevertheless from a data security point of view it is important to separate user and internal data.

ALGORITHM: A computational procedure.

APPLICATION: A routine or set of routines performing some specialized user-oriented function eg. payroll calculation.

ARBITRARY DISTRIBUTION: The placing of records in the available data space without regard to any ordering criteria internal to the record.

ARBITRARY PLACEMENT: See ARBITRARY DISTRIBUTION.

AREA(CODASYL): A named logical subdivision of the addressable storage space which may contain occurrences of records and SETS (or parts of SETS) of various types. AREAS may be processed exclusively by a particular RUN-UNIT or accessible to all.

ARITHMETIC OPERATORS: The ARITHMETIC OPERATORS are plus ('+'), minus ('–'), divide ('/'), multiply ('x') and exponentiate ('*').

ARRAY: An n-dimensional collection of data items all having the same characteristics.

ASSOCIATIVE MEMORY: Storage in which data is identified by its value not by its address. It provides a much faster way of searching for data meeting complex criteria than conventional storage which has addressing related to physical storage.

ASSOCIATIVE TRANSACTION: Processing which is automatically invoked when some DATA ITEM or ELEMENT changes value.

ATTRIBUTE: The characteristics of an ENTITY.

BACKOUT: The process of returning a DATABASE to the condition applying prior to some unit of processing ie. reversing all changes made by that unit of processing.

BACKUP: see DATABASE COPY (cf. RECOVERY, RESTART).

BATCH PROCESSING: The term is derived from the batching of input data received over a period of time and pertains to the technique of accumulating a number of similar input items prior to processing them.

BDAM (IBM): BASIC DIRECT ACCESS METHOD.

BENCHMARK: This is a test designed to evaluate the performance of some aspect of the computer hardware or software.

BINARY SEARCH: A method of searching an ordered table or file. The process involves successively halving the area of search by examining the mid-point value until the required value is found.

BINDING(TIME): Linking the specific data types required by the application program with the data as physically stored in the DATABASE.

BLOCK: The unit of physical data transfer between the CPU and secondary storage. It will contain one or more logical records.

BOOLEAN ALGEBRA: The use of algebraic notation to express logical relationships. The operators are Conjunction (AND), Disjunction (OR) and Negation (NOT).

BUCKET: An area of secondary storage which can hold one or more synonym records and will be referred to as a unit by some addressing algorithm (cf. HOME BLOCK).

BUFFER: A temporary store for DATA UNITS.

CALL: The command available in most standard programming languages to pass parameters to and activate a subprogram.

CANDIDATE KEY (Relational): A key that uniquely identifies a TUPLE, it may be chosen as the PRIMARY KEY.

CANONICAL SCHEMA: This is a data model which essentially represents the inherent structure of the data. It is therefore totally independent of the software and hardware mechanisms used to represent and manipulate the data.

CARDINALITY (Relational): The number of TUPLES in a relation.

CELL: Contiguous storage locations.

CHAIN: A technique for establishing a relationship between records of a SET. Pointers can link each record to is successor and/or its predecessor. It is possible to reach all records in the chain from any record.

CHAINED FILE: A file where the records do not have to be in any physical order because each record contains a POINTER to the 'next' logical record.

CHECKPOINT: The writing of a record to a secondary storage medium (usually the LOG FILE) signifying that the DATABASE was logically intact at the time of writing. This can be used later to reconstruct the DATABASE and defines a point from which the program(s) may be restarted.

CHECKPOINT/RESTART: See CHECKPOINT.

CHILD: A term used in hierarchical structures to denote an immediate dependent of a record or segment. (cf. PARENT)

CIRCULAR FILE: See RING FILE.

CIPHERING: This is a technique for rendering sensitive information unreadable both to DBMS users without the cipher key and also for external dumps of the DATABASE.

CODASYL: Conference of Data Description Languages. As its activities with the COBOL language were drawing to a close, it began developing a set of machine and manufacturer independent languages for DATABASE management. It was planned to incorporate the DML in the COBOL language. The scope of the work has been extended to include a DATA DICTIONARY concept.

COMMAND: An instruction for directing the processing of a program.

COMMON DATA: Information elements common to a given information class.

COMMUNITY OF DATA: All the data shared by all the users of a DATABASE.

COMPACTION: See COMPRESSION.

COMPOSITE ATTRIBUTE (Relational): This is an ATTRIBUTE composed of more than one simple ATTRIBUTE.

COMPOSITE PRIMARY KEY (Relational): This is a PRIMARY KEY made up from a COMPOSITE ATTRIBUTE.

COMPOSITION: See RELATIONAL ALGEBRA.

COMPRESSION: This is a technique for reducing the space occupied by a DATA UNIT eg. a record, to a minimum. Various methods are in common use. Two examples are:
- the record will be treated as a data string, all repeating characters will be supressed
- the record will be treated as a series of fields, all numeric fields will be packed and all leading zeroes and trailing blanks will be supressed.

Space reduction of ca. 50% is quite normal.

CONCATENATE: This term simply means 'linking together', thus a concatenated KEY is a KEY composed of a number of separate fields.

CONCEPTUAL SCHEMA: The description of the overall logical structure of a DATABASE.

CONJUNCTION: See BOOLEAN ALGEBRA.

CONTENT ADDRESSABLE STORE: A secondary storage device which achieves a high retrieval rate by using a technique of sequentially scanning the stored values rather than by the use of hardware addressing.

CONTENTION: See DEADLY EMBRACE.

CONVERSATION: The dialogue between a terminal and an online program.

CURRENCY: The position(s) established by the application program in the DATABASE.

DATA: A general expression for any bit combination representing a value and/or identification.

DATA ADMINISTRATOR: The person whose job it is to control the enterprise's data descriptions and their relationship to each other.

DATA AGGREGATE(CODASYL): A named collection of DATA ITEMS within a record.

DATA ANALYSIS: A detailed investigation of the enterprise's data, with the object of identifying all DATA ITEMS and their relationships, eliminating redundancy, and thus rationalizing the control over the data.

DATABASE:
1. A generalized, common and integrated collection of interrelated data containing controlled data redundancy whose purpose is to serve one or more applications.
2. (CODASYL)
   It consists of all record, SET and AREA occurrences under the control of a single SCHEMA.

DATABASE ADMINISTRATOR: A person or persons responsible for analysing an enterprise's data requirements, and for defining, organizing and protecting the DATABASE(s) and contents.

DATABASE COPY: This is the act of writing out the state of the DATABASE at some instant in time to a secondary storage medium eg. tape, for the purpose of reconstructing a DATABASE should some irrecoverable error occur.
No modifications to the DATABASE may be made during this process.

DATABASE DUMP: See DATABASE COPY.

DATABASE INTEGRITY: This is the protection of the data from concurrent updating (see DATA INTEGRITY).

DATABASE KEY (CODASYL): The unique identifier assigned by the DBMS to each and every record occurrence in the DATABASE.

DATABASE MANAGEMENT SYSTEM: The collection of software designed to control the activities of the DATABASE efficiently and to protect it from misuse. Typically a DBMS package would contain such additional features as a Report Writer, a query language, recovery software, a DATA DICTIONARY and a TP Monitor or at least interfaces to these products.

DATABASE PROCEDURE: A routine, usually written by (or for) the DBA, which is included via a USER-EXIT in the DBMS and is automatically invoked when needed.

DATA DESCRIPTION LANGUAGE (CODASYL): The language used to describe the full DATABASE structure (and also the USER-VIEWS in some DBMSs).

DATA DICTIONARY: A catalogue of all data types, records and DATABASES giving their names, characteristics, structures and relations to each other. Sometimes the data types description includes source, user and ownership information. Some DBMSs have an integrated DATA DICTIONARY, which can be an enormous advantage.

DATA ELEMENT: See DATA ITEM.

DATA FIELD: See DATA ITEM.

DATA INDEPENDENCE: The concept of separating the definitions of the logical and physical data structures, thus avoiding the problem of changes to the physical DATABASE affecting existing programs.

DATA INTEGRITY: The concept that all DATABASES must be protected against accidental or deliberate damage either of a physical or logical nature.

DATA ITEM: The smallest unit of named data.

DATA MANIPULATION LANGUAGE (CODASYL): The language used in the application program which causes data to be moved between the program and the DATABASE. The DML is not a self-contained language but has to be embedded in some host language.

DATA PRIVACY: The concept that units of data may only be retrieved and altered by those users who have the proper authority.

DATA SECURITY: See DATA PRIVACY.

DATA UNIT: A generic term indicating a particular collection of data; it may be a DATA ITEM, a DATA AGGREGATE, a SET or a DATABASE.

DBA: See DATABASE ADMINISTRATOR.

DDL: See DATA DESCRIPTION LANGUAGE.

DEADLOCK: See DEADLY EMBRACE.

DEADLY EMBRACE: The situation where two or more users are 'stalled' because they are competing for the same

	resources and none may proceed until one of the others has released its resources.
DEGREE (Relational):	The number of DOMAINs within a relation.
DERIVED DATA ITEM:	A DATA ITEM which has no independent existence but is generated by the DBMS.
DEVICE MEDIA CONTROL LANGUAGE (CODASYL):	The language used to specify the storage of data at the physical level, including control of space on each device, overflow, buffering and paging.
DIALOGUE:	A generic term indicating a planned man-machine interaction.
DICTIONARY:	See DATA DICTIONARY.
DIFFERENCE (Relational):	See RELATIONAL ALGEBRA.
DIRECT ACCESS:	The storage and retrieval of data which is totally independent of any previously held position in the data. The ACCESS TIME may be considered constant.
DIRECTORY:	A primitive form of DATA DICTIONARY used internally in some DBMSs. It holds the relationship information between DATA ITEMS.
DISJUNCTION:	See BOOLEAN ALGEBRA.
DISTRIBUTED DATABASE:	A DATABASE which can be dynamically allocated to have different parts residing on different computers in the network.
DISTRIBUTED FREE SPACE:	Space left empty at intervals over the database during loading to accommodate future insertions.
DMCL:	See DEVICE-MEDIA CONTROL LANGUAGE.
DML:	See DATA MANIPULATION LANGUAGE.
DOMAIN (Relational):	Groups of like data upon which a relation is defined.
DUAL LOGGING:	An feature offered by most DBMSs writing the logged information to two separate LOG FILES thus offering enhanced safety.
DYNAMIC STORAGE ALLOCATION:	A storage allocation technique in which memory is assigned temporarily from a pool to a RUN UNIT. Until the RUN UNIT returns the memory to the pool, it remains one of its resources.

EMBEDDED POINTER: POINTERS attached to the records themselves rather than in an INDEX or DIRECTORY.

ENTITY: Something of interest to the enterprise or its activities, about which data is stored.

ENTITY IDENTIFIER: A key which uniquely identifies an ENTITY or the data associated with the ENTITY.

ENTITY NAME: The symbol by which the ENTITY is known.

ENTITY STREAM: All ENTITIES of a particular type.

EXPLICIT: Implies the direct specification of characteristics of the DATA-UNIT.

EXTENT: A contiguous area of data storage.

EXTERNAL SCHEMA: See SUBSCHEMA.

FIELD: See DATA ITEM.

FILE: A set of records having logical interrelationships.

FIRST NORMAL FORM: See NORMAL FORM.

FLAT FILE: A two-dimensional ARRAY of DATA-ELEMENTS ie. a file with neither hierarchical nor network relationships.

FLUSH(ING): This is the activity associated with a CHECKPOINT or closing the DBMS down when the changes to the DB still held in the I/O buffers are written out to the files. A log record will normally also be written.

FOREIGN KEY (Relational): This is an ATTRIBUTE of relation R1 that is not the PRIMARY KEY of R1 but is the PRIMARY KEY of relation R2.

FREE SPACE BIT MAP: A technique for managing free space by using one bit to indicate whether or not free space above a certain size is available in each block. It should only be used for files with one constant length record type because with VARIABLE LENGTH records or different record lengths only those blocks containing sufficient space for the largest record size are noted in the bit map. Thus all smaller free space areas are underused.

FREE SPACE CHAIN:
1. In DBMSs where free space within a block stays fragmented because no effort is made to

combine the space made available via deletes and record 'shrinkage', there is usually a free space anchor point at the beginning of the block pointing to the first free space fragment. The first four bytes of each free space fragment contain a pointer to the next free space fragment in the block.

2. Instead of using a FREE SPACE LIST to indicate which blocks contain free space, a series of pointers can be used to link these blocks (usually in LIFO order). It has the disadvantage that it is almost impossible to gain an overall impression of the free space distribution.

FREE SPACE LIST: A technique for managing free space within a file or database by entering the size of the available space in each block in a list.

FULLY INVERTED ATTRIBUTE: See INVERTED FILE.

FUNCTIONAL DEPENDENCE: An ATTRIBUTE A of a relationship is FUNCTIONALLY DEPENDENT on an ATTRIBUTE B of the same relationship if the ATTRIBUTE A has no more than one value of ATTRIBUTE B associated with it.

$R.A \rightarrow R.B$

GRANULARITY: This is a measure of the size of the DATA ITEMS in the record. Fine GRANULARITY means that the fields are small. This is advantageous for DATA INDEPENDENCE but the disadvantage is that it can have a negative impact on performance.

HASHING: See RANDOMIZING.

HEAD OF LIST: This is the record which occupies the first place in the list.

HEURISTIC: Pertaining to methods of investigation using inductive reasoning based on experience (trial-and-error) to obtain a solution to a problem.

HIERARCHICAL STRUCTURE: See HIERARCHY.

HIERARCHY: A relationship between DATA UNITS in which

some are subordinate to others in an inverted tree structure, such that one DATA UNIT has no PARENT and all others have exactly one PARENT. The maximum number of levels allowed differs from one DBMS to the next.

HIT RATE: That percentage of records of a file or DATABASE which are accessed in a given run. (cf. ACTIVITY RATIO)

HOME ADDRESS: See HOME BLOCK.

HOME BLOCK: That block which a record has been logically assigned to. When more records are assigned to a block than it can accommodate, the excess will be placed in an adjacent (or overflow) block. Pointers link all SYNONYMS usually in ascending key sequence.

HOME BUCKET: See HOME BLOCK.

HOMONYM: A term used in DATA DICTIONARY work, meaning something with the same name, but a different meaning.

HOST (PROGRAMMING) LANGUAGE: A programming language in which the DBMS DML commands are embedded.

IDENTIFIER: A DATA ITEM or ITEMS which uniquely identify an occurrence of a DATA UNIT.

IMAGE:
1. BEFORE A copy of a block/record immediately prior to a change being made.
2. AFTER A copy of a block/record immediately after a change has been made.

IMPLICIT: Conditions implied but not plainly stated.

INCESTUOUS RELATIONSHIP: See INVOLUTED RELATIONSHIP.

INDEPENDENCE: See DATA INDEPENDENCE.

INDEX: An ARRAY, usually in the form of a file containing key/keypointer pairs, used to locate records rapidly.

INDEXED SEQUENTIAL FILE: The data file is sequentially ordered on the PRIMARY KEY. An INDEX based on the PRIMARY KEY enables the records to be rapidly retrieved.

As the data is in sequence, the INDEX has only to hold the highest (or lowest) key value from each data block.

INDEX TABLE: See INDEX.

INFORMATION: The AGGREGATE of all that is known about an ENTITY occurrence.

INTEGRITY: See DATA INTEGRITY.

INTERLOCK: See DEADLY EMBRACE.

INTERNAL SCHEMA: See STORAGE SCHEMA.

INTERSECTION (Relational): See RELATIONAL ALGEBRA.

INTERSECTION DATA: In an M:M relationship, data associated with a specific occurrence of the relationship. This data only has meaning in conjunction with this relationship occurrence.

INVERTED FILE: The data file is in no particular sequence because no PRIMARY KEY can be defined. An INDEX is constructed for each key defined thus enabling complex queries to be resolved without accessing the data file. This INDEX also provides a number of alternative processing paths. Because the data file is unsequenced, each INDEX must contain entries for every value (cf. INDEXED SEQUENTIAL FILE).

A fully INVERTED FILE has all its values held in INDEXES. This is usually unnecessary and the overhead of index maintenance detracts greatly from performance. It is therefore normal practicc to select only those DATA ITEMS that are absolutely required. This is known as a partially INVERTED FILE.

INVERTED LIST: See INVERTED FILE.

INVOLUTED RELATIONSHIP: This is a relationship where the OWNER of the SET is also a MEMBER of the same SET.

ISAM(IBM): INDEX SEQUENTIAL ACCESS METHOD.

JOIN: See RELATIONAL ALGEBRA.

JOURNALLING: See LOG FILE.

KEY: A DATA ITEM or ITEMS used to identify a

	record, but not necessarily uniquely (cf. PRIMARY and SECONDARY KEY)
KEY COMPRESSION:	A technique for reducing the space occupied by the keys in the INDEX.
KEY TRANSFORM:	See RANDOMIZING.
LFU (Least Frequently Used):	A technique for identifying that DATA UNIT in a storage area (buffer) which is to be overwritten when the buffer is full and space is required, by establishing which DATA UNIT has been least frequently used (cf. LRU).
LINKAGE:	A mechanism for connecting DATA UNITS to each other.
LINKED LIST:	An ordered set of DATA ITEMS with each member pointing to its successor in the list (cf. CHAIN).
LIST:	See LINKED LIST.
LISTING ORDER:	See ORDERING RULES.
LOCAL VIEW:	See USER VIEW.
LOCATION MODE (CODASYL):	The techniques used by a DBMS to allocate DATABASE KEYS to records.
LOG FILE:	A file maintained by the DBMS containing all requests made to the DATABASE, checkpoint information and sometimes also user written messages. The main purpose of this file is to enable the DATABASE to be reconstructed should the DATABASE integrity be compromised. This file can also contain information for security audit purposes.
LOGICAL DATABASE:	See USER VIEW.
LOGICAL READ:	A read command issued by the program which can be satisfied by data already available in the I/O buffer.
LOGICAL RECORD:	A record as seen by the user. The DATA ITEMS may be drawn from different actual records. The USER VIEW dictates what the contents of the LOGICAL RECORD will be.
LOGICAL VIEW:	See USER VIEW.

LRU (Least Recently Used): A technique for identifying that DATA UNIT in a storage area (buffer) which is to be overwritten when the area is full and space is required, by establishing which DATA UNIT has been least recently used (cf. LFU).

MEMBER (CODASYL): A record within a SET, a dependent of the OWNER of the SET.

MULTIPLE-KEY RETRIEVAL: Retrieval of a record or records which satisfy complex search criteria, consisting of a number of key/key value combinations linked with Boolean operators.

MULTIPROCESSING: Pertaining to the simultaneous execution of two or more programs by a network of linked computers (processors).

MULTIPROGRAMMING: Pertaining to the concurrent execution of two or more programs by a single computer.

MULTITASKING: Pertaining to the concurrent execution of two or more tasks.

MULTITHREADING: Pertaining to the concurrent execution of a REENTRANT program by more than one RUN UNIT.

MULTIUSER: Pertaining to the ability of a software package to serve a number of users concurrently.

NAVIGATION: The process by which a program establishes POSITION in the DATABASE and then moves through the DATABASE structure by following the ACCESS PATHS.

NETWORK STRUCTURE: A relationship between DATA UNITS in which some are subordinate to others, such that some are OWNERS and others MEMBERS where each MEMBER may have more than one OWNER (cf. HIERARCHY).

NON-KEY ATTRIBUTE (Relational): An ATTRIBUTE may be so described if it does not constitute part (or the whole) of the PRIMARY KEY.

NORMAL FORM (Relational):

1. FIRST NORMAL FORM (1NF) is the reduction of each value of each TUPLE to non-decomposable (atomic) elements ie. each row/

column position contains only a simple value, never a set of values.

2. SECOND NORMAL FORM (2NF). Problems arise with 1NF because ATTRIBUTES are not fully FUNCTIONALLY DEPENDENT on the same PRIMARY KEY. This can lead to ambiguities when manipulating TUPLES in 1NF. To overcome this difficulty the ATTRIBUTES should be split into a series of TUPLES where each non-key ATTRIBUTE is fully FUNCTIONALLY DEPENDENT on the PRIMARY KEY. This is SECOND NORMAL FORM.
N.B. a 1NF relation that is not in 2NF must have a COMPOSITE PRIMARY KEY.

3. THIRD NORMAL FORM (3NF). Unfortunately 2NF also has its problem namely TRANSITIVE DEPENDENCE. Thus a 3NF relation is described as a relation in 2NF with every non-key ATTRIBUTE nontransitively dependent on the PRIMARY KEY.
Another definition of 3NF (not involving 1NF and 2NF) is: a normalised relation in which every determinant is a CANDIDATE KEY.

NORMALIZATION: The reversable process of reducing complex relationships ie. reducing complex data structures to FLAT FILES. The object is to free relationships from undesirable interactions (cf. NORMAL FORM).

OCCURRENCE (CODASYL): A specific instance of the value of a DATA UNIT.

OFF-LINE PROCESSING: See BATCH PROCESSING.

ON-LINE PROCESSING: Processing that reacts directly to any input (cf. BATCH PROCESSING).

OPERATORS: See ARITHMETIC and BOOLEAN OPERATORS.

ORDERING RULE:

1. FIFO (First-in First-out).
The first record entered into a list will be the first one retrieved ie. they will be retrieved in the same order that they were stored.

2. LEXICOGRAPHIC.
   The records will be ordered in the list on the value of some DATA ITEM.
3. LIFO (Last-in First-out).
   The last record entered into a list will be the first one retrieved ie. they will be retrieved in the reverse order to that they were stored in.

OVERFLOW: This is the condition when the HOME BLOCK is no longer capable of accommodating a new occurrence of a record. It may be accommodated in a neighbouring block or in an area reserved for such cases normally at the end of the file.

OWNER RECORD (CODASYL): A record which determines the existence of a SET and upon which all MEMBERS are dependent.

PADDING: Data extended with some default character; numeric with leading zeroes; alpha and alphanumeric with trailing blanks.

PAGE(CODASYL): A physical block containing records.

PAGING: This is a technique central to the operation of virtual storage operating systems whereby each program is split into a series of blocks (pages). A program is allocated a much smaller area of main storage than the whole program actually requires. Thus the main memory appears to be much larger that it is.
(As main memory is becoming ever cheaper the necessity for optimal use of this resource will decrease).

PARENT: A term used in hierarchical relationships to denote the immediate ancestor of a record (cf. CHILD).

PERMUTATION: See RELATIONAL ALGEBRA.

PHYSICAL READ: The transfer of a BLOCK of data from secondary storage to the I/O buffers.

PHYSICAL RECORD: See BLOCK.

PLEX STRUCTURE: See NETWORK STRUCTURE.

POINTER: This is the address of a DATA UNIT. It may be in absolute, relative or symbolic form.

POSITION: See CURRENCY.

PRIMARY KEY:
1. This is the key that determines the order in which the records will be physically stored. It need not be unique but often is.
2. (Relational). A key that uniquely identifies a TUPLE not necessarily composed of a single ATTRIBUTE.

PROGRESSIVE OVERFLOW: This is a technique for handling OVERFLOW with direct access methods. It does not require pointers because an overflow record is placed in the next higher block in which space is available. It can be retrieved by a forward serial search from the HOME BLOCK.

PROJECTION (Relational): See RELATIONAL ALGEBRA.

QUERY: The formal statement of a retrieval request.

QUERY LANGUAGE: A simply constructed, easy to use interactive language used to interrogate the DATABASE. Some QUERY LANGUAGES also allow DATABASE modification.

RANDOM ACCESS: See DIRECT ACCESS.

RANDOM DISTRIBUTION: See RANDOM PLACEMENT.

RANDOMIZING: A DIRECT ADDRESSING technique in which each PRIMARY KEY value is converted into a relative file address. The aim is to distribute the records uniformly over the available data space.

RANDOM PLACEMENT: The distributing of records uniformly across a data space, without regard for any DATA ITEM internal to the record occurrence.

RANDOM PROCESSING: Processing data in a random sequence.

RECORD(CODASYL): A named collection of data ELEMENTS.

RECOVERY: This is a feature available with most DBMSs. It returns the DATABASE to a physically consistent state after some hard- or software failure. Different techniques have been evolved to cater for the different sorts of failure. Different approaches have been adopted by the various DBMSs: some rely heavily on TP Monitor facilities, others not at all (cf. ROLLFORWARD, CHECKPOINT, TRANSACTION, WARM and COLD RESTART).

RECURSIVE RELATIONSHIP (CODASYL): See INVOLUTED RELATIONSHIP.

REDUNDANCY: The storage of the same DATA ITEM type in more than one record type. Ideally no data should be stored more than once. Due to hardware restrictions it is necessary to introduce the concept of 'controlled redundancy'. This means allowing some redundancy in order to achieve acceptable performance.

RE-ENTRANT: An ATTRIBUTE of a routine or program that allows one copy to be used concurrently by more than one RUN UNIT. This requires that no RUN UNIT change the body of the code.

RELATION: A two-dimensional array of DATA ITEMS.

RELATIONAL ALGEBRA: One of the two DMLs proposed for RELATIONAL DATABASES. It offers the same processing power as in RELATIONAL CALCULUS. The commands are:

1. COMPOSITION.
   This command combines relations with common DOMAINS. Relations can only be COMPOSED if they can also be JOINed.
2. DIFFERENCE.
   This command creates a relation which is composed of only those relations found in one of the relations but not in the other.
3. INTERSECTION.
   This command selects common TUPLES of stated relations.
4. JOIN.
   This command takes two relations as arguments and forms a new relation by concatenating the TUPLES of each relation whenever a specified condition applies.
5. PERMUTATION.
   This command reorders the TUPLES of a relation.

6. PROJECTION.
   This command returns only specified columns of a relation and eliminates all duplicates.
7. RESTRICTION.
   This command selects only those TUPLES of a relation which satisfy a given condition.
8. SELECTION.
   This command selects those TUPLES satisfying certain criteria.
9. UNION.
   This command combines relations where all the DOMAINS are common; duplicates are discarded.

RELATIONAL CALCULUS: One of the two DMLs proposed for RELATIONAL DATABASES. It offers the same processing power as in RELATIONAL ALGEBRA. The commands are:

1. CLOSE terminates the retrieval of TUPLES singly.
2. DELETE removes a defined relation from the DATABASE.
3. DROP removes a relation definition from the data dictionary.
4. HOLD indicates that a retrieved TUPLE may be modified.
5. GET retrieves the defined relations into a work area.
6. OPEN starts returning the TUPLES singly to the user instead of returning complete relations.
7. PUT inserts the work area contents to the DATABASE.
8. RANGE temporalily changes the relation name.
9. RELEASE indicates that the 'held' TUPLES will not be modified.
10. UPDATE modifies the DATABASE as defined in the work area.

RELATIONAL DATABASE: This is simply a DATABASE in which the USER VIEW can be in at least THIRD NORMAL FORM and RELATIONAL CALCULUS and/or

ALGEBRA are available for RELATION manipulation.

REORGANIZATION: This is a technique for optimizing performance by rationalizing the space occupied by the DATABASE. It is achieved by unloading the DATABASE and then loading it again. Some DBMSs seldom require reorganisation runs to be performed, as they continuously reorganise themselves. Others have no order so cannot be reorganised. The great disadvantage of a formal REORGANIZATION, apart from the computer time involved, is that the DATABASE must be taken off-line for it. It is also usually necessary when the database structure is modified.

REPORT GENERATOR: See REPORT WRITER.

REPORT WRITER: A software package with a simple yet powerful language for producing reports. Usually many reports can be produced in one pass of the file or DATABASE.

RESEQUENCE: This is simply ordering the records on some key, to speed up sequential processing on this key. This should not be confused with REORGANIZATION.

RESPONSE TIME: The time elapsing between the last character of the input message leaving the terminal and the first character of the reply reaching the terminal.

RESTART:

1. WARM.
   This describes the ability of a DBMS to recover automatically from a soft or hardware failure.
2. COLD.
   Starting the DBMS running such that no reference is made to the conditions applying when the DBMS was stopped.

RESTRICTION: See RELATIONAL ALGEBRA.

RESTRUCTURE: This is an activity involved with introducing new record types into the DATABASE structures or introducing new DATA ITEM types into a record or even just changing the characteristics of a DATA ITEM. There are great differences between the DBMSs in the ease with which changes can be made.

RING: See RING STRUCTURE.

RING FILE: A file organisation used in highly volatile environments. New records overwrite the oldest. Thus the file never overflows.

RING STRUCTURE: A LIST of linked records, with the last record in the list linked to the first record thus forming a RING.

ROLLBACK: This is a RECOVERY technique using the actual DATABASE and the LOG FILE (or work file for TRANSACTIONS).
It applies the BEFORE IMAGES from the LOG FILE to the DATABASE thus returning the DATABASE to an earlier status.

ROLLFORWARD: This is a RECOVERY technique using a DATABASE COPY and the LOG FILE. It applies the AFTER IMAGES from the LOG FILE to the DATABASE COPY thus bringing the DATABASE forward to a later status.

ROOT: The base node of an inverted tree structure.

RUN UNIT (CODASYL): The execution of a program. Each RUN UNIT is a separate ENTITY serviced by the DBMS with its own user work areas etc.

SCHEMA(CODASYL): The complete description of AREAS, records, ELEMENTS and SETS constituting a DATABASE.

SECONDARY INDEX: This is an INDEX composed of one or more DATA ITEMS normally but not necessarily non-unique, which offers rapid resolution of complex queries because only the INDEXES have to be consulted and also alternative entry points into the DATABASE.

SECONDARY KEY: See SECONDARY INDEX.

SECOND NORMAL FORM: See NORMAL FORM.

SECURITY: The protection of the DATABASE from unauthorised access, it can take the form of:
- password security,
- sign-on security,
- resource access security.

SELECTION (Relational): See RELATIONAL ALGEBRA.

SENSITIVITY: When a program is limited to a certain subset of the DATA ITEM types, it is said to be sensitive to only these types.

SEQUENTIAL FILE: A file organised such that a record can only be accessed by first reading all records preceding it in the file. It is not possible to insert a record into the file directly; the file must be copied record for record and the new record inserted in the relevant position.

SEQUENTIAL PROCESSING: Accessing records in ascending order on some key value. This does not have to be SEQUENTIAL FILE.

SEQUENTIAL RETRIEVAL: See SEQUENTIAL PROCESSING.

SERIAL PROCESSING: Accessing records in physical sequence.

SERIAL RETRIEVAL: See SERIAL PROCESSING.

SERIALLY REUSABLE: A characteristic of a routine or program which allows a single copy of the code to be used by a series of RUN UNITS. The restriction is that the present RUN UNIT must finish processing before the next one may start (cf. REENTRANT).

SET(CODASYL): A named collection of record types. It represents a 1:M relationship between the OWNER record type and the MEMBER record type(s).

SET SELECTION (CODASYL): The process whereby the appropriate occurrence of a SET type is determined.

SIBLING: A term used in hierarchical relationships to denote occurrences of the different record types under the same PARENT occurrence. (cf. TWIN)

SINGULAR SET(CODASYL): A SET apparently without an OWNER. The OWNER is declared to be the 'system'. It is used to provide a simple non-hierarchical DATABASE.

SPACE MANAGEMENT FUNCTION: See FREE SPACE.

STRUCTURE DATA: Internal DBMS data used to define the relationships between DATA ITEMS.

SUBSCHEMA(CODASYL): A program oriented subset of the SCHEMA. (cf. USER VIEW).

SYNONYM:
1. A term used in DATA DICTIONARY work, meaning something with the different name, but the same meaning.
2. In DIRECT ACCESS methods, all records that map to the same HOME BLOCK are called SYNONYMS.

SYNONYM CHAIN: This is a technique used in DIRECT ACCESS methods of linking all records that map to the same address (HOME BLOCK).

TABLE: See ARRAY.

TELEPROCESSING: This is the processing of data from a remote terminal linked to the computer by telecommunications lines.

TEMPORARY AREA: See DYNAMIC STORAGE ALLOCATION.

THIRD NORMAL FORM: See NORMAL FORM.

TP MONITOR: This is a software package that removes the problems associated with telecommunication hardware from the user program. A TP Monitor is designed to effectively control a heterogeneous mix of terminal types, and interface the user program with a DBMS or a file ACCESS METHOD.

TRANSACTION: A TRANSACTION is a logical unit of work as seen by the user. It will often consist of a DIALOGUE between the terminal user and the computer consisting of a number of exchanges of information.

TRANSITIVE DEPENDENCE (Relational): This is the situation where an ATTRIBUTE although fully FUNCTIONALLY DEPENDENT on a PRIMARY KEY has a further dependence on another ATTRIBUTE:

ie. if $R.A \rightarrow R.B$ and $R.B \rightarrow R.C$
then $R.A \rightarrow R.C$

	N.B. R.A → R.B	means that in the binary relation R(A,B) B is FUNCTIONALLY DEPENDENT on A.

TRANSPARENCY: See DATA INDEPENDENCE.

TRANSPARENT DATA: Internal STRUCTURE DATA attached to the record but not seen by the user.

TRANSPOSED FILE: Such files are only suitable for sequential processing, where not all fields of each record are required for processing. Records are not stored as contiguous DATA UNITS; all DATA ITEMS of the same type are collected together in VECTORS.

TRAVERSE: See NAVIGATION.

TREE STRUCTURE (INVERTED): See HIERARCHY.

TUPLE (Relational): A group of related DATA ITEMS.

TWIN: A term used in hierarchical relationships to denote two or more occurrence of the same record type under the same PARENT occurrence (cf. SIBLING).

UNION (Relational): See RELATIONAL ALGEBRA.

USER VIEW: That subset of a database structure available to a particular program.

VARIABLE LENGTH RECORD:

1. A file or DATABASE containing a number of different record types each with a different but fixed length.
2. A file or DATABASE where the records of the same type may have different lengths, but an occurrence never changes its length.
3. A file where each record occurrence can take on a new length (within certain limits eg. block size) each time it is modified.
   The last definition is the correct definition – the others are only subsets of it.

VECTOR (CODASYL): A one-dimensional ordered collection of DATA ITEMS, all of which have identical characteristcs.

VIRTUAL DATA: See DERIVED DATA.

VOLATILE: An adjective describing a file or DATABASE with a high rate of insertion and/or deletion activity.

VSAM: VIRTUAL SEQUENTIAL ACCESS METHOD.

Appendix III: Report Writers, TP Monitors and Data Dictionaries with Interfaces of the DBMSs

Product type	product	ADABAS	IDMS	IMS	DATACOM	TOTAL	S2000
Report Writers	CULPRIT		X	X	X	X	
	MARK IV	X	X	X		X	
	EASYTRIEVE	X	X			X	
	The Data Analyser	X		X		X	
TP Monitors	Intercomm	X	X			X	X
	Betacomm			X		X	
	CICS	X	X	X	X	X	X
	Com-plete	X					
	DATACOM/DC				X		
	Environ/1	X				X	
	IMS/DC		X	X			
	SHADOW II	X	X	X		X	X
	TASKMASTER	X	X	X	X	X	X
	TSO	X	X			X	
	WESTI		X		X	X	X

product type	product	ADABAS	IDMS	IMS	DATACOM	TOTAL	S2000
Data Dictionary	DATA–MANAGER	X	X	X		X	
	LEXICON		X	X		X	
	CINCOM–DD					X	
	IMS–DD			X			
	DATA CATALOGUE			X			
	UCC TEN			X			
	ADABAS DD	X					
	DATACOM/DD				X		
	CONTROL 2000						X
	IDMS–IDD		X				
	smallest mainframe	370/ 135	370/ 115	370/ 138	370/ 125	370/ 115	370/ 135
	MEMORY (OS) (minimum)	200K	200K		50K *	50K	256
no. of installed systems June 1981		850+	1000+	circa 2100	350	2700*	450*

* all hardware types

Software	operating system	ADABAS	IDMS	IMS	DATACOM	TOTAL	S2000
	OS	X	X	X	X	X	X
	OS/VS1	X	X	X	X	X	X
	SVS	X	X	X	X	X	X
	MVS	X	X	X	X	X	X
	DOS	X	X	X	X	X	X
	DOS/VS	X	X	X	X	X	X
	DOS/VSE	X	X	X	X	X	X
	VM/CMS	X			X	X	X
	edos		X				
	BS1000	X	X			X	
	BS2000	X	X				
	BS3000	X	X				
Hardware							
	360/370	X	X	X	X	X	X
	4300	X	X	X	X	X	X
	Series 30	X	X	X	X	X	X
	compatible hardware	X	X	X	X	X	X

Appendix IV: Manuals Available from the DBMS Vendors

1. ADABAS
   - 1.1 ADABAS Utilities Manual
   - 1.2 ADABAS Commands Reference Manual
   - 1.3 ADABAS Design Guide
   - 1.4 ADABAS Performance Optimization Guide
   - 1.5 DBA Reference Manual
   - 1.6 DBA Policies and Procedures
   - 1.7 Messages and Codes Manual
   - 1.8 ADAMINT Reference Manual
   - 1.9 ADACOM Reference Manual
   - 1.10 ADASCRIPT+ Reference Manual
   - 1.11 NATURAL LANGUAGE Reference Manual
   - 1.12 Programmer's Guide for TP Applications
2. DATACOM/DB
   - 2.1 DATACOM/DB Users' Guide
3. IDMS
   - 3.1 IDMS Sequential Processing Facility
   - 3.2 IDMS Error Messages and Codes Guide
   - 3.3 IDMS Concepts and Facilities
   - 3.4 IDMS Installation and Operation Guide
   - 3.5 IDMS Utilities
   - 3.6 IDMS Database Design and Definiton Guide
4. IMS
   - 4.1 IMS/VS System Application Design Guide or
     IMS/VS Data Base Administration Guide
   - 4.2 IMS/VS Application Programming Reference Manual or
     IMS/VS Application and Programming: Design and Coding
   - 4.3 IMS/VS Utilities
   - 4.4 IMS/VS Messages and Codes
   - 4.5 IMS/VS Primer and Appendices
   - 4.6 IMS/VS Performance Monitoring and Tuning Guide
   - 4.7 IMS/VS-VSAM Interface Guide
   - 4.8 IMS/VS PTF2 Recovery Restart
   - 4.9 IMS/VS System Programmer Reference Manual
   - 4.10 IMS/VS Message Format Services User's Guide
   - 4.11 OS/VS Virtual Storage Acces Method Programmer's Guide
   - 4.12 OS/VS2 Access Method Services
   - 4.13 VSAM Primer and Reference

5. SYSTEM 2000
   - 5.1 Language Specification Manual
   - 5.2 Product Support Manuals
   - 5.3 Messages and Codes
6. TOTAL
   - 6.1 TOTAL Database Administration Reference Manual
   - 6.2 TOTAL Application Programming Reference Manual
   - 6.3 TOTAL Loader/Unloader Utilities
   - 6.4 TOTAL Print/Modify and Statistics Reference Manual
   - 6.5 SOCRATES Users' Manual
   - 6.6 TOTAL Installation Guide
   - 6.7 TOTAL-INTERCOMM Interface Reference Manual
   - 6.8 TOTAL-CICS Interface Reference Manual

Appendix V: The Addresses of the DBMS Vendors

1 – USA
2 – FRG
3 – UK
4 – Norway

ADABAS

1 Software AG of North America, Inc.,
11800 Sunrise Valley Drive,
Reston,
Virginia 22091.

2 Software AG,
Hilpertstr. 20,
D-61 Darmstadt.

3 ADABAS Software Ltd.,
3 Hallam Way,
Hallam,
Derbyshire DE7 6LA.

DATACOM/DB

1 Applied Data Research, Inc.,
8515 Greenville Av.,
Dallas,
Texas 75243.

	2 Applied Data Research (ADR) Software-Entwicklung und Vertrieb GmbH, Hauptstr. 21, D-4000 Duesseldorf 13. 3 Computer Program Products, London.
IDMS	1 Cullinane Corporation, 20 William Street, Wellesley, Massachusetts 02181. 2 ADV/Orga F.A. Meyer GmbH., Kurt-Schuhmacher-Str. 241, D-2940 Wilhelmshaven. 3 Scientific Control Systems Ltd., Sanderson House, 49–57 Berners Street, London WIP 4AQ.
IMS	1 IBM Corporation, 1133 Westchester Avenue, White Plains, New York 10604.
SYSTEM 2000	1 MRI Systems Corporation, P.O. Box 9968, 12675 Research Boulevard, Austin, Texas 78766. 2 INTEL SEMICONDUCTOR GmbH, MRI Systems, Mainzer Str. 75, D-6200 Wiesbaden. 3 MRI has no offices in the UK.
TOTAL	1 Cincom Systems, Inc. 2300 Montana Avenue Cincinnati Ohio 45211. 2 Cincom Systems GmbH Heinrichstr. 169, D-4000 Duesseldorf. 3 Cincom Systems International SA, St. Ives House,

St. Ives Road,
Maidenhead,
Berkshire SL6 1QS.

The addresses of futher Software Products:

DATAMANAGER (Data Dictionary)	1	Management Systems and Programming, 133 Mount Auburn Street, Cambridge, Massachusetts 02138,
	2	MSP Software Products GmbH, Ellebecker Weg 11. D-2084 Rellingen 1.
	3	Mangement Systems and Programming, 71 Gloucester Place, London W1H 3PF.
204 (DBMS)	1	Computer Corporation of America, 575 Technology Square, Cambridge, Massachusetts 02139.
SIBAS (DBMS)	1	Shipping Research Services, Inc., 205 S. Whiting Street, Alexandria, Virginia 22304.
	4	SRS Information Systems Division, Haugerudsenteret, Oslo 6.
MARK IV (DMS)	1	Informatics Inc., Software Products, 21050 Vanowen Street, Canoga Park, California 91304.
	2	Informatics GmbH., Postfach 2363, Louisenstr. 128, D-6380 Bad Homburg.
	3	Informatics (UK) Ltd., Ferranti House, 102 College Road, Harrow, Middlesex HA1 1BQ.
RAMIS II (DMS/DBMS)	1	Mathematica Products Group, Princeton Station Office Park, P.O. Box 2392, Princeton, New Jersey 08540.

2 Prognos A.G.,
Steingraben 42,
CH-4011 Basel.

3 Mathematica Products Group,
Kent House
Market Place,
London W1N 7AJ.

INQUIRE (DBMS)

1 Infodata Systems Inc.,
Information Products Division,
5205 Leesburg Pike,
Falls Church, Virginia 22041.

3 Software Implementations Ltd.,
VLI House,
68–69 St. Martins Lane
London WC2N 4JS.

REACT (DBMS)

1 Cybertech Data Systems
3000 Diamond Park
Dallas, Texas 75247

Further addresses of interest:

ACM Association for Computing Machinery,
1133 Avenue of the Americas,
New York, N.Y. 10036,
USA.

ACM Order Department,
P.O. Box 12105,
Church Street Station,
New York, N.Y. 10249,
USA.

Addison-Wesley Publishing Co.,
Reading, Massachusetts,
USA.

AFIPS Publishers Inc.,
210 Summit Avenue,
Montvale, N.J. 07645,
USA.

AUERBACH Publishers Inc.,
6560 North Park Drive,

Pennsauken, N.J. 08109,
USA.

British Computer Society,
29 Portland Place,
London W1N 4AP,
England.

Computer Sciences Corporation,
El Segundo, California,
USA.

DATAMATION,
35 Mason St.,
Greenwich, CT 06830,
USA.

Datapro 70,
Datapro Research Corporation,
1805 Underwood Boulevard,
Delran, N.J. 08075,
USA.

Dept. of Supply and Services,
Government of Canada,
Technical Services Branch,
Ottawa, Ontario,
Canada.

Hayden Publishing Co., Inc.,
50 Essex St.,
Rochelle Park, N.J. 07662,
USA.

Gesellschaft fuer Mathematik und
Datenverarbeitung,
Abteilung fuer Informationswesen,
Postfach 1240,
D-5205 St. Augustin 1,
FRG.

GUIDE International,
Mr. S. Hill,
Smith, Bucklin and Associates,
One Illinois Center,
111E Wacker Drive,
Chicago, Illinois 60601,
USA.

IFIP Administrative Data Processing Group,
6 Stadhouderskade,
Amsterdam 1013,
The Netherlands.

INFOTECH Information Ltd.
Nicholson House,
Maidenhead,
Berkshire,
England.

Learned Information Ltd.
Besselsleigh Road,
Abingdon,
Oxford OX13 6EF,
England.

McGraw-Hill Inc.,
1221 Avenue of the Americas,
New York, N.Y. 10020,
USA.

National Technical Information Service,
Springfield, Virginia,
USA.

NCC Publications,
The National Computing Centre Ltd.,
Oxford Road,
Manchester M1 7ED,
England.

North-Holland Publishing Co.,
P.O. Box 103,
Amsterdam,
The Netherlands.

Performance Development Corp.,
1101 State Road, Bldg., M,
Princeton, N.J. 08540,
USA.

Petrocelli Books, Inc.,
384 Fifth Avenue,
New York, N.Y. 10018,
USA.

Prentice-Hall Publishing Co.,
Englewood Cliffs, N.J.
USA.

QED Information Sciences, Inc.,
141 Linden Street,
Wellesley, Massachusetts 02181,
USA.

SHARE Inc,
Suite 750,
25 Broadway,
New York, NY 10004,
USA.

SYNERGETICS CORP.,
One DeAngelo Drive,
Bedford,
Massachusetts 01730
USA.

University Computing Co.,
8303 Elmbrook Street,
Dallas,
Texas 75247,
USA.

U.S. Department of Commerce,
National Bureau of Standards,
Washington D.C. 20234.
USA.

John Wiley & Sons Ltd,
Wiley – Interscience Series,
605 Third Avenue,
New York, NY 10158,
USA.

Appendix VI: Database Literature

TODS	Transactions on Database Systems.
Comm.ACM	Communications of the ACM.
SIGMOD/ SIGFIDET	The ACM Special Interest Group on the Management of Data.
ACM	Association of Computing Machinery
BCS	British Computer Society

ANSI/SPARC.

1. ANSI/X3/SPARC Study Group on Database Management Systems 'Interim Report', FDT (Bulletin of ACM-SIGMOD) 7,No.2,pp1-30 (1975).

2. ANSI/SPARC Study Group on Database Management Systems, 'Interim Report', Bulletin of ACM SIGMOD 7,No.21,p140 (1975).

3. D.A.Jardine (editor), 'The ANSI/SPARC DBMS Model', North-Holland, Amsterdam, Netherlands (1977)

4. F.Manola, 'An Evaluation of the New CODASYL and ANSI/SPARC Database Proposals', Data Base Technology, Infotech State of the Art Report, England, (1978).

5. D.Tsichritzis and A.Klug (eds.), 'The ANSI/X3/SPARC DBMS Framework - Report of the Study Group on Database Management Systems', AFIPS Press, Montvale, USA, (1977).

CONCEPTS and TUTORIALS.

6. CODASYL Systems Committee, 'Introduction to Feature Analysis of Generalized Database Management Systems', Comm.ACM 14,No.5,pp308-318 (May 1971).

7. E.F.Codd, 'Normalized Data Base Structure: A Brief Tutorial' ACM-SIGFIDET Workshop on Data Description, Access and Control, pp 1-17 (November 1971).

8. C.J.Date, 'An Introduction to Database Systems', Addison-Wesley, Reading, Massachusetts, USA. (1977).

9. S.M.Deen, 'Fundamentals of Data Base Systems' Macmillan, London, England (1977).

10. G.C.Everest,
'The Objectives of Database Management',
4th International Symposium on Computer and Information Sciences (COINS IV),
Plenum Publishing Corp., New York, USA. (Dec 1972).

11. R.W.Engels,
'A Tutorial on Data Base Organisation'
Technical Report TR.00.2004,IBM Corporation, (March 1970).
(Topics covered:-storage structures,accessing methods and data independence)

12. W.Kent,
'The Primer of Normal Forms',
Technical Report TR 02.600,
IBM Corporation, San Jose,Cal., USA, (April 1978).

13. P.G.Raymont,
'Tutorial Introduction to the DBTG Report',
BCS Conference on the April 1971 Report, pp 29-52, (Oct. 1971)

14. J.Rissanen,
'The Theory of Relations for Databases - A Tutorial Survey'
IBM Research Lab., San Jose, California, USA (April 1978).

15. J.Sandberg,
'A Primer on Relational Data Base Concepts',
IBM Systems Journal 20,No.1,pp 23-40, (1981).

16. R.F.Schubert,
'Basic Concepts in Data Base Management Systems'
Datamation 18,No.7, (July 1972).

GENERAL.

17. CODASYL Systems Committee,
'Feature Analysis of Generalized Database Management Systems',
ACM (May 1971).

18. CODASYL Systems Committee,
'A Survey of Generalized Database Management Systems'
ACM. (May 1969).

19. D.S.Appleton,
'What Data Base Isn't',
Datamation 23,No.1 (January 1977).

20. R.Ashany and M.Adamowicz,
'Data Base Systems'
IBM Systems Journal 15,No.3, pp 253-263 (1976).

21. C.W.Bachman,
'The Programmer as Navigator',
Comm.ACM 16,No.11, pp 653-658 (November 1973).

22. R.A.Bassler and J.J.Logan,
'The Technology of Data Base Management Systems',
College Reading Inc., P.O.Box 2323,
Arlington, Virginia 22202 (1974).
A collection of useful and interesting DBMS articles.

23. J.S.Blanchard
'We Bet Our Company on Data Base Management',
Datamation 20,No.9 (September 1974).

24. R.G.Canning,
'Problem Areas in Data Management',
EDP Analyzer 12,No.3 (March 1974).

25. D.A.Jardine,
'Data Base Management Systems: A Look at Concepts and State of the Art',
Datamation 22,No.4,(April 1976).

26. D.G.Keene and J.O.Lacy,
'VSAM Dataset Design Parameters',
IBM System Journal 13,No.3,pp 186-212 (September 1974).

27. J.Martin,
'Computer Data Base Organisation',
Prentice-Hall, New Jersey, USA, (1975).

28. J.Martin,
'The Principles of Data Base Management',
Prentice-Hall, New Jersey, USA, (1976).

29. E.Nahouraii, A.F.Cardenas and O.Brooks,
'An Approach to Data Communications Between Different Generalized DBMSs',
Research Report TR 03.104,
IBM Corporation, Palo Alto (May 1976).

30. R.G.Parsons,A.G.Dale and C.V.Yurkanan,
'Data Manipulation Language Requirements',
The Computer Journal 17,No.2,pp 99-103, (1974).

31. K.D.Reside and J.Seiter,
'Evolution of an Integrated Data Base',
Datamation 20,No.9 (September 1974).

32. M.E.Senko, E.B.Altman, M.M.Astrahan and P.L.Fedher,
'Data Structure and Accessing in Data Base Systems',
IBM Systems Journal 12,No.1,pp30-94 (1973).

33. M.E.Senko,
'Records, Relations, Sets, Entities and Things',
Information Systems, Vol.1,pp 3-13 (1975).

34. T.B.Steel Jr.,
'Database Standardization: A Status Report',

ACM-SIGMOD International Conference on Management of Data, 1975, pp 149-156(1975).

35. D.C.Tsichritzis and F.H.Lochovsky, 'Hierarchical Data-base Management; a Survey', ACM Computing Surveys 8,No.1,pp105-123 (1976).

36. T.F.Walton, 'Communications and Data Management', Wiley & Sons,New York, USA.

37. E.Wong and K.Youssefi, 'Decomposition Strategy for Query Processing', ACM TODS 1,No.3,pp223-241 (September 1976).

CODASYL DBMS PROPOSALS.

38. CODASYL DATA DESCRIPTION LANGUAGE COMMITTEE, 'Journal of Development 1978', Canadian Government, Ottawa (1978).

39. CODASYL. 'COBOL Database Facility Proposal', Canadian Government, Ottawa (1973).

40. CODASYL. 'COBOL Journal of Development 1976, Canadian Government, Ottawa (1976).

41. CODASYL. 'Data Base Task Group, October '69 Report' ACM (1969).

42. CODASYL. 'Data Base Task Group, April '71 Report' ACM (1971).

43. CODASYL. 'Data Base Task Group Subset Language Specification' (August 1971).

44. CODASYL Data Description Language Committee, 'Journal of Development' (June 1973).

45. R.G.Canning. 'The Debate on Data Base Management' EDP Analyser 11,No.3 (March 1973).

46. R.G.Canning, 'What's Happening with CODASYL-type DBMS?', EDP Analyser 12,No.10 (October 1974).

47. C.J.Date, 'An Architecture for High Level Language Database Extensions' ACM-SIGMOD 1976 pp 101-122 (1976).

48. E.G.Dee,
'Aspects of Data Base Management Towards a Data Base Language'
Data Processing (March-April 1971).

49. R.W.Engels,
'An Analysis of the April 1971 Data Base Task Group Report'
1971 ACM-SIGFIDET Workshop on Data Description
Access and Control.

50. R.L.Frank and E.H.Sibley,
'CODASYL Database Group Report - An Illustrative Example'
University of Michigan, USA.
Department of Industrial and Operations Engineering (Feb.1973)

51. S.P.Ghosh and P.Sakti,
'Data Base Organisation for Data Management',
Acedemic Press, San Francisco, USA (1977).

52. T.R.Heywood,
'The IBM Position on the CODASYL DBTG Proposal',
BCS Conference on the April 71 Report, pp81-103 (Oct.1971).

53. M.H.Kay,
'An Assessment of the CODASYL DDL for use in the Relational Schema',
Data Base Description, B.C.M.Douque and G.M.Nijssen (editors),
North-Holland, Amsterdam, Netherlands, pp 199-214 (1975).

54. W.Kent,
'Describing Information (Not Data, Reality?)',
Technical Report TR 03.012,
IBM Corporation, San Jose, Calif., USA (May 1976).

55. P.J.H.King
'Some Comments on the DBTG Report',
BCS Conference on the April 71 Report, pp 53-74 (Oct 1971).

56. J.R.Lucking,
'A Brief Summary of the CODASYL DBTG Report',
BCS Conference on the April 71 Report, pp 3-28 (Oct 1971).

57. T.W.Olle,
'An Analysis of the Shortcomings in the Schema DDL with an Outline of Proposed Improvements',
Proceedings ofthe IFIP TC-2 Special Working Conference on the CODASYL DDL,
North-Holland, Amsterdam, Netherlands, (1975).

58. T.W.Olle,
'An Assessment of how the CODASYL DBTG Proposal Meets the GUIDE-SHARE Requirements',
Norwegian Computer Center (April 1972).

59. T.W.Olle,
'The CODASYL Approach to Database Management',
Wiley Interscience Series, Wiley & Sons, New York, USA. (1978).

60. K.A.Robinson,
'An Analysis of the Uses of the CODASYL Set Concept'
Data Base Description, B.C.M.Douque and
B.C.M.Douque and G.M.Nijssen (editors), pp169-182.
North-Holland, Amsterdam, Netherlands, (1975).

61. H.Schenk,
'Implementation Aspects of the CODASYL DBTG Proposals',
Database Management,
J.W.Klimbie and K.L.Koffeman (editors), pp339-412.
North-Holland, Amsterdam, Netherlands. (1974).

62. E.H.Sibley,
'The CODASYL Database Approach: A Cobol Example
of Design and Use of a Personnel File',
NBSIR 74-500, Institute of Computer Sciences and Technology.

63. R.W.Taylor and R.L.Frank,
'CODASYL Data-base Management Systems'
ACM Computing Surveys 8,No1, pp 67-104 (1976).

64. R.W.Taylor,
'Observations on the Attributes of Sets',
Data Base Description, B.C.M.Douque and G.M.Nijssen (eds.),
B.C.M.Douque and G.M.Nijssen (editors), pp73-84.
North-Holland, Amsterdam, Netherlands, (1975).

65. W.J.Waghorn,
'The DDL as an Industry Standard?',
Proceedings of the IFIP TC-2 Special Working
Conference on the CODASYL DDL, pp121-167.
North-Holland, Amsterdam, Netherlands, (1975).

66. T.Warren,
'Feature Analysis of CODASYL Database Management Systems',
AD-A014 972/4WC, National Technical Information Service (1975)

DATABASE ADMINISTRATION (DBA).

67. 'The Data Base Administrator' GUIDE Information Management Group,
GUIDE International (November 1972).

68. 'The Database Administrator Today'
GUIDE International (1975).

69. R.G.Canning,
'The Data Administrator Function',
EDP Analyser 10,No.11 (November 1972).

70. R.M.Curtice,
'Standards and Procedures for the Data Base Administration
Functions',
Arthur.D.Little, Inc., (1978).

71. J.J.Florentin,
'New Era of the DBA',
Computing p13 (January 1974).

72. J.R.Lucking,
'The Database Administrator: His Role and His Needs',
Data Base Management pp557-572 Infotech Information (1973).

73. J.K.Lyon,
'The Data Base Administrator',
Wiley Interscience Publications, J.Wiley & Sons. New York USA.

74. J.K.Lyon,
'The Role of the Database Administrator',
Database 3,No.4,pp11-12. (ACM)

75. R.L.Peck,
'The Data Base Administrator',
Eurocomp Conference Proceedings (1974).

76. R.W.Taylor,
'Data Administration and the DBTG Report',
ACM SIGMOD/SIGFIDET Conference 1974, pp 431-444 (1974).

77. E.W.Yasaki,
'The Many Faces of the DBA',
Datamation 23,No.5,pp75-79 (May 1977).

DATABASE DESIGN AND IMPLEMENTATION.

78. L.Aspinal, B.K.Alfred and T.W.Rogers,
'Adaptability to Change in Large Data Base Information Retrieval Systems',
IBM,UK Scientific Centre (April 1972).

79. R.G.Canning.
'The Cautious Path to a Data Base',
EDP Analyser 11,No.6 (June 1973).

80. R.G.Canning.
'Creating the Corporate Data Base',
EDP Analyser 8,No.2 (February 1970).

81. R.G.Canning.
'Technical Support for an MIS',
EDP Analyser 7,No.11 (November 1969).

82. A.F.Cardenas and J.Sagamang,
'Doubly-chained Tree Database Organisation - Analysis and Design Strategies',
The Computer Journal 20,No.1, pp 15-26 (1977).

83. L.J.Cohen,
'Data Base Considerations and Implementation Techniques',
Data Management (September 1972).

84. D.Comer
'The Difficulty of Optimum Index Selection',
Purdue University (September 1977).

85. D.E.Cuozzo and J.F.Kurtz,
'Building a Base for Data Base: A Management Perspective'
Datamation 19,No.10,pp71-75 (October 1973).

86. R.M.Curtice,
'Access Mechanisms and Data Structure Support in Data Base Management Systems',
QED Information Sciences,Massachusetts,USA.

87. R.M.Curtice,
'Planning for Data Base Systems',
QED Information Sciences,Massachusetts,USA (1976).

88. T.R.Finneran and J.S.Henry,
'Structured Analysis for Data Base Design',
Datamation 23,No.11,pp 99-113 (November 1977).

89. L.Frank,
'Designing for Intersystem Independence',
Datamation 27,No.4,pp203-206 (April 1981).

90. A. Gabay,
'A Data Base and its Management',
Computer Management Vol 7,pp 35-40 (May 1972).

91. G.E.Huhn,
'The Data Base in a Critical On-line Business Environment'
Datamation 20,No.9, pp 52-56 (September 1974).

92. P.E.Jones,
'Data Base Design Methodology: A Logical Framework',
QED Information Sciences,Massachusetts,USA (1976).

93. B.K.Kahn,
'A Review of Systems Analysis and Data Base Design Techniques'
ISDOS Working Paper No.129 The University of Michigan, (Nov.1975).

94. C.J.Lewis,
'Understanding Database and Data Base',
Journal of System Management (September 1972).

95. V.Y.Lum,
'Multi-attribute Retrieval with Combined Indexes'
Comm. ACM 13,No.11 (November 1970).

96. V.Y.Lum and H.Ling,
'An Optimization Problem in the Selection of Secondary Keys'
Proc. 1971 ACM National Conference 26, pp 349-356 (1972).

97. J.K.Lyon,
'An Introduction to Database Design',
John Wiley & Sons, New York, USA (1971).

98. R.A.McLaughlin,
'Building a Database',
Datamation 18,No.7,(July 1972).

99. J.K.Mullin,
'Retrieval Update Speed Tradeoffs Using Combined Indices',
Comm.ACM 14,No.12, (December 1971).

100. R.L.Nolan,
'Computer Data Bases. The Future is Now',
Harvard Business Review pp 98-114 (September 1973).

101. J.A.van der Pool,
'Optimum Storage Allocation for Initial Loading of a File',
IBM Journal of Research & Development,
16,No.6,pp579-586, (Nov 1972).

102. J.A.van der Pool,
'Optimum Storage Allocation for a File with Open Addressing',
IBM Journal of Research & Development,
17,No.2,pp106-114, (March 1973).

103. G.F.Price,
'The Ten Commandments of Data Base',
Data Management, pp 14-23 (May 1972).

104. M.Schkolnick,
'Secondary Index Optimization',
ACM-SIGMOD International Conference on the Management of Data, May 1975, pp 186-192 (1975).

105. M.E.Senko,
'Conceptual Schemas, Abstract Data Structures, Enterprise Descriptions',
International Computer Symposium 1977,
E.Morlet and D.Ribbens (editors), pp 85-102,
North-Holland, Amsterdam, Netherlands, (1977).

106. D.G.Severance and J.Carlis,
'A Practical Approach to Selecting Record Access Paths'
ACM Computing Surveys 9,No.4, pp 259-272,(December 1977).

107. S.W.Sherman and R.S.Brice,
'Performance of a Database Manager in a Virtual Memory System'
ACM TODS 1,No.4, pp 317-343 (Dec.1976).

108. H.E.Sibley and A.G.Merton,
'Implementation of a Generalized Data Base Management System within an Organisation',
Management Informatics, pp21-31 (February 1973).

109. P.M.Stocker and P.A.Dearnley,
'A Self-organising Database Management System',
Database Management,
J.W.Klimbie and K.L.Koffeman (editors), pp 337-348,
North-Holland, Amsterdam, Netherlands, (1974).

110. M.Stonebraker,
'The Choice of Partial Inversions and Combined Indices',
International Journal of Computer and
Information Sciences 3,No.2 (1974).

111. C.P.Wang and H.H.Wedekind,
'Segment Synthesis in Logical Data Base Design',
IBM Journal of Research and Develop., 19,No.1 (1975)

112. G.Wiederhold,
'Database Design',
McGraw-Hill, New York (1977).

113. P.C.Yue and C.K.Wong,
'Storage Cost Considerations in Secondary Index Selection'
International Journal of Computer and
Information Sciences 4,No.4 (1975).

114. R.T.Yeh, N.Roussopoulos and P.Chang
'Data Base Design An Approach and Some Issues'
Technical Report SDBEG-4,
University of Texas in Austin,Austin,Texas (1978).

DBMS EVALUATION and SELECTION.

115. 'Data Base Management Systems' Infotech State of the Art Report
including:- ADABAS, IDMS, IMS, S2000 and TOTAL.

116. 'International Data Base Directory' Eurisdic's European Scientific
Information Referral Working Group,Learned Information Ltd.

117. Performance Development Corporation reports on the following DBMSs
ADABAS, IDMS, IMS, S2000 and TOTAL, from
QED Information Sciences,Massachusetts,USA.

118. Reports on ADABAS, IMS and S2000 in English from the
Gesellschaft fuer Mathematik and Datenverarbeitung, W.Germany.

119. 'Selection and Aquisition of Data Base Management Systems'
CODASYL Systems Committee, (March 1976).

120. 'Six DBMSs: Feature Analysis and User Experience'
NBS Technical Note 887, US Department of Commerce.

121. R.G.Canning.
'The Current Status of Data Management',
EDP Analyser 12,No.2 (February 1974).
ADABAS and SYSTEM 2000 are examined.

122. R.G.Canning,
'Trends in Data Management, 1',
EDP Analyzer 9,No.5 (May 1971).
TOTAL etc are examined.

123. R.G.Canning,
'Trends in Data Management, 2',
EDP Analyzer 9,No.6 (June 1971).
IMS/2 etc are examined.

124. A.F.Cardenas,
'Analysis and Performance of Inverted Data Base Structures'
Comm.ACM 18,No.5, pp 253-263 (May 1975).

125. L.J.Cohen,
'Database Management Systems',
QED Information Sciences, Massachusetts, USA. (1978).

126. J.C.Cullen, D.J.Neal and M.A.Prince,
'A Survey Of Data Base Programming Systems',
BP Computer Dept., Systems Development Division,
Report No.305 (September 1971).

127. B.Davis
'The Selection of Database Software',
The National Computer Centre, Manchester, England. (1977).

128. J.P.Fry and E.H.Sibley,
'Evaluation of Data-base Management Systems',
ACM Computing Surveys 8,No1,pp 17-42 (1976).

129. D.A.Jardine (editor),
'Data Base Management Systems',
SHARE Working Conference on DBMSs,
Noth-Holland, Amsterdam, Netherlands, (1973).

130. I.R.Palmer,
'Database Systems: A Practical Reference',
QED Information Sciences, Massachusetts, USA. (1975).

131. I.R.Palmer,
'Whose Database for Us?',
Computing, pp10-13, (November 1973).

132. S.L.Prendergast,
'Selecting a Data Management System',
Computer Decisions (August 1972).

133. R.G.Ross,
'Evaluating Data Base Management Systems',
Journal of System Development (Jan 1976).

134. D.Smith,
'Data Base Management System Selection Procedure',
19th. Annual College and University Machine Records
Conference (May 1974).

135. C.J.Testa and J.Laube,
'How do you Chose a Data Base Management System? Carefully '
Infosystems (January 1975).

136. R.G.Treanor,
'Data Management: Fact or Fiction',
Database 3,No.1, pp17-25

DATA COMPRESSION.

137. D.A.Marron and P.A.D. de Maine,
'Automatic Data Compression'.
Comm. ACM 10,No.11 (November 1967).

DATA DICTIONARIES/DIRECTORIES

138. 'Data Dictionary Systems Working Party Report'
British Computer Society/DDSWP (1977).

139. R.G.Canning,
'The Data Dictionary/Directory Function',
EDP Analyser 12,No.11 (1974).

140. R.G.Canning,
'Installing a Data Dictionary',
EDP Analyser 16,No.1 (1978).

141. H.C.Lefkovits,
'Data Dictionary Systems',
QED Information Sciences, Massachusetts, USA. (1977).

142. R.A.Nerad,
'The Data Dictionary in Data Management',
Infotech State of the Art Report (1973).

143. I.B.McCrickick and R.B.Goldstein,
'What do Data Administrators Really Do?',
Datamation 26,No.8, pp131-134 (August 1980)

144. G.Schussel,
'The Role of the Data Dictionary,
Datamation 23,No.6,(June 1977).

145. P.P.Uhrowczik,
'Data Dictionaries/Directories',
Comm.ACM 12,No.4, pp 332-350 (1973).

DATA ENCRYPTION.

146. H.Katzan,Jr.,
'The Standard Data Encryption Algorithm',
Petrocelli Books, New York, USA (1978).

147. M.G.Rocke,
'The Need for Data Code Control',
Datamation 19,No.9, pp105-107, (September 1976).

148. D.J.Sykes,
'Protecting Data by Encryption',
Datamation 22,No.8, pp81-85, (August 1976).

DATA INDEPENDENCE.

149. 'Data Independence in Data Base Systems'
Datamation 21,No.4,(April 1975).

150. C.J.Date and P.Hopewell,
'File Definition and Logical Data Independence',
ACM-SIGFIDET Workshop on Data Description,
Access and Control, pp 117-138 (November 1971).

151. M.Stonebraker,
'A Functional View of Data Independence',
ACM-SIGFIDET Workshop on Data Description, Access and Control,
pp 139-168 (November 1971).

152. A.J.Collmeyer,
'Implications of Data Independence on the Architecture of DBMSs'
ACM-SIGFIDET Workshop on Data Description,
Access and Control, pp 307-321 (1972).

153. C.J.Date and P.Hopewell,
'Storage Definition and Physical Data Independence',
ACM-SIGFIDET Workshop on Data Description,
Access and Control, pp 139-168 (November 1971).

DATA STRUCTURES AND SEARCH TECHNIQUES

154. 'When are Pointer Arrays Better than Chains'
Proceedings of the ACM Annual Conference (November 1974).

155. C.W.Bachman,
'Data Structure Diagrams',
Data Base 1,No.2, pp 4-10 (1969).

156. C.W.Bachman,
'The Data Structure Set Model',
ACM SIGMOD Debate 'Data Models: Data Structure Set vs.
Relational,R.Rustin editor, pp1-10, (May 1974).

157. C.W.Bachman
'The Evolution of Storage Structures',
Comm.ACM 15,No.7, pp 628-634 (July 1972).

158. C.W.Bachman,
'Implementation Techniques for Data Structure Sets',
Database Management Systems, D.A.Jardine - editor, pp 147-257,
North Holland, Amsterdam, Netherlands, (1974).

159. W.Buchholz,
'File Organisation and Addressing',
IBM System Journal 2,No.2 (1963).
North-Holland, Amsterdam, Netherlands, (1974).

160. W.D.Climenson,
'File Organisation and Search Techniques',
Annual Review of Information Science and Technology Vol. 1,
J.Wiley and Sons, New York, USA. (1966).

161. G.D.Dodd
'Elements of Data Management Systems',
ACM Computing Surveys 1,No.2,pp 117-133 (June 1969).

162. C.P.Earnest,
'A Comparison of the Network and Relational Structure Models'
Technical Report, Computer Science Corp., (April 1974).

163. J.Earley,
'Towards an Understanding of Data Structures',
Proceedings of the 1970 ACM-SIGFIDET Workshop on
Data Description Access and Control. ACM (April 1971).

164. R.Gerritsen,
'A Preliminary System for the Design of DBTG Data Structures'
Comm.ACM 18,No.10,pp 551-557 (October 1975).

165. G.D.Held,
'Storage Structures for Relational DBMSs',
Memorandum No.ERL-M533, Univ.of Calif.,Berkeley (Aug.1975).

166. D.Hsiao and F.Harary,
'A Formal System of Information Retrieval from Files',
Comm.ACM 13,No.2, (February 1970).

167. S.T.March and D.Severance,
'The Determination of Efficient Record Segmentation and Blocking
Factors for Shared Data Files',
ACM TODS 2,No.3, pp 279-296 (September 1977).

168. F.M.Mitoma and K.B.Irani,
'Automatic Database Schema Design and Optimization',
International Conference on Very Large
Databases, pp 286-321 (1975).

169. G.M.Nijssen,
'Data Structuring in the DDL and the Relational Model',
Database Management,
J.W.Klimbie and K.L.Koffeman (editors), pp 363-384,
North-Holland, Amsterdam, Netherlands. (1974).

170. T.W.Olle,
'Data Structuring Facilities in Commercially Available DBMS',
Computer Bulletin, pp20-22 (September 1974).

171. M.E.Senko,
'Data Structures and Data Accessing in Data Base Systems Past Present and Future',
IBM Systems Journal 16,No.3, pp 208-257 (1977).

DBMS TOOLS.

172. P.P.Chen and S.B.Yao,
'Design and Performance Tools for Data Base Systems',
International Conference on Very Large Databases pp 3-15 (1977).

173. R.M.Curtis,
'Some Tools for DBMS Development',
Datamation 20,No.7,pp102-106 (July 1974).

DISTRIBUTED DATABASES and MINI DBMSs.

174. 'Operational and Technological Issues in Distributed Data Bases'
Data Base Management,
Auerbach Pub. Inc., New Jersey, USA. (1977).

175. G.A.Champine,
'Six Approaches to Distributed Data Bases',
Datamation 23,No.5,pp 69-72 (May 1977).

176. R.N.Canaday
'A Back-end Computer for Data Base Management',
Comm.ACM 17,No.10,pp 575-582 (October 1974).

177. R.G.Canning,
'Distributed Data Systems',
EDP Analyzer 14,No.6 (June 1976).

178. W.W.Chu and G.Ohlmacher,
'Avoiding Deadlocks in Distributed Data Bases',
ACM National Conference pp 156-160 (Nov.1974).

179. R.A.Davenport,
'Distribution of Centralized Data Bases',
Computer Journal 21,No.1, pp 7-13 (February 1978).

180. G.Floam,
'Putting a Data Base on a Mini ',
Datamation 22,No.6, (June 1976).

181. P.G.Hebalkan and C.Tung,
'Design Considerations for Distributed Data Base Systems'
IBM Research Report, 965-IBM-03, (1977).

182. E.Manning and R.Peebles,
'System Architecture for Distributed Data Management',
Computer pp 40-47 (January 1978).

183. F.J.Maryansky,
'A Survey of Development in Distributed Data Base Management Systems',
Computer pp 28-38 (February 1978).

184. P.Morris and D.Sagalowicz,
'Managing Network Access to a Distributed Data Base',
Berkley Workshop on Distributed Data Management and Computer Networks,LBL-6416, pp58-67 (May 1977).

185. I.Palmer,
'Distributed Data Bases',
Infotech State of the Art Report (November 1976).

186. A.B.Whinston and C.W.Holsapple,
'DBMS for Micros',
Datamation 27,No.4,pp165-167. (April 1981).

GUIDE-SHARE DBMS PROPOSALS.

187. GUIDE-SHARE Database Task Force,
'Database Management System Requirements'
SHARE Inc., New York, USA, (1971).

188. 'Requirements for a Database Management System'
Joint SHARE and GUIDE Database Requirements Group, (Nov. 1971)

189. R.G.Canning,
'The Debate on Data Base Management'
EDP Analyser 11,No.3 (March 1973).

190. G.C.Everest and E.H.Sibley,
'A Critique of the GUIDE-SHARE DBMS Requirement',
1971 ACM-SIGFIDET Workshop on Data Description, Access and Control, pp 93-112, ACM (November 1971).

PRIVACY INTEGRITY and SECURITY.

191. P.A.Alsberg, G.G.Belford and S.R.Brunch,
'Synchronization and Deadlock',
CAC, Doc.No.185, Univ of Illinios (Mar.1976).

192. L.A.Bjork,
'Generalized Audit Trail Requirements and Concepts for Database Applications',
IBM Systems Journal 14,No.3, pp 229-245 (1975).

193. P.S.Browne.
'Data Privacy and Integrity: An Overview',
1971 ACM-SIGFIDET Workshop on Data Description Access and Control. ACM (November 1971).

194. D.D.Chamberlin, R.F.Boyce and I.L.Traiger,
'A Deadlock-free Schema for Resource Locking in a Data Base Environment',

Information Processing 74, IFIP Congress August 1974, pp 340-343, North-Holland, Amsterdam, Netherlands, (1974).

195. E.G.Coffman, M.J.Elphick and A.Shoshani,
'System Deadlocks',
ACM Computing Surveys 3,No.2,pp67-78 (1971).

196. R.M.Curtice,
'Integrity in Data Base Systems',
Datamation 23,No.5,pp64-68 (May 1977).

197. A.L.Dean 1971 ACM-SIGFIDET Workshop on Data
'Data Privacy and Integrity Requirements for On-line Data Management Systems' 1971 ACM-SIGFIDET Workshop on Data Description,Access and Control. ACM (November 1971).

198. D.E.Denning and P.J.Denning,
'Data Security',
ACM Computing Surveys 11,No.3,pp227-249 (September 1979).

199. D.E.Denning, P.J.Denning and M.D.Schwartz,
'The Tracker: A Threat to Statistical Data Base Security'
ACM Transactions on Database Systems 4,No.1,pp76-96 (1979).

200. K.P.Eswaran, J.N.Gray, R.A.Lorie and I.L.Traiger,
'On the Notions of Consistency and Predicate Locks in a Relational Database System',
Comm.ACM 19,No.11,pp624-634 (November 1976).

201. J.J.Florentin,
'Consistence Auditing of Data Bases',
Computer Journal 17,No.1,pp 52-58 (February 1974).

202. B.M.Fossum,
'Database Integrity as Provided for by a Particular DBMS'
Database Management, pp271-288,
J.W.Klimbie and K.L.Koffeman (editors),
North-Holland, Amsterdam, Netherlands, (1974).

203. J.Gosden,
'The Conceptual Requirements for a Management Information Data Bank',
Information Processing 1971,
North Holland, Amsterdam, Netherlands, (1972).

204. J.N.Gray, R.A.Lorie, G.F.Putzolu and I.L.Traiger,
'Granularity of Locks and Degrees of Consistency In a Shared Data Base',
Research Report RJ1606, IBM Corporation, USA (1976).

205. N.Habermann,
'Prevention of System Deadlock',
Comm.ACM 12,No.7,pp373-377, (July 1969).

206. J.W.Havender,
'Avoiding Deadlock in Multi-tasking Systems',
IBM Systems Journal 7,No.1,pp74-87 (1968).

207. D.A.Hawley, J.S.Knowles and E.E.Tozer,
'Database Consistency and the CODASYL DBTG Proposals'
Computer Journal 18,No.3,pp206-212 (1975).

208. L.J.Hoffman
'Modern Methods for Computer Security and Privacy',
Prentice-Hall, New Jersey, USA, (1977).

209. R.C.Holt,
'Comments on Prevention of System Deadlocks',
Comm.ACM 14,No.1,pp36-38 (January 1971).

210. R.C.Holt,
'On Deadlock in Computer Systems',
Technical Report CSRG-6, Computer Systems Research Group,
University of Toronto, Canada, (January 1975).

211. R.C.Holt,
'Some Deadlock Properties of Computer Systems',
ACM Computing Surveys 4,No.3,pp179-196 (September 1972).

212. J.H.Howard,
'Mixed Solutions for the Deadlock Problem',
Comm.ACM 16,No.7,pp427-430 (July 1973).

213. J.Martin
'Security, Accuracy and Privacy in Computer Systems',
Prentice-Hall, New Jersey, USA, (1973).

214. N.Minsky,
'Intentional Resolution of Privacy Protection in Data Base
Comm.ACM 19,No.3,pp148-159 (1976).

215. J.E.Shemer and A.J.Collmeyer,
'Database Sharing: A Study of Interference,
Roadblock and DeadLock',
1971 ACM-SIGFIDET Workshop on Data Description
Access and Control. ACM (November 1971).

216. C.Wood,E.B.Fernandez and R.C.Summers
'Database Security: Requirements, Policies and Models'
IBM Systems Journal 19,No.2,pp229-252 (1980).

RANDOMIZING ALGORITHMS.

217. A.V.Aho, J.E.Hopcroft and J.D.Ullman,
'The Design and Analysis of Computer Algorithms',
Addison-Wesley, Massachusetts, USA. (1975).

218. I.F.Blake and A.G.Konheim,
'Bigger Buckets are (are not) Better',
Journal of the ACM 24,No.4,pp591-606 (October 1977).

219. B.Carter,
'The Reallocation of Hash-coded Tables',
Comm.ACM 16,No.1,pp11-14 (Jan.1973).

220. S.P.Ghosh and V.Y.Lum,
'An Analysis of Collisions When Hashing by Division',
Information Systems 1,No.1,pp15-22 (1975).

221. V.Y.Lum,
'General Performance Analysis of Key-to-Address Transformation Methods Using an Abstract File Concept'
Comm.ACM 16,No.10,pp603-612 (Oct.1973).

222. V.Y.Lum, P.S.T.Yuen and M.Dodd,
'Key-to-address Transform Techniques: A Fundamental Performance Study on Large Existing Formatted Files,
Comm.ACM 14,No.4,pp228-239 (April 1971).

223. R.Morris,
'Scatter Storage Techniques',
Comm.ACM 11,No.1, (January 1968).

224. G.D.Nott,
'Hashing Functions' G.D.Nott,
Computer Journal 18,No.3,pp 216-278 (1975).

225. W.W.Peterson,
'Addressing for Random Access Storage',
IBM Journal of Research and Development 1,No.2, (April 1957).

226. D.Severance and R.Duhne,
'A Practitioner's Guide to Addressing Algorithms',
IBM Systems Journal 12,No.4,pp 332-350 (1973).
and Comm.ACM 19,No.6,pp314-326 (1976).

RELATIONAL MODEL.

227. 'Derivable, Redundancy and Consistency of Relations Stored in Large Data Banks',
Research Report RJ599,
IBM Corporation, San Jose, Calif., USA (August 1969).

228. A.V.Aho, C.Beeri and J.D.UllMan,
'The Theory of Joins in Relational Databases',
18th IEEE Symposium on Foundations of Computer Science, (1977).

229. M.M.Astrahan et al,
'A History and Evaluation of System R',
Research Report RJ2843,
IBM Corporation, San Jose, California, USA, (June 1980).

230. M.M.Astrahan et al,
'System R: A Relational Approach to Database Management'
ACM TODS 1,No.2,pp97-137,(June 1976) and
Research Report RJ1738,
IBM Corporation, San Jose, California, USA, (Feb. 1976)

231. M.W.Blasgen et al,
'System R: An Architectural Overview',
IBM Systems Journal 20,No.1,pp 41-62, (1981).

232. D.D.Chamberlin,
'Relational Data Base Management Systems',
ACM Computing Surveys 8,No.1,pp43-66 (March 1976).

233. P.P.Chen,
'The Entity Relationship Model, Toward a Unified View of Data'
ACM TODS 1,No.1, pp9-36, (March 1976).

234. E.F.Codd,
'Access Control for Relational DBS',
BCS Symposium on Relational DB Concepts, (April 1973).

235. E.F.Codd,
'A Data Base Sublanguage Founded on the Relational Calculus'
1971 ACM-SIGFIDET Workshop on Data Descrition,
Access and Control. ACM (November 1971).
and IBM Research Report RJ893.

236. E.F.Codd,
'Further Normalization of the Data Base Relational Model',
Data Base Systems,Courant Computer Science Symposia Series,
Vol.6, R.Rustin editor, pp33-64,
Prentice-Hall, New Jersey, USA, (May 1972).
Research Report RJ909, IBM CORP., San Jose, Ca., USA. (Apr. 1971).

237. E.F.Codd,
'Implementation of Relational Data Base Management Systems'
FDT, Quarterly Bulletin of ACM-SIGMOD 7, pp 3-4 (1975).

238. E.F.Codd,
'Recent Investigations in Relational Data Base Systems'
Information Processing 74, IFIP Congress, pp 1017-1021,
North-Holland, Amsterdam, Netherlands, (1974).

239. E.F.Codd,
'Relational Algebra',
Data Base Systems,Courant Computer Science Symposia Series,
Vol.6, R.Rustin editor,
Prentice-Hall, New Jersey, USA, (May 1972).

240. E.F.Codd,
'A Relational Model of Data for Large Shared Data Banks'
Comm.ACM 13,No.6,pp 377-387 (June 1970).

241. E.F.Codd,
'Relational Completeness of Data Base Sublanguages',

Research Report RJ987,
IBM Corporation, San Jose Calif, USA, (March 1972) and
Data Base Systems,Courant Computer Science Symposia Series,
Vol.6, R.Rustin editor, pp 65-98,
Prentice-Hall, New Jersey, USA, (May 1972).

242. E.F.Codd,
'Seven Steps to Rendezvous with the Casual User',
Proceedings of the IFIP TC-2 Special Working Conference
on Data Base Management Systems April 1974,
North-Holland, Amsterdam, Netherlands, (1974).

243. E.F.Codd and C.J.Date,
'Interactive Support for Non-programmers: the Relational and
Network Approaches',
1974 ACM-SIGMOD Debate: 'Data Models: Data Structure
Set vs. Relational', R.Rustin editor, pp 13-41, (1974).

244. C.J.Date,
'Relational Data Base Concepts',
ACM Computing Surveys 8,No.1,pp 43-66 (March 1976).

245. C.J.Date,
'Relational Data Base Systems: A Tutorial',
4th International Symposium on Computer and Information
Sciences (COINS IV),
Plenum Publishing Corp., New York, USA. (Dec 1972).

246. C.J.Date and E.F.Codd,
'The Relational and Network Approaches: Comparison of the
Application Programming Interfaces',
ACM-SIGMOD Debate 'Data Models: Data Structure Set vs.
Relational' R.Rustin editor, pp 85-113 (1974).

247. E.Dee, W.Hilder,P.J.H.King and E.Taylor,
'COBOL Extensions to Handle a Relational Data Base',
BCS Working Party No.5, (October 1973).

248. C.Deheneffe, H.Hennebert and W.Paulus,
'A Relational Model for a Data Base',
Proceedings of the IFIP TC-2 Special Working Conference
on Data Base Management Systems
North-Holland, Amsterdam, Netherlands,(1974).

249. R.Y.Fadous and J.Forsyth,
'Finding Candidate Keys for Relational Data Bases',
ACM-SIGMOD Conference, pp203-210, (May 1975).

250. L.R.Gotlieb,
'Computing Joins of Relations',
ACM-SIGMOD Conference (May 1975).

251. P.A.V.Hall,
'Optimization of Simple Expressions in Relational Data Base
Expressions',
IBM Journal of Research and Development (May 1976).

252. I.J.Heath
'Unacceptable File Operations in a Relational Database',
1971 ACM-SIGFIDET Workshop on Data Description,
Access and Control. ACM (November 1971).

253. G.Held and M.Stonebraker,
'Networks, Hierarchies and Relations in Data Base Management Systems',
ACM Pacific regional Conference, pp 1-9, (April 1975).

254. W.Kim,
'Relational Database Systems',
ACM Computing Surveys 11,No.3,pp 185-211, (September 1979).

255. M.F.Korns,
'Halfway to a Relational Data Base',
Datamation 22,No.5 (May 1976).

256. A.S.Michaels, B.Mittman and C.R.Carlson,
'A Comparison of the Relational and CODASYL Approaches to Data-Base Management',
ACM Computing Surveys 8,No.1,pp 125-150, (March 1976).

257. M.G.Notley,
'The Peterlee IS/1 System',
IBM UK Scientific Centre Report UKSC-0018, (March 1972).

258. R.M.Pecherer,
'Efficient Evaluation of Expressions in a Relational Algebra'
ACM Pacific 75 Regional Conference,pp 45-49 (April 1975).

259. H.A.Schmid and J.Swenson,
'On the Semantics of the Relational Data Model',
ACM-SIGMOD Conference, (May 1975).

260. D.Smith and J.Smith,
'Relational Database Machines',
Computer 12,No.3,pp 28-38, (March 1979).

261. J.M.Smith and P.Chang,
'Optimizing the Performance of a Relational Algebra Data Base Interface',
Comm.ACM 18,No.10,pp 568-579, (October 1975).

262. A.J.Strand,
'The Relational Approach to the Management of Data Bases',
Information Processing 71, IFIP Congress, pp 901-904,
North-Holland, Amsterdam, Netherlands, (1971).

263. S.J.P.Todd,
'Implementation of the Join Operator in Relational Data Bases'
IBM UK Scientific Centre,Note No.15, Peterlee, England.

264. S.J.P.Todd,
'Peterlee Relational Test Vehicle PRTV - a Sytem Overview'
IBM Systems Journal 15,No.4,pp285-308 (1976).

265. S.J.P.Todd,
'Relational Database Research at the IBM UK Scientific Centre Peterlee, a Survey 1970-1977',
Report UKSC-93, IBM UK Ltd., Hants., England (Dec. 1977).

266. D.C.Tsichritzis,
'A Network Framework for Relational Implementation'
Proceedings of the IFIP TC-2 Special Working Conference on the CODASYL DDL
North-Holland, Amsterdam Netherlands, (1975).

267. R.S.S.Wee,
'Problems in the Dynamic Sharing of Data in a Relational Data Base Environment',
IBM UK Scientific Centre Report UKSC-0067, (August 1975).

268. R.E.Westgaard,
'A COBOL Data Base Facility for the Relational Data Model'
ACM Pacific Regional Conference, pp 132-139, (April1975).

269. V.K.M.Whitney,
'Relational Data Management System(RMDS)',
General Motors (October 1972) GMR-1273.

270. V.K.M.Whitney,
'RDMS: A Relational Data Management System',
4th International Symposium on Computer and Information Sciences (COINS IV),
Plenum Press, New York, USA. (December 1972).

271. M.M.Zloof,
'Query-by-Example: A Data Base Language',
IBM Systems Journal 16,No.4,pp324-343 (1977).

REORGANIZATION and RECOVERY.

272. J.N.Gray et al,
'The Recovery Manager of a Data Management System',
Research Report RJ2623,
IBM Corporation, San Jose, California, USA, (August 1979).

273. B.Schneiderman,
'Optimum Data Base Reorganisation Points',
Comm.ACM 16,No.6,pp 352-365 (June 1973).

274. J.S.M.Verhofstad,
'Recovery Techniques for Database Systems',
ACM Computing Surveys 10,No.2,pp 168-193 (June 1978).

275. M.V.Wilkes,
'On Preserving the Integrity of Databases',
The Computer Journal 15,No.3,pp 191-194.

276. S.B.Yao, K.S.Das and T.J.Teorey,

'A Dynamic Database Reorganisation Algorithm',
TODS 1,No.2,pp 159-174 (June 1976).

REPORTS ON SPECIFIC DBMSs.

277. F.Aschim and P.Boone
'SIBAS, An Implementation of the Codasyl Data Base Concept'
Management Informatics 2,No.3 (June 1973).

278. D.Burns,
'A Self-Sufficient ROBOT',
Computing, p9 (November 1973).

279. F.Johnson,
'The TOTAL Picture',
Data Processing (July/August 1975).

280. D.Kapp and J.F.Leben,
'IMS Programming Techniques - a Guide to Using DL/I',
van Nostrand, New York, USA. (1978).

281. W.C.McGee,
'The Information Management System IMS/VS
Part I:General Structure and Opertion',
IBM Systems Journal 16,No.2, pp 84-95, (1977).

282. W.C.McGee,
'The Information Management System IMS/VS
Part II:Data Base Facilities',
IBM Systems Journal 16,No.2, pp 96-122, (1977).

283. W.C.McGee,
'The Information Management System IMS/VS
Part III:Batch Processing Facilities',
IBM Systems Journal 16,No.2, pp 123-135, (1977).

284. W.C.McGee,
'The Information Management System IMS/VS
Part IV:Data Communication Facilities',
IBM Systems Journal 16,No.2, pp 136-147, (1977).

285. W.C.McGee,
'The Information Management System IMS/VS
Part V:Transaction Processing Facilities',
IBM Systems Journal 16,No.2, pp 148-168, (1977).

286. R.F.Schubert,
'IDMS',
BCS Syposium on Implementation of CODASYL Data Base
Management Proposals (October 1974).

TRENDS in DBMS

287. C.W.Bachman,
'Advances in Data-base Technology',
Infotech State of the Art Tutorial, (December 1977).

288. C.W.Bachman,
'Trends in Database Management',
Proceedings of AFIPS National Computer Conference 1975,
Vol 44,pp 569-575, AFIPS Press, Montvale, USA, (1975).

289. A.Blaser and H Schmutz,
'Data Base Research: A Survey',
Research Report TR 75.10.009,
IBM Heidelberg Scientific Center, Heidelberg, FRG (1975).

290. V.Chvalovsky,
'Anything New In Database Technology',
Datamation 22,No.4, (April 1976).

291. R.M.Curtice,
'The Outlook for Data Base Management',
Datamation 22,No.4, (April 1976).

292. G.C.Everest.
'The Future of Data-base Management',
ACM-SIGMOD Workshop on Data Description, Access and Control,
May 1974, pp 445-462 (1974).

293. G.M.Nijssen,
'On the Gross Architecture for the Next Generation of Database Management Systems'
IFIP Conference Proceedings, 1977, pp 327-335,
North-Holland, Amsterdam, Netherlands (1977).

294. T.W.Olle,
'Current and Future Trends in Data Base Management Systems'
Information Processing 74, IFIP Congress, August 1974
Vol.5, pp 998-1006,
North-Holland, Amsterdam, Netherlands (1974).

295. R.G.Ross,
'Assessment of Current Data Base Trends',
Data Base Monograph No. 5, R.M.Curtice, Editor,
QED Information Sciences,Massachusetts,USA (1977).

296. R.F.Schubert,
'Directions in Data Base Management Technology',
Datamation 20,No.9, (September 1974).

WORDS OF CAUTION.

297. T.Gilb,
'Data Base Software: A Sceptical Viewpoint and some Alternatives',
Management Informatics,pp227-234 (October 1973).

298. A.C.Patterson,
'Database Hazards',
Datamation 18,No.7,pp48-50 (July 1972).

299. M.J.Smith,
'Aspects of Database Management. A Cautious Approach',
Data Processing (March-April 1971).

LITERATUR in DEUTCHER SPRACHE.

300. 'Eine Auswahl von Datenbank-Management-Systeme'
online/adi-nachrichten, (2/1978).

301. 'Datenbank Systeme: Konzepte und Modelle' Teuber Studienbuecher Informatik, Stuttgart (1977).

302. B.Adam,
'Kriterien zur Auswahl von Datenbank Systemen',
online/adi-nachrichten, (2/1978).

303. M.Bauer,
'Methodische Auswahl eines Datenbanksystems' M.Bauer,
online/adi-nachrichten, (2/1978).

304. M.Bauer,
'Wann ist eine Datenbank sinnvol?',
online/adi-nachrichten, (2/1978).

305. M.Bauer,
'Das Zusammenspiel Datenbank und TP-Systeme.',
online/adi-nachrichten, (11/1976).

306. H.J.Doerfel,
'Datenbank Systeme - Pro und Kontra' H.J.Doerfel,
online/adi-nachrichten, (2/1978).

307. R.Durchholz
'Das Datenmodell bei Codd',
Technical Report No.69 (July 1972),
Gesellschaft fuer Mathematik und Datenverarbeitung.

308. M.Plesch and J.Griese,
'Eigenschaften von Datenbanken - ein Vergleich',
Angewandte Informatik, pp 489-498, (November 1972).

309. K.Schroeder,
'Vergleich der Verweistechnik: Adresskettung contra Indextabellen'
Angewandte Informatik pp 145-153 (April 1972).

310. M.Schwiersch,
'Sinn und Grenzen von Data Dictionaries',
online/adi-nachrichten, (3/1979).

311. H.J.Skron,
'Methoden der Strukurierung von Datenbanken',
Angewandte Informatik (May 1975).

312. Z.Sokolovsky,
'Bemerkungen zur Benutzeradaequanz Formatierter Datenbanksysteme'
online/adi-nachrichten, (1-2 1978).

313. Z.Sokolovsky,
'Die Funktion des Datenbank-Administrators im EDV-Betrieb'
Informatik-Fachberichte, Vol.15,
Organisation von Rechenzentren, Springer, Berlin. (1977).

314. H.Wedekind,
'Datenbank Systeme',
Bibliographisches Institute, Mannheim, Vol.1 (1974), Vol.2 (1976).

315. H.Wedekind,
'Stand der Datenbankentwicklung',
online/adi-nachrichten, (2/1978).

316. C.A.Zehner,
'Datenbank Systeme oder Traditionelle Datenverarbeitung'
Management Zeitschrift IO 45,No.10 (1976).

Bei Fragen zur Produktsicherheit wenden Sie sich bitte an:
If you have any questions regarding product safety,
please contact:

Walter de Gruyter GmbH
Genthiner Straße 13
10785 Berlin
productsafety@degruyterbrill.com